Telemedicine in the ICU

Matthew A. Koenig
Editor

Telemedicine in the ICU

Springer

Editor
Matthew A. Koenig, MD, FNCS
Neuroscience Institute
The Queen's Health Systems
Honolulu, HI
USA

ISBN 978-3-030-11568-5 ISBN 978-3-030-11569-2 (eBook)
https://doi.org/10.1007/978-3-030-11569-2

This Springer imprint is published by the registered company Springer Nature Switzerland AG
The registered company address is: Gewerbestrasse 11, 6330 Cham, Switzerland

Preface

The story of telemedicine in the ICU starts back in Cleveland, Ohio, in 1975 when the Department of Anesthesiology at the University Hospitals of Cleveland (UH), affiliated with Case Western Reserve University Medical School, installed a two-way audiovisual link between UH and Forest City Hospital (FCH). At the time, FCH was a 102-bed private hospital in Cleveland that was operated by African-American physicians and served a largely African-American patient population. FCH was on the verge of bankruptcy when the project began and had few specialists on the medical staff to treat patients in the seven-bed ICU. Engineers at Case Western Reserve University built a novel telemedicine link that enabled specialists from UH to consult on patients in the operating room, neonatal nursery, and ICU at FCH. In the first publication of its kind in 1977, lead author Betty Lou Grundy, MD, an intensivist at UH, described the ICU telemedicine technology as follows:

> A mobile color camera at FCH is connected to cabling in the ICU by nurses without the aid of a technician. Upon activation, the camera is remotely controlled by the consultant. Video signals are transmitted by wide-band helium-neon laser or by microwave. The UH consultant has control of the transmission mode. He views the FCH ICU on a 19-inch color screen. Two 9-inch monochrome screens on the unit at FCH allow users there to see both the UH consultant and themselves as they appear on camera. Audio signals are transmitted by cable; sound level is adjustable at UH and FCH [1].

The tele-ICU model would now be described as a centralized tele-ICU command center with a single spoke site, closed architecture, and portable telemedicine end point at the originating site [2]. The program included a scheduled care delivery model with once-daily rounding and no continuous, proactive, or reactive patient monitoring. Despite these limitations, the technology and workflow were surprisingly contemporary with synchronous audiovisual telecommunications, remote far-end camera control, a mobile telemedicine cart, and multidisciplinary nurse-driven telemedicine bedside rounds.

> At noon each day, a nurse at Forest City Hospital positioned and activated the mobile camera unit, whereupon the University Hospitals consultant controlled the camera remotely (pan, tilt, zoom, focus, iris aperture). The nurse reported on those patients to be seen and noted the consultant's initial suggestions. She then moved the camera out of the relative

> privacy of the nursing station and from bedside to bedside, introducing physician and patient via the telemedicine link. The consultant observed patients and conversed with those well enough to speak, often making additional recommendations of care on the basis of information gained during audiovisual contact [3].

The study authors included anecdotal responses and survey data on the acceptance of ICU telemedicine from the perspective of the FCH patients, private attending physicians, and nursing staff. According to the authors, most patients were satisfied with the telemedicine program and were able to make personal connections with the consulting remote intensivists.

> A surprisingly direct patient/physician relationship was often established via the telemedicine link. Several patients smiled and waved at the consultant from a distance as the mobile camera unit was being moved around the ICU. Patients frequently thanked the remote consultant for visiting. They often inquired as to the consultant's welfare and made solicitous personal comments [1].

The project ran into significant problems, however, in building relationships with the ICU nursing staff and private attending physicians. The UH intensivists sought to build a trusting relationship between the FCH and UH providers through several important actions. The first was creating a requirement that both the patient and the attending physician consent to having the patient seen by the tele-intensivist prior to first patient contact. The second was to invite the nurses, house staff, and attending physicians to participate during bedside telemedicine rounds. The third was to have all of the UH intensivists visit FCH in person at least once prior to telemedicine visits and to set up a weekly on-site educational conference so the originating site providers and distant site providers could have regular in-person meetings. Despite these efforts, the communication between the UH and FCH providers was adversely impacted by cultural and staffing considerations.

> The attitudinal survey revealed that many of the private physicians at FCH were not well acquainted with telemedicine. Most of them regarded inadequate communication within FCH and between FCH and UH as the most serious handicap to the project. They thought the potential of telemedicine as an educational tool was great and had not been adequately exploited. Some physicians expressed resentment at the idea that they might be offered advice from the 'Ivied Tower,' but several thought attending physicians should attend the telemedicine ICU rounds more often [1].

The UH tele-intensivist functioned in a consultant role to make suggestions on patient care, but the private attending physician still retained autonomy to decide whether or not to heed this advice. Because the attending physician rarely attended bedside rounds, it was typically up to the bedside nurse or house officer to relay recommendations from the tele-intensivist to the private physician. Over the 18-month period that the program continued from 1975 to 1977, the tele-intensivists performed 1548 remote consultations for 395 patients. They made a total of 3267 treatment recommendations during this period, but only 30% of these recommendations were carried out by local staff at FCH [2].

> Almost all of the consultant's contact, in person or by telemedicine, was with nursing personnel who could not implement suggestions for medical care without orders from Forest City physicians. Relationships between facilities were hampered by these manpower constraints; opportunities for face-to-face discussion either in person or via interactive television were rare [2].

Aside from having to chart new territory with the telemedicine technology, the UH tele-intensivists also had to navigate an uncertain regulatory landscape before issues related to proxy credentials, telemedicine privileges, clinical guidelines for appropriate use of telemedicine, and malpractice coverage were defined and resolved. The UH consultants were also careful not to initiate discussions of inter-hospital transfer for ICU patients at FCH unless the private attending physician first requested that transfer be considered. In addition, the tele-intensivist had to be mindful not to recommend tests and procedures that were not available locally at FCH. Reading between the lines of the published account, one can surmise that the first tele-intensivists had to walk an ethical fine line between their duty to provide appropriate patient care and the political landscape.

> The question of professional liability for telemedicine consultants in anesthesiology was explored by a lawyer and by the liability insurance carrier for the University anesthesiologist group. No precedents were found. Though the insurance carrier agreed to cover the anesthesiologists' telemedicine consultations for the price of one additional anesthesiologist's liability insurance premium per year, many University anesthesiologists remained concerned about medicolegal risks, partly because the standards of care at the small hospital differed in some respects from the standards of care in the critical care units at the tertiary care facility [3].

These pioneering tele-intensivists also faced economic uncertainties created by a combination of very high initial costs for the technology and infrastructure, lack of payer reimbursement for professional fees, and unknown return on investment. As with many tele-ICU programs, the first tele-ICU was funded by the grant support from the US federal government which paid for the equipment and training but did not reimburse for the physician time.

> Development and installation of the original hardware cost approximately $100,000 and maintenance costs were approximately $35,000 for the 18-month period. Because the system was also used for consultations in the operating room and newborn nursery, we allotted one-third of these costs to the critical care project – $12.72 per intensive care bed/day… We did not assess costs of physician services; these were either donated by the University Hospitals consultants or paid through Public Health Service grant support [3].

In 2018 dollars, the original telemedicine equipment would have cost a budget-busting $468,412.00, which is almost ten times the start-up cost per monitored bed at this point. Understandably, the cost of the project led to significant problems with sustainability after the conclusion of grant funding, especially in a financially strapped hospital on the verge of bankruptcy. In fact, the project ultimately concluded 6 weeks before FCH closed its doors in 1977.

Another challenge faced by investigators in this first tele-ICU project was the ability to obtain reliable data and analyze it in a way to determine the impact of telemedicine on metrics like mortality, complication rates, and length of stay. Because the tele-intensivists were unable to directly intervene in patient care and their recommendations were variably enacted by the treating physicians, the impact of the program was difficult to measure. In fact, there was at least a correlation between the implementation of tele-intensivist recommendations and patient mortality such that patients were more likely to die when the tele-intensivist's recommendations went unheeded.

> Though in-hospital mortality (7%) remained stable, outcome varied directly with the impact of telemedicine on patient care. Patients for whom a greater proportion of consultant's suggestions were implemented were more likely to survive and less likely to be left with new permanent disability [3].

The vivid and detailed narrative descriptions of the first tele-ICU program in the two initial publications [1, 3], in many ways, reinforce how much and how little has changed over the past 40 years. Many of the same challenges and uncertainties that were present in 1975 – malpractice coverage and reimbursement, project implementation, high start-up cost, questionable financial and clinical benefits, lack of concrete metrics of success, cultural barriers to adoption, technological problems, integration into bedside care pathways, acceptance by on-site personnel, and role confusion – will sound very familiar to the readers of this book. It is striking how many of these issues remain unresolved today. In fact, these same issues are the backbone of the book you are about to read, and each of the ensuing chapters will focus on these areas.

Although many issues with tele-ICU have remained constant over the past 40 years, much has changed as well. After the conclusion of the first landmark tele-ICU project, at least as far as the medical literature reflects, tele-ICU then underwent a long period of dormancy stretching into the late 1990s. By that time, computer and network technology had advanced far enough that early electronic medical records, remote telemetry monitors, and video-teleconferencing technologies enabled the centralization of medical care. In 1997, a group of intensivists from the Johns Hopkins Hospital began a tele-ICU coverage of a ten-bed surgical ICU in a hospital in Northern Virginia [4]. In this intervention, tele-intensivists provided around-the-clock coverage of the remote ICU from home computers which included synchronous video teleconsultation with the patients, rounds with the ICU staff, and remote access to lab results and diagnostic imaging.

This experience with tele-ICU led to the founding of the company VISICU in 1998 by two intensivists from the Johns Hopkins. By 2004, the VISICU concept included simultaneous management of patients in multiple ICUs by a tele-intensivist at a centralized location along with some rudimentary proactive patient monitoring [5]. This set the stage for what would now be called a centralized tele-ICU model with open architecture and a preemptive care delivery model within a hub-and-spoke network. Further, the development of the flagship eICU® product then led to Philips acquiring VISICU in 2007 with subsequent domination of the tele-ICU market through much of the previous decade.

The last 10 years have seen significant expansion in the number of tele-ICU programs, technology platforms, and provider networks as well as increasing adoption from healthcare organizations and providers. In addition, the jointly released guideline on tele-ICU operations from the American Telemedicine Association and the Society of Critical Care Medicine [6] has helped to clarify standards of practice and make tele-ICU more mainstream. Finally, changes in US regulation and payment for tele-ICU services have continued to evolve in more supportive ways, including proxy credentialing, creation of the Interstate Medical Licensure Compact, and release of the G0508 code for telemedicine-based critical care from the Centers for Medicare and Medicaid Services.

Telemedicine has been considered the "future of medicine" for so long that it has quietly transformed into the *present of medicine*, particularly in the ICU. As tele-ICU programs continue to evolve, hospital administrators and providers now face important choices and challenges related to practice models, staff roles, regulatory and legal issues, technology and design features, and payment models. Organizations considering investment in new ICU telemedicine programs need to be aware of the different staffing models, the challenges of building homegrown programs versus contracting for services, and the impact of state laws and payer policies on the reimbursement for tele-ICU services. These issues will be reviewed in Part I of "Telemedicine in the Intensive Care Unit."

Although the practice of telemedicine in the ICU has been growing over the last 40 years, high-quality evidence for the impact of telemedicine on patient outcomes, quality and safety metrics, and patient satisfaction have lagged behind. Part II of the book will review the current state of the evidence for and against ICU telemedicine based on clinical trials, before-and-after implementation studies, and observational data. In addition, this section will review the potential costs and savings associated with building a new tele-ICU program to assist with business planning. Finally, appropriate metrics for tracking and improving the quality of telemedicine practice and the patient experience will be discussed.

Part III of the book will dive deeper into specific use cases for telemedicine in the ICU including well-established practices like telestroke as well as emerging telemedicine programs in pediatrics and cardiac intensive care. This section also reviews the use of telemedicine technologies for early treatment of declining patients with sepsis and prehospital coordination with paramedics and first responders. The use of telemedicine to bring medical specialists to the bedside for consultation in general ICUs will also be discussed.

The focus of this book will be on the implementation of ICU telemedicine programs with particular attention to practical issues faced by providers and hospital administrators who are leading new telemedicine programs. This book is the most current, comprehensive review published to date and will serve as a practical guide to building tele-ICU programs. I hope you learn as much by reading it as I did editing this book. I will close this introduction with the final words from the first tele-ICU publication in 1977.

> Present problems of telemedicine in critical care stem less from inadequate technology than from inadequate ways of using available systems. Technical innovations can free us from limitations of time and space only when we develop innovative professional and administrative patterns of use [1].

Honolulu, HI, USA Matthew A. Koenig

References

1. Grundy BL, Crawford P, Jones PK, Kiley ML, Reisman A, Pao YH, Wilkerson EL, Gravenstein JS. Telemedicine in critical care: an experiment in health care delivery. JACEP 1977;6:439–44.
2. Reynolds HN, Rogove H, Bander J, McCambridge M, Cowboy E, Niemeier M. A working lexicon for the tele-intensive care unit: we need to define tele-intensive care unit to grow and understand it. Telemed J E Health 2011;17(10):773–82.
3. Grundy BL, Jones PK, Lovitt A. Telemedicine in critical care: problems in design, implementation, and assessment. Crit Care Med 1982;10(7):471–5.
4. Rosenfeld BA, Dorman T, Breslow MJ, Pronovost P, Jenckes M, Zhang N, Anderson G, Rubin H. Intensive care unit telemedicine: alternate paradigm for providing continuous intensivist care. Crit Care Med 2000;28:3925–31.
5. Breslow MJ, Rosenfeld BA, Doerfler M, Burke G, Yates G, Stone DJ, Tomaszewicz P, Hochman R, Plocher DW. Effect of a multiple-site intensive care unit telemedicine program on clinical and economic outcomes: an alternative paradigm for intensivist staffing. Crit Care Med 2004;32(1):31–8.
6. Davis TM, Barden C, Dean S, Gavish A, Goliash I, Goran S, Graley A, Herr P, Jackson W, Loo E, Marcin JP, Morris JM, Morledge DE, Olff C, Rincon T, Rogers S, Rogove H, Rufo R, Thomas E, Zubrow MT, Krupinski EA, Bernard J. American Telemedicine Association guidelines for TeleICU operations. Telemed J E Health 2016;22(12):971–80.

Contents

Contributors

Christian D. Becker Westchester Medical Center Health Network, Valhalla, NY, USA

New York Medical College, Department of Medicine, Division of Pulmonary, Critical Care and Sleep Medicine, Valhalla, NY, USA

Jordana Bernard Policy and Public Affairs for InTouch Health, Santa Barbara, CA, USA

Brendan G. Carr Department of Emergency Medicine, Thomas Jefferson University, Philadelphia, PA, USA

Sherita N. Chapman Department of Neurology and Karen S. Rheuban Center for Telehealth, University of Virginia Health System, Charlottesville, VA, USA

John Chuo Clinical Pediatrics, Children's Hospital of Philadelphia, Philadelphia, PA, USA

Bart M. Demaerschalk Mayo Clinic College of Medicine and Science, Rochester, MN, USA

Robert Derrett III University of Minnesota, Minneapolis, MN, USA

Marcus C. Divers Department of Neurology and Karen S. Rheuban Center for Telehealth, University of Virginia Health System, Charlottesville, VA, USA

M. Elizabeth Wilcox Department of Medicine (Respirology), University Health Network, Toronto, ON, Canada

Interdepartmental Division of Critical Care Medicine, University of Toronto, Toronto, ON, Canada

Spyridon Fortis Pulmonary, Critical Care and Occupation Medicine, University of Iowa Hospitals and Clinics, Center for Comprehensive Access & Delivery Research & Evaluation (CADRE), Iowa City VA Health Care System, Iowa City, IA, USA

Mario Fusaro Westchester Medical Center Health Network, Valhalla, NY, USA

New York Medical College, Department of Medicine, Division of Pulmonary, Critical Care and Sleep Medicine, Valhalla, NY, USA

Alexis S. Gilroy Jones Day, Washington, DC, USA

Matthew R. Goede University of Nebraska Medical Center, Veterans Affairs VISN 23 Regional Tele-ICU Associate Medical Director, Omaha, NE, USA

Carley M. Howard Draddy Pediatric Telehealth and Special Projects, Children's Hospital of Greenville Health System, Greenville, SC, USA

Ann Marie Huffenberger Penn Medicine Center for Connected Care, University of Pennsylvania Health System, Philadelphia, PA, USA

Emily K. Hurst Avera eCARE, Sioux Falls, SD, USA

Henry Ford Health System, Detroit, MI, USA

Asad Latif Johns Hopkins University School of Medicine, Department of Anesthesiology and Critical Care Medicine, Johns Hopkins Medicine, Armstrong Institute for Quality and Patient Safety, Baltimore, MD, USA

Yuxiu Lei Department of Pulmonary and Critical Care Medicine, Lahey Hospital and Medical Center, Burlington, MA, USA

Timothy N. Liesching Department of Pulmonary and Critical Care Medicine, Lahey Hospital and Medical Center, Burlington, MA, USA

Tufts University School of Medicine, Boston, MA, USA

A. Clinton MacKinney Department of Health Management and Policy, University of Iowa College of Public Health, Iowa City, IA, USA

Atul Malhotra Division of Pulmonary, Critical Care, and Sleep Medicine, UC San Diego Health, San Diego, CA, USA

Niels D. Martin Division of Traumatology, Surgical Critical Care & Emergency Surgery, Perelman School of Medicine at the University of Pennsylvania, Philadelphia, PA, USA

S. David McSwain Pediatric Critical Care Medicine, Telehealth Optimization, Medical University of South Carolina, Charleston, SC, USA

Nicholas M. Mohr Department of Emergency Medicine, University of Iowa Carver College of Medicine, Iowa City, IA, USA

Department of Anesthesia Division of Critical Care, University of Iowa Carver College of Medicine, Iowa City, IA, USA

Emma C. Nash Department of Emergency Medicine, University of Iowa Carver College of Medicine, Iowa City, IA, USA

Christopher M. Palmer Department of Anesthesiology, Division of Critical Care, Division of Emergency Medicine, Washington University School of Medicine in St. Louis, St. Louis, MO, USA

Haydon M. Pitchford Department of Neurology and Karen S. Rheuban Center for Telehealth, University of Virginia Health System, Charlottesville, VA, USA

Jayant K. Raikhelkar Department of Medicine, Division of Cardiovascular Medicine, University of Chicago School of Medicine, Chicago, IL, USA

Jayashree Raikhelkar Emory University School of Medicine, Atlanta, GA, USA

Nagarajan Ramakrishnan Department of Critical Care Medicine, Apollo Hospitals, Chennai, India

Venktesh R. Ramnath Critical Care Telemedicine Outreach, Division of Pulmonary, Critical Care, and Sleep Medicine, UC San Diego Health, San Diego, CA, USA

H. Neal Reynolds University of Maryland School of Medicine, Baltimore, MD, USA

R Adams Cowley Shock Trauma Center, Baltimore, MD, USA

Kimberly L. Rockwell Jones Day, Boston, MA, USA

Herbert J. Rogove Residential Connected Health, New York, NY, USA

Mark Romig Johns Hopkins University School of Medicine, Department of Anesthesiology and Critical Care Medicine, Johns Hopkins Medicine, Armstrong Institute for Quality and Patient Safety, Baltimore, MD, USA

Adam Sapirstein Johns Hopkins University School of Medicine, Department of Anesthesiology and Critical Care Medicine, Johns Hopkins Medicine, Armstrong Institute for Quality and Patient Safety, Baltimore, MD, USA

Dana Schinasi Pediatric Emergency Medicine, Telehealth Programs, Ann & Robert H. Lurie Children's Hospital of Chicago, Chicago, IL, USA

Corey S. Scurlock Westchester Medical Center Health Network, Valhalla, NY, USA

New York Medical College, Department of Anesthesiology, Department of Medicine, Valhalla, NY, USA

Brian Skow Avera eCARE, Sioux Falls, SD, USA

Andrew M. Southerland Department of Neurology and Karen S. Rheuban Center for Telehealth, University of Virginia Health System, Charlottesville, VA, USA

Rebecca Stamm Clinical Nursing Systems, The Hospital of the University of Pennsylvania, University of Pennsylvania Health System, Philadelphia, PA, USA

Sanjay Subramanian Division of Critical Care, Department of Anesthesiology, Washington University School of Medicine in St. Louis, St. Louis, MO, USA

Ricardo Teijeiro Instituto Nacional de Ciencias Medicas y Nutrición Salvador Zubirán, Mexico City, Mexico

Department of Medicine (Respirology), University Health Network, Toronto, ON, Canada

Ramesh Venkataraman Department of Critical Care Medicine, Apollo Hospitals, Chennai, India

Part I
Tele-ICU Practice Models

Chapter 1
The Tele-ICU: Formative or Out-of-Date or Both? Practice Models and Future Directions

H. Neal Reynolds

Basic Issues

The American Hospital Association 2014 annual survey [1, 2] noted that the USA has 5686 hospitals. Essentially all acute care hospitals have at least one ICU with nearly 55,000 critically ill patients cared for each day. From 2006 to 2010, the number of critical care beds in the USA increased 15%, from 67,579 to greater than 80,000 [3]. ICU care is expensive and generally estimated as 30% of total hospital costs [4].

History of the Tele-ICU

Historically, the tele-ICU concept is approaching the half century mark. The tele-ICU was first conceptualized in the 1970s by Grundy [5, 6]. Subsequently, the tele-ICU concept and reality has grown rapidly following the first commercial system installation in Norfolk, Virginia, in 2000 [7, 8]. The initial drivers for the expansion of the tele-ICU evolved from a shortage of intensivists [9–13], a general physician misdistribution [14, 15], recognized value of intensivists [16–19], and pressure from the private business sector LeapFrog recommendations [20]. An extensive review of the tele-ICU experience from 2004 through 2013, completed by Coustasse [21], included more than 35 studies over a 9-year period which revealed the following: 16 studies demonstrated shortened ICU length of stay (LOS), 11 studies showed greater adherence to "best practice" protocols, 7 studies demonstrated improved

H. N. Reynolds (✉)
University of Maryland School of Medicine, Baltimore, MD, USA

R Adams Cowley Shock Trauma Center, Baltimore, MD, USA
e-mail: NReynolds@SOM.UMARYLAND.EDU

M. A. Koenig (ed.), *Telemedicine in the ICU*,
https://doi.org/10.1007/978-3-030-11569-2_1

financial performance of the ICU, 4 found greater teamwork or "team-ness," and 5 studies described "improved patient care" without further specification. The recent tele-ICU literature further supports significantly reduced mortality based upon two meta-analyses [22, 23]. The process literature is now being followed by calls promoting the tele-ICU as the preferred business model [24–28]. However, despite an initial rapid expansion of tele-ICU of 101% per year from 2003 to 2007, the subsequent growth rate has declined to 8% per year between 2006 and 2010 [29]. The concept, process, and recommendations have now been formalized in the American Telemedicine Association Tele-ICU guidelines [30].

Pressures for Change in the Tele-ICU

Evolving patterns in Medicare reimbursement including "pay for performance," "value-based purchasing," "Hospital Readmission Reduction Program" [31], "population health," and Accountable Care Organizations [32] are all driving the focus away from inpatient care. Consequently, hospital-based telemedicine initiatives may be more focused on remote patient monitoring [33] or the Patient-Centered Medical Home [34].

There is no explicit CMS direct physician reimbursement for tele-ICU services, at least as those services are most commonly provided [35, 36]. It is hard to accumulate the mandatory 30 minutes or greater time for the remote physician who is making sequential 3–5 minute visits, trying to create the necessary documentation, while covering a large volume of patients. Evolution to alternative billing by the minute, such as billing for anesthesia time [37], may be an alternative, but currently no such impetus exists. Consequently, the tele-ICU often exists as a recognized cost center for a hospital and justified by the hoped-for cost savings generated including shorter LOS. However, the cost and benefit ratio remains unclear. Kumar [38] in a 21-year retrospective review and seven-facility prospective study found that the first year of implementation can cost from $50,000 to $100,000 per monitored bed and *could* save $3000 or *could* cost $5600 per ICU patient. Others [39] have cited even more pessimistic estimates, suggesting a 24% daily cost increase and as much as 43% increase cost per case and ineffectiveness for the less sick. However, the same group found value for the sicker patient populations. As is cited in other articles [40], support of a tele-ICU program is dependent upon many variables beyond simple finances, including personal disposition of the current hospital CEO or resistance of internal hospital groups. Ultimately, internal hospital support may be CEO personality-dependent based on his or her perceptions of "doing what is best for the patient" versus population-based impact versus caring for the "sicker patients." Nonetheless, commercial markets project a "sturdy" growth for the tele-ICU from a US$500 million marketplace in 2015 to $2.5 billion market predicted by 2024 with greater global growth already at $1.2 billion in 2015 rising to $5.8 billion in the same time frame [41].

Of the ongoing expenses after initial implementation, physician and advanced practice provider staffing is the largest fraction. The University of Massachusetts study reported ongoing yearly staffing costs of almost $2.3 million (72%) of a total

$3.1 million annual operating costs [25]. When initially conceived, the tele-ICU was to be intentionally placed in a location that is remote from the physical ICUs so that the intensivists could be available to all covered ICUs. With mounting cost pressures and intermittent needs of "hands" on-site, some may adopt hybrid models with the tele-ICU immediately adjacent to the system-led ICU such as the Eastern Maine Medical Center Model [42]. Finally, there is always generic pressure from industry for change. According to Kaiser Permanente Medical Group, 86% of CEOs consider themselves "disrupters" with technology being the major disruptive force and some moving rapidly forward, others proceeding with caution [43].

Pressures Against Change in the Tele-ICU

There are three general types of changes with evolution of the tele-ICU. The first would be evolving "TO" the tele-ICU, the second would be evolving to "DIFFERENT" tele-ICU technology, and the third would be "ABANDONING" the technology altogether.

Regarding the first type of reluctance to evolve to the tele-ICU, physicians may be "Luddites" to a degree. The Luddites allegedly protested "industrialization" fearing time spent in learning new technology would be wasteful and the technology could replace their jobs [44]. Perhaps more relevant is the concept of "Neo-Luddites" – those who would slow the advancement of technology in favor of a return to the simpler life [45]. Kruse [46] has nicely tabulated organizational and staff reluctance to adoption of telemedicine in general. The leading organizational barrier is cost, whereas the reluctance from staff centers around staff being "technically challenged" and a general "resistance to change."

Regarding evolution to a different tele-ICU model, once tele-ICU technology is selected and installed, there will be administrative reluctance to abandon expensive legacy technology despite being outdated, cumbersome, and slow. Typical installation for the leading vendor product is about $50,000 per monitored bed. Subsequently, once a technology is learned, the consumer may be reluctant to learn yet another technology [47].

Finally, closure of current tele-ICU programs does occur. The prime driver for closure is likely to be the balance of expense versus perceived benefit. It is virtually impossible to currently find data defining the frequency of tele-ICU closure much less driving forces leading to closure.

The Business of Technology

The homogeneity of tele-ICU technology stems from litigation launched by the founding vendor, apparently intended to control the growth of competition in the early 2000s [48]. As a result, there was essentially no growth in competition, allowing a single vendor to take a dominant hold of the market for a decade. Although the patent infringement case was dismissed in 2010 [49], one vendor was left with the leading market share. As a result, most studies of the structured tele-ICU care delivery model employ Philips/VISICU® technology. The leading tele-ICU technology went live in 2000 [50] and is largely unchanged since that time except for some updates. As part of the initial patent application, the acronym "eICU®" became a registered trademark [51]. As a consequence of dominating the market share and registering the name "eICU®," this registered trademark became the common street name for any tele-ICU program and was perceived as synonymous with all tele-ICUs.

Subsequently, an effort evolved to educate the medical public on decision points when designing a tele-ICU [42]. A lexicon for the tele-ICU was written [52] to provide users with the breadth of characteristics necessary when deciding on a system. From that lexicon, two concepts had staying power: (1) centralized versus decentralized design and (2) open architecture versus closed architecture. The "centralized" model for the tele-ICU describes the Philips/VISICU® model with a remote "bunker" staffed "continuously" with connectivity to one or more ICUs. By comparison, the "decentralized" tele-ICU does not have a distinct "bunker," but rather, care providers are positioned at sites of convenience such as private offices, home, or operating from mobile devices [53]. "Closed architecture" versus "open architecture" refers to the connectivity of the technology. Closed architecture is defined by dedicated lines such as T3 lines from a "bunker" to the medical facility limiting point-to-point access to only those within the "bunker." "Open architecture" describes a system supporting access to the remote patient from many sites and ultimately mandates internet connectivity.

Personnel Staffing the Tele-ICU

The Physician Supply

American Association of Medical Colleges (AAMC) posted the 2016 update [54] regarding predicted physician supply and demand. Although not focused on critical care medicine (CCM), the estimated shortfall of physicians by 2025 is predicted to range from 61,700 to 98,700 and could be as high as 125,200 under worst-case scenarios. By 2030, over 20% of the US population will be older than 65 years of age, the population known to be the greatest consumers of healthcare services and critical care services.

Reports in the early 2000s [9, 11] suggested a manpower undersupply of critical care physicians of around 30,000. A more recent Health Resources Services Administration (HRSA) study/prediction actually suggests an oversupply of critical care physicians by the year 2025 [55]. Recently, a trend has evolved with more medical students choosing emergency medicine (EM) residencies and many doing an additional critical care fellowship. Data from the National Residency Matching Program [56] indicates that, from 2000 to 2015, there has been a near-doubling of

EM residency training programs from 971 to 1821. With nearly 100% match rate, predictions are for a near-doubling of EM physicians entering the workplace. In 2009, the American Board of Internal Medicine (ABIM) and the American Board of Emergency Medicine [57] established a pathway for EM physicians to gain concurrent board certification in CCM and EM [58, 59]. Currently, there are approximately 20 US programs with combined EM and CCM training. Additionally, the number of pulmonologists seeking combined pulmonary-CCM training has risen 17% per year from 118 to 135. New pathways to achieve critical care board certification have evolved for EM-trained physicians that include surgical critical care (boards from the American Board of Surgery [ABS]), neurocritical care (certified by the United Council for Neurologic Subspecialties), and an anesthesia pathway (American Board of Anesthesiology). Ultimately, there appears to be a major easing of the shortage of critical care capable physicians on the horizon.

Traditional Tele-ICU Coverage

At the initiation of the first commercial tele-ICU program, the intent was to provide 24/7/365 physician and nursing coverage remotely as diagramed in Fig. 1.1.

This staffing paradigm has proven challenging. Because there was a national shortage of intensivists, it had been equally challenging to staff the tele-ICU programs. At any given time, a long list of tele-ICU intensivist jobs is readily available [60–63]. As is true of much of the staffing in the tele-ICU, it is impossible to determine the current tele-ICU physician need, positions that go unfilled, or longevity of the tele-ICU physician. However, the presence of literature supporting alternative staffing models supports the belief that there is currently a shortage of bedside *and* tele-ICU intensivists.

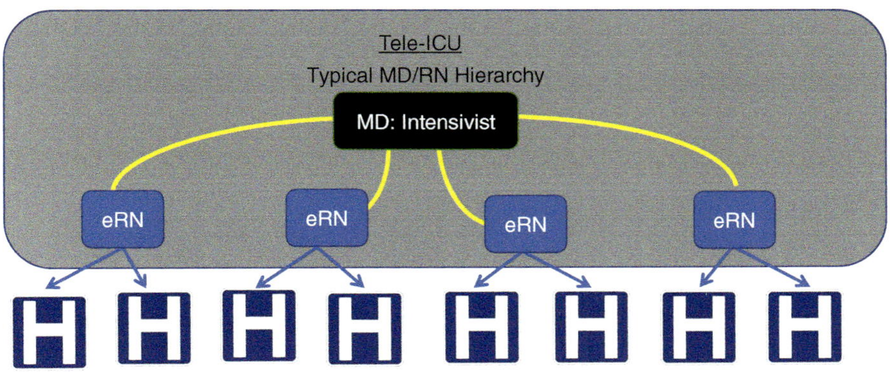

Fig. 1.1 Traditional tele-ICU staffing model with the physician intensivists supervising care through trained tele-ICU critical care nurses

Staffing the Tele-ICU with Non-intensivist Physicians

LeapFrog has promoted the adoption of bedside intensivists when possible and the tele-ICU when the intensivists cannot be physically available. Due to the current paucity of trained intensivists, LeapFrog [64] has promoted alternative staffing models to include:

Physicians board-certified in medicine, anesthesiology, pediatrics, emergency medicine, or surgery, and who have:

- *Completed training prior to the availability of a subspecialty certification in critical care; and*
- *Provided at least six weeks of full-time ICU care each year.*

Others have proposed that hospitalists [65, 66] with additional training and intensivist backup could direct critical care services in some community hospitals. The benefit of this "pyramidal hierarchy" lies in the ability of a single intensivist to cover even more ICU beds with nursing staff managing the majority of monitoring and screening and non-intensivist physicians managing more complex issues and able to write orders with overall intensivist oversight (Fig. 1.2).

Staffing the Tele-ICU with Advanced Care Providers

There has been a relatively recent movement to employ advanced care providers in the physical ICU [67–69] particularly when under the direction of a trained intensivist. Therefore, extension of this same staffing model to the tele-ICU would seem equally feasible. The benefit of advanced care providers is the ability to give therapeutic orders while avoiding hiring higher-cost non-intensivist physicians (Fig. 1.3).

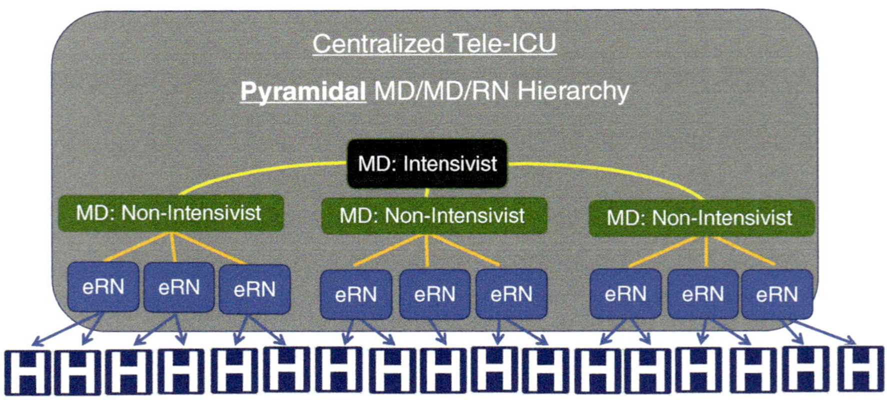

Fig. 1.2 Alternative tele-ICU staffing model leveraging an intensivist over a greater number of patients/hospitals with the use of non-intensivist physicians providing the direct supervision over trained tele-ICU critical care nurses

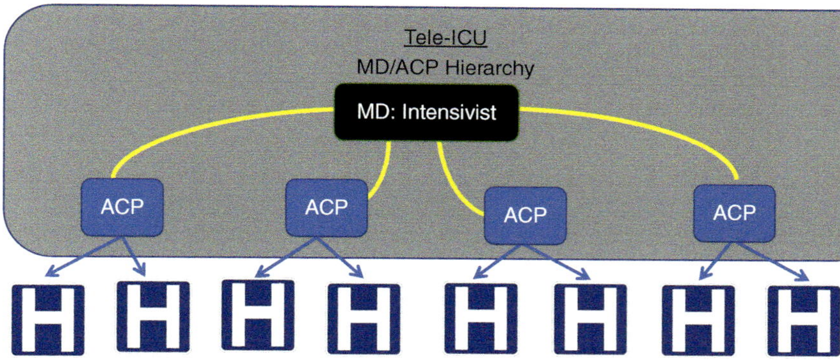

Fig. 1.3 Alternative tele-ICU staffing model employing advanced care providers (ACPs) supervised by intensivists

Clinical Coverage Options

A flexible tele-ICU program may be able to offer various coverage models with some option of cost savings. The highest level of coverage with 24/7/365 remote monitoring may be best suited for rural facilities with no on-site intensivist or pulmonary coverage whatsoever. For programs with existing on-site daytime coverage, the tele-ICU could go live during evening hours only. Tele-ICU nursing options could also be independently tailored to the needs of a particular ICU (Fig. 1.4). Certain options exist combining the evening-only tele-ICU coverage for the week days and the 24/7 intensivists for the weekends.

Turning "Night to Day"

Perhaps the most innovative evolution of staffing is to ensure that the care providers are always working during their personal daytime shift. There is data suggesting that nighttime providers may be less experienced, and outcomes could be impacted [70]. There is significant physiologic impact upon the "shift worker" manifesting as sleep disturbances, increased accidents and injuries, and social isolation for nurses [71, 72] and physicians [73]. The concept of "turning night to day" was most recently promulgated from Emory University in Atlanta. The program links US-based tele-ICU programs with a tele-ICU program at the Royal Perth Hospital on the west coast of Australia. The Australian site is 12–13 time zones from the east coast of the USA [74–77]. Functionally, the US facility receives nighttime coverage from Australian providers who are working during their respective daytime shift and vice versa. Ultimately, all care providers are working during their daytime providing night coverage half a world away. A similar program has been in existence for several years with Avera eCare®. The Avera eCare® links to Tel Aviv, Israel,

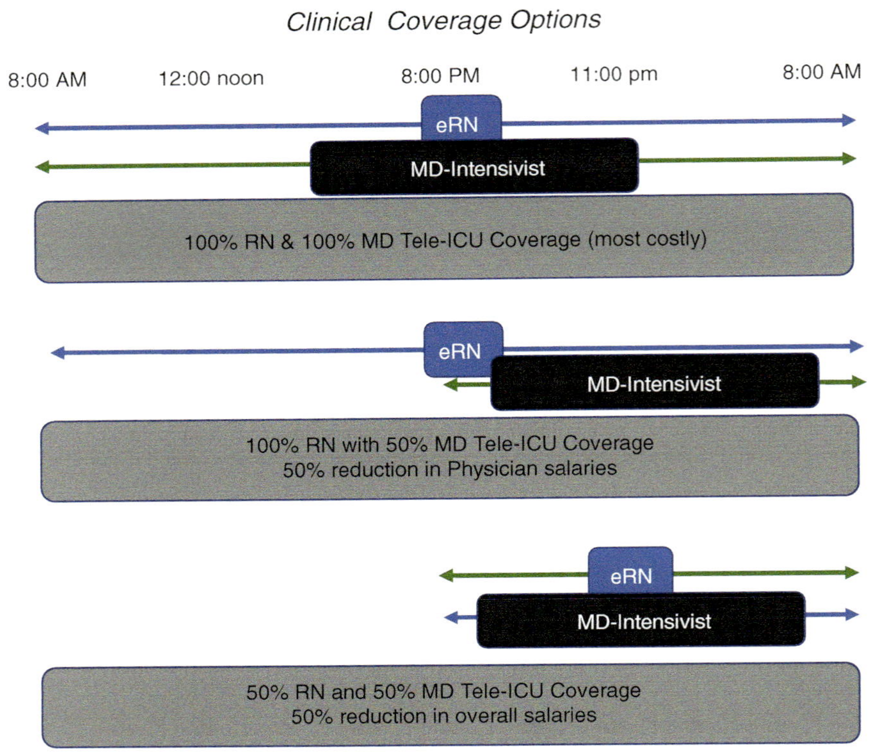

Fig. 1.4 Options for hours of coverage and personnel

which is 8 hours later than the South Dakota home site of Avera eCare. The Tel Aviv tele-intensivists provide tele-ICU coverage during the night hours in Sioux Falls, South Dakota (Fig. 1.5).

Business Models

Fundamental questions of the ultimate business model for the tele-ICU exist. Should the tele-ICU continue as an independent entity within a medical system, evolve to a stand-alone program outside the medical system, or be incorporated into a larger telemedicine program. Designing for the present or future mandates considerations of vertical or horizontal scaling [78]. "Horizontal scaling" [79] also known as "scaling out," in business, means adding more discrete but different service lines. Alternatively, "vertical scaling" [80], also known as "scaling up," translates to increasing the capacity of existing entities or service lines. An example of a horizontal scaling model could be adding alternative services to the tele-ICU such as neurology, postoperative care, pharmacology support services, palliative care services,

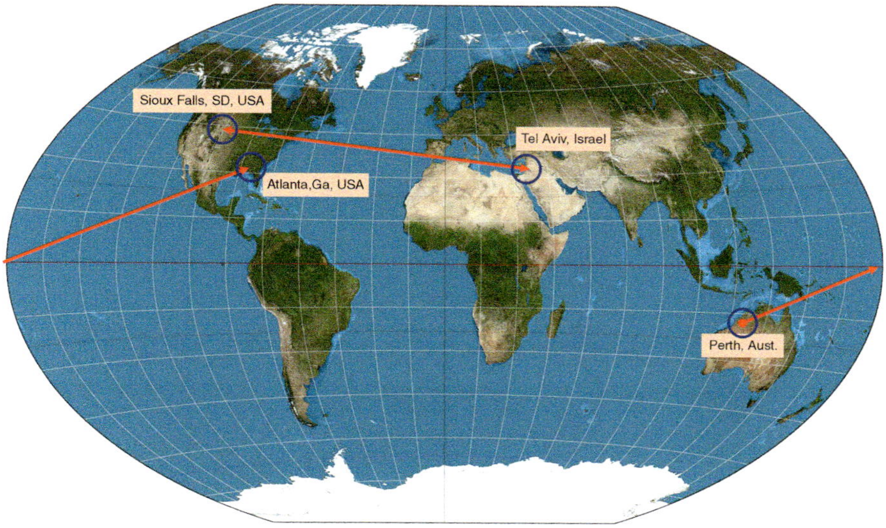

Fig 1.5 "Turning night into day": extremely remote coverage of tele-ICUs (map modified from Google Maps)

and behavioral health – all based from a telemedicine center that subsumes the tele-ICU.

In some cases, with horizontal scaling, tele-ICU programs or programs beginning with other focuses have evolved to "virtual hospitals." An example of horizontal scaling is Avera eCare [81] – a virtual hospital in Sioux Falls, South Dakota, which evolved initially from a consult service then to a tele-ICU-focused program. The Avera tele-ICU, now more generally known as Avera eCare, includes eCorrectional Care, eBehavioral Care, eEmergency Care, ePharmacy, eSchool Health, eSenior Care, eSpecialty Consultations, and eHospitalist programs. Similarly, the virtual hospital at Intermountain Healthcare in Utah incorporates 35 individual telemedicine programs including tele-ICU, tele-neonatal consultations, telestroke, behavioral health evaluations, and other services [82, 83]. In Chesterfield, Missouri, the Mercy Virtual Care Center exists in a stand-alone, four-story building providing tele-ICU, telestroke, tele-sepsis, tele-hospitalists, and remote patient monitoring for homebound patients with chronic illnesses all while touting "no beds" [84]. The Mercy facility is a 125,000-square-foot, $54 million-dollar structure working to meet or exceed the CMS goals of reducing cost of care and keeping patients out of the brick-and-mortar hospitals [85].

Forces that drive the development of vertical scaling are essentially the same as the forces that drove the initial development of the tele-ICU: *shortage of intensivists*. Programs desiring to establish a tele-ICU program may discover that they are not able to recruit intensivists to staff a "bunker" when using the centralized model. Consequently, an organization may have deployed the hardware and software technology but seek physician and nursing coverage from elsewhere. Corporate tele-

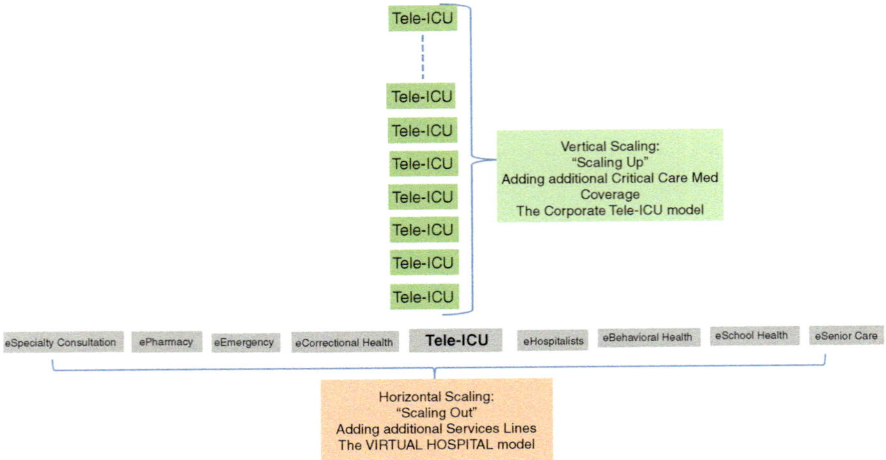

Fig. 1.6 Vertical and horizontal scaling of telemedicine programs either initially based upon the tele-ICU concept or subsequently incorporating tele-ICU into a larger scaled program

ICU has evolved and is currently doing business such as Advanced ICU Care® which is advertised to be the "first external tele-ICU solution" providing the "manpower" when "manpower" is not otherwise available. The Advanced ICU Care program has installations in at least 65 hospitals and health systems, sites in at least 24 states, five operations centers (plus three special arrangements), and a staff of 140 focused clinicians [86] (Fig. 1.6).

The concept of scaling up or out is presented here as if these are independent entities. In fact, a horizontally scaled program may be requested to provide more of an established service – that is, to vertically scale within a horizontally scaled program.

Recently, one group in the state of Maryland proposed a different horizontal scaling model for the extension of critical care services (Fig. 1.7) from "the scene" through emergency transport to the Emergency Department, operating room, and the ICU [87]. Maryland was the first state with a statewide trauma program and a statewide helicopter medical evacuation program [88] with a long-established infrastructure that includes the Maryland Institute for Emergency Medical Services System. Since most critical care services pass through the Emergency Department environment and with the lines between the Emergency Department and the ICU becoming blurred, this could represent horizontal scaling from the Emergency Department or the ICU. The concept was to begin critical care with active physician input beginning at the scene, continuing through all phases of transport, and into the hospital. The direct benefit is immediate physician input to care and a degree of continuity of care. An ancillary benefit is the creation of documentation directly without the risk of translational changes via handoffs among many care providers.

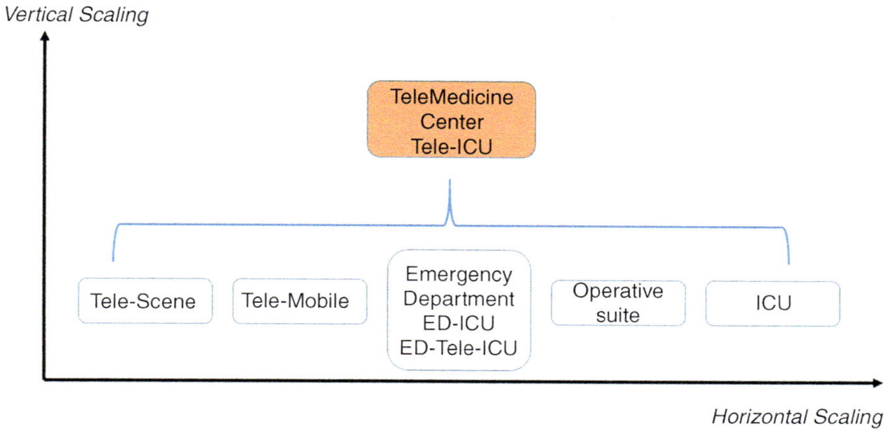

Fig. 1.7 Horizontal scaling of the tele-ICU into the realm of scene care, the mobile environment, through the Emergency Department and operative suite until arrival in the ICU

Project ECHO®

Project ECHO® (Extension for Community Health Outcomes) was launched in 2003 with the intention to "de-monopolize" medical knowledge and improve quality of care to the underserved. Initially focused on a single disease entity, hepatitis C, the program has expanded to de-monopolize knowledge for at least 100 different disease states in over 31 countries. The concept is simple. Experts at a "hub" could share information with remote care providers in a *case-presentation* or *question-and-answer* format on a weekly basis using the "hub-and-spoke" capabilities [89, 90].

The tele-ICU was initially established on a hub-and-spoke model. While not all current tele-ICU models are based on this functional model, those that are could spread and share medical knowledge using Project ECHO® concepts. Currently, there are no tele-ICU programs providing the Project ECHO® Model (personal communication, ECHO Institute); however, there are significant hub-and-spoke programs that do share knowledge such as:

1. EMS/Trauma – University of Utah
2. Burn and Soft Tissue Injury – University of Utah
3. Integrated Care – Northeast Ohio Medical Center (NEOMED)
4. Long-Term Care – University of Rochester
5. 10 ECHO projects providing for quality improvement training

Now in the era of "population health," medical centers are responsible to keep their community of patients healthy. The tele-ICU model, particularly if expanded into a horizontally scaled program, is ideally suited and situated to educate a community of healthcare providers, improve quality of care, and support the "Patient-Centered Medical Home."

Unanswered Questions

There remains a series of unanswered questions regarding the tele-ICU. The following is not meant to be an all-inclusive list but rather raises a few concerns or thoughts.

1. The ideal structure has never been defined. There are no comparative studies of centralized versus decentralized tele-ICU programs.
2. The best staffing model has never been defined. There are no studies that guide which clinician type is the most cost-effective and/or clinically effective.
3. The coverage model remains to be defined. Is the 24/7/365 model better than 12/7/365 with in-person intensivists during daytime hours? Are there programs that only require weekend coverage versus programs that only require nighttime coverage? Would the episodic consultation model/demand response model be adequate in some cases?
4. With a changing "manpower supply," is there indeed a "manpower" shortage – which was the primary driver for the evolution of the tele-ICU – or will the newer HRSA projections correctly predict an eventual oversupply?
5. Conversely, does the tele-ICU solve the manpower shortage or just exacerbate the demand as programs try to meet the LeapFrog guidelines?
6. What is the best business model? Judging from the success of programs that have chosen horizontal or vertical scaling, remaining as an isolated tele-ICU may not be the most optimal design.
7. When will hospital-based tele-ICU programs become part of the "population health" initiative and assume community education as a priority, i.e., the ECHO Model?

Summary

The tele-ICU concept and process is now well established and highly functional. Long-term viability may be dependent upon adopting different staffing models, different functional models, or different business models. With the apparent domination of a single tele-ICU product line, many will assume that there is *only* a single product line. Those new to the technology should learn the variables (lexicon) and make investments and staffing decisions based upon new business models, flexibility of design that accounts for the "manpower" availability, needs of the "manpower," and the overall programmatic goals. The world no longer has just one "Black Sedan."

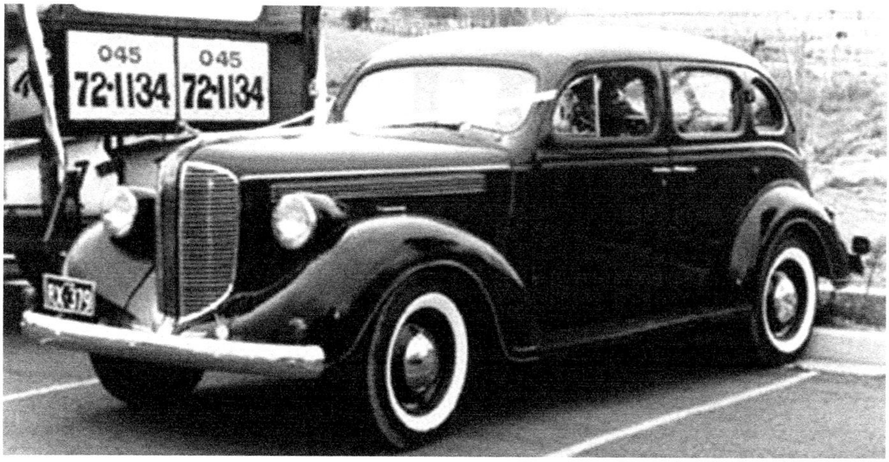

Conflicts of Interest H. Neal Reynolds: No conflicts of interest relevant to information presented in this chapter. H. Neal Reynolds has served on the Research Board for InTouch Health, owns stock options with InTouch Health, and has spoken at the annual InTouch Health Scientific Forum.

References

1. Health Forum, LLC. American Hospital Association Hospital Statistics, 2015 (2014 Survey Data). Chicago: American Hospital Association. p. 2015.
2. Critical care statistics. http://www.sccm.org/Communications/Pages/CriticalCareStats.aspx. Accessed 8/28/2018.
3. Wallace DJ, Angus DC, Seymour CW, Barnato AE, Kahn JM. Critical care bed growth in the United States. A comparison of regional and national trends. Am J Respir Crit Care Med. 2015;191(4):410–6.
4. Chalfin D, Cohen L, Lambrinos J. The economics and cost-effectiveness of critical care medicine. Intensive Care Med. 1995;21:952–61.
5. Grundy BL, Crawford P, Jones PK, et al. Telemedicine in critical care: an experiment in health care delivery. JACEP. 1977;6(10):439–44.
6. Grundy BL, Jones PK, Lovitt A. Telemedicine in critical care: problems in design, implementation, and assessment. Crit Care Med. 1982;10(7):471–5.
7. Rosenfeld BA, Dorman T, Breslow MJ, et al. Intensive care unit telemedicine: alternate paradigm for providing continuous intensivist care. Crit Care Med. 2000;28:3925–31.
8. Breslow MJ, Rosenfeld BA, Doerfler M, Burke G, Yates G, et al. Effect of a multiple-site intensive care unit telemedicine program on clinical and economic outcomes: an alternative paradigm for intensivist staffing. Crit Care Med. 2004;32:31–8.
9. Angus DC, Kelley MA, Schmitz RJ, Whiet A, Popovich J. Current and projected workforce requirements for care of the critical ill and patients with pulmonary disease: can we meet the requirements of an aging population? JAMA. 2000;284:2762–70.

10. Health Resources and Services Administration Report to Congress: the critical care workforce: a study of the supply and demand for critical care physicians. https://www.mc.vanderbilt.edu/documents/CAPNAH/files/criticalcare.pdf. Accessed 8/29/2018.
11. Kelley MA, Angus DC, Chalfin DB, et al. The critical care crisis in the United States: a report from the profession. Crit Care Med. 2004;32:1219–22.
12. Grover A. Critical care workforce: a policy perspective. Crit Care Med. 2006;34(Suppl):S7–S11.
13. Krell K. Critical care workforce. Crit Care Med. 2008;36:1350–3.
14. Kirch DG. President and CEO of the American Association of Medical Colleges. How to fix the doctor Shortage. Wall Street; January 4, 2010.
15. Health care Workforce Distribution and Shortage Issues in Rural America, National Rural Health Association, March 2003. https://www.ruralhealthweb.org/getattachment/Advocate/Policy-Documents/HealthCareWorkforceDistributionandShortageJanuary2012.pdf.aspx?lang=en-US. Accessed 8/27/2018.
16. Reynolds HN, Haupt MT, Carlson R. Impact of critical care physician staffing on patients with septic shock in a University Medical Care Unit. JAMA. 1988;260(33):3446–50.
17. Li TC, Phillips MC, Shaw L, et al. On site physician staffing in a community hospital intensive care unit: impact on test and procedure use and on patient outcome. JAMA. 1984;252:2023–7.
18. Young M, Birkmeyer J. Potential reduction in mortality rates using an intensivist model to manage intensive care units. Eff Clin Pract. 2000;3:284–9.
19. Engoren M. The effect of prompt physician visits on intensive care unit mortality and cost. Crit Care Med. 2005;33:727–32.
20. http://www.leapfroggroup.org: Four leaps in hospital quality, safety and affordability. Accessed 8/27/2018.
21. Coustasse A, Deslich S, Bailey D, Paul D. A business case for tele-intensive care units. Perm J. 2014;18(4):76–84.
22. Young LB, Chan PS, Lu X, Nallamothu BK, Sasson C, Cram PM. Impact of telemedicine intensive care unit coverage on patient outcomes: a systematic review and meta-analysis. Arch Intern Med. 2011;171(6):498–506.
23. Wilcox ME, Adhikari NK. The effect of telemedicine in critically ill patients: systematic review and meta-analysis. Crit Care. 2012;16(4):R127.
24. Deslich S, Coustasse A. Expanding technology in the ICU: the case for the utilization of telemedicine. Telemed J E Health. 2014;20(5):1–8.
25. New England Healthcare Institute, Massachusetts Technology Collaborative. Critical care, critical choices: the case for Tele-ICUs in intensive care. Westborough: Massachusetts Technology Park Corporation; 2010. https://www.nehi.net/publications/19-critical-care-critical-choices-the-case-for-tele-icus-in-intensive-care/view. Accessed 8/27/2018.
26. Rufo B. Tele-ICU positive return on investment. Health Aff. 2009;28(6):1859–60. https://www.ncbi.nlm.nih.gov/pubmed/19887429. Accessed 8/28/2018.
27. NEHI Report: Tele-ICU poised for major growth in health care informatics. 11-18-2013. https://www.healthcare-informatics.com/news-item/nehi-report-tele-icu-poised-major-growth. Accessed 8/28/2018.
28. Lilly CM, McLaughlin JM, Zhao H, Baker SP, UMass Memorial Critical Care Operations Group, et al. A multi-center study of ICU telemedicine reengineering of adult critical care. Chest. 2014;145(3):500–7.
29. Kahn JM, Cicero BD, Wallace DJ, Iwashyna TJ. Adoption of intensive care unit telemedicine in the United States. Crit Care Med. 2014;42(2):362–8. https://www.ncbi.nlm.nih.gov/pmc/articles/PMC3947050/. Accessed 7/11/2018.
30. Guidelines for the Tele-ICU, 2014. American Telemedicine Association. http://www.learnicu.org/SiteCollectionDocuments/Guidelines-ATA-TeleICU.pdf. Accessed 6/7/2018.
31. Linking quality to payment. https://www.medicare.gov/hospitalcompare/linking-quality-to-payment.html. Accessed 6/5/2018.
32. Populations, Population Health, and the Evolution of Population Management: Making Sense of the Terminology in US Health Care Today. Institute of Healthcare Improvement.

http://www.ihi.org/communities/blogs/population-health-population-management-terminology-in-us-health-care. Accessed 6/5/2018.
33. Remote patient monitoring/center for connected health. http://www.cchpca.org/remote-patient-monitoring. Accessed 6/5/2018.
34. Herendeen N, Deshpande P. Telemedicine and the patient centered medical home. Pediatr Ann. 2014;43(2):e28–32.
35. Critical Care Visits and Neonatal Intensive Care (Codes 99291 and 99292) https://www.cms.gov/Outreach-and-Education/Medicare-Learning-Network-MLN/MLNMattersArticles/downloads/MM5993.pdf. Accessed 6/5/2018.
36. Reynolds HN. "Remote Critical Care Services" in Coding and Billing: 6th Edition. Editors: George Sample, M.D. and Todd Dorman, M.D. Published by the Society of Critical Care Medicine (in press for 2014).
37. Calculating time units for anesthesia coding and billing. 4-4-2016. http://mbmps.com/calculating-time-units-for-anesthesia-billing-and-coding/. Accessed 6/5/2018.
38. Kumar G, Falk DM, Bonello RS, et al. The costs of critical care telemedicine programs: a systematic review and analysis. Chest. 2013;143(1):19–29.
39. Franzini L, Sail KR, Thomas EJ, et al. Cost and cost-effectiveness of a Tele-ICU program in six intensive care units in a large healthcare system. J Crit Care. https://www.ncbi.nlm.nih.gov/entrez/eutils/elink.fcgi?dbfrom=pubmed&retmode=ref&cmd=prlinks&id=21376515. Accessed 6/5/2018.
40. Reynolds HN, Bander JJ. Options for Tele-ICU design: Centralized vs De-Centralized and other considerations: It is not just another Black Sedan. Crit Care Clin. 2015;31:335–50.
41. Tele-Intensive Care Unit (ICU) Market Analysis By Component (Hardware, Software), By Type (Intensivist, Co-managed, Open, Open With Consultants) And Segment Forecasts To 2024. https://www.grandviewresearch.com/industry-analysis/tele-intensive-care-unit-icu-market. Accessed 6/5/2018.
42. Reynolds HN, Bander J, McCarthy M. Different systems and formats for Tele-ICU coverage. Designing a Tele-ICU system to optimize functionality and investment. Crit Care Nurs Q. 2012;35(4):1–14.
43. KPMG: Growing pains US CEO outlook. https://home.kpmg.com/content/dam/kpmg/us/pdf/2018/05/kpmg-ceo-outlook-2018.pdf. Accessed 7/11/2018.
44. Luddites https://en.wikipedia.org/wiki/Luddite. Accessed 7/11/2018.
45. Neo-Luddites https://en.wikipedia.org/wiki/Neo-Luddism. Accessed 7/11/2018.
46. Kruse CS, Karem P, Shifflett K, Vegi L, Ravi K, Brooks M. Evaluating barriers to adopting telemedicine worldwide: a systematic review. J Telemed Telecare. 2018;24(1):4–12. https://pdfs.semanticscholar.org/720a/fd525473897ebd663500bb5596ee85bf95d5.pdf. Accessed 7/11/2018.
47. Waddell K. How to get people 4 to embrace technological change. 6/2016. https://www.theatlantic.com/technology/archive/2016/06/how-to-get-people-to-embrace-technological-change/488720/. Accessed 7/11/2018.
48. Cerner Sues Firm, Alleges Patent Misuse. November 17, 2004. http://www.bizjournals.com/kansascity/stories/2004/11/15/daily24.html. Accessed 8/28/2018.
49. Cerner Prevails in Patent Dispute. https://www.bizjournals.com/kansascity/stories/2009/12/07/daily44.html. Accessed 8/28/2018.
50. Checking in on the Country's First Tele-ICU: 15 years later. https://www.beckershospital-review.com/healthcare-information-technology/checking-in-on-the-country-s-first-tele-icu-15-years-later.html. Accessed 8/24/2018.
51. U.S. Patent and Trademark Office Reaffirms VISICU's Novel Central Monitoring ICU Process. https://www.businesswire.com/news/home/20070615005268/en/VISICU-eICU-Patent-Reaffirmed. Accessed 7/16/2018.
52. Reynolds HN, Rogove H, Bander JJ, McCambridge M, Cowboy E, Niemeier M. A working lexicon for the tele-intensive care unit: we need to define tele-intensive care unit to grow and understand it. Telemed J E Health. 2011;17(10):773–83.

53. Reynolds EM, Grojovski A, Wright T, Foster M, Reynolds HN. Utilization of robotic "remote presence" technology within North American intensive care units. Telemed J E Health. 2012;18(7):1–9.
54. Dall T, West T, Chakrabarti R, Iacobucci W. The complexities of physician supply and demand: projections from 2013 to 2025. https://www.aamc.org/download/458082/data/2016_complexities_of_supply_and_demand_projections.pdf. Accessed 8/28/2018.
55. HRSA Work Force. Health workforce projections: critical care physicians and nurse practitioners https://bhw.hrsa.gov/sites/default/files/bhw/health-workforce-analysis/research/projections/critical-care-fact-sheet.pdf. Accessed 8/28/2018.
56. National Residency matching program. http://www.nrmp.org/match-data/nrmp-historical-reports/. Accessed 8/28/2018.
57. ACEP 5 alternative pathways to board certification in critical care medicine. https://www.acep.org/criticalcare-faq/. Accessed 8/28/2018.
58. EM-CCM Fellowships. http://emccmfellowship.org/. Accessed 8/28/2018.
59. ABIM offers opportunity for Triple Board Certification in IM, EM, and CCM. https://www.abim.org/certification/policies/combined-training/internal-medicineemergency-medicine-critical-care-medicine/overview.aspx. Accessed 8/28/2018.
60. Physician Tele-ICU jobs. Glassdoor.com. https://www.glassdoor.com/Job/physician-tele-icu-jobs-SRCH_KO0,18.htm. Accessed 7/11/2018.
61. Tele-ICU Medical Director Jobs. Indeed.com https://www.indeed.com/q-Tele-Icu-Medical-Director-jobs.html. Accessed 7/11/2018.
62. 13 Best Physician Tele-ICU jobs. Simplyhired.com https://www.simplyhired.com/search?q=physician+tele+intensivist&job=AglfDDP6S0zU_6FJhQS5UISBNl0A8XsOmm4Yz3bzwdQ1q7EoER7hqA. Accessed 7/11/2018.
63. Tele-ICU Critical Care Physicians Jama.Careers http://jama.careers.adicio.com/jobs/tele-icu-critical-care-physicians-long-island-ny-106022278-d. Accessed 7/11/2018.
64. LeapFrog Hospital Survey: Fact sheet-ICU Physician Staffing 4/1/2016. http://www.leapfroggroup.org/sites/default/files/Files/IPS%20Fact%20Sheet.pdf. Accessed 7/11/2018.
65. Nelson B. Alternative healthcare models aim to boost sagging critical-care workforce. The Hospitalist. 2012(10). https://www.the-hospitalist.org/hospitalist/article/125073/alternative-healthcare-models-aim-boost-sagging-critical-care-workforce. Accessed 8/28/2018.
66. Siegal EM, Dressler DD, Dichter JR, Gorman MJ, Lipsett PA. Training a hospitalist workforce to address the intensivist shortage in American hospitals: a position paper from the Society of Hospital Medicine and the Society of Critical Care Medicine. Crit Care Med. 2012;40(6):1952–6.
67. Gershengorn HB, Johnson MP, Factor P. Use of non-physician provides in the adult intensive care unit. Critical care perspectives. Am J Respir Crit Care Med. 2012;185(6):600–5.
68. Garland A, Gershengron HB. Staffing in the ICU: Physicians and alternative staffing models. Chest. 2013;143(1):214–21. https://doi.org/10.1378/chest.12-1531.
69. Buchman TG, Coopersmith CM, Meissen WH, Grabenkort WR, Bakshi V, Hiddleson CA, Gregg SR. Innovative interdisciplinary strategies to address the intensivist shortage. Crit Care Med. 2017;45(2):298–304.
70. Hayley B, Gershengorn HB, Scales DC, Kramera A, Wunsch H. Nighttime extubations are associated with worse outcomes for U.S. Intensive Care Unit Patients. Oral presentation at the American Thoracic Society Symposium, 2016.
71. Berger AM, Hobbs BB. Impact of shift work on the health and safety of nurses and patients. J Oncol Nurs. 2006;10(4):465–71.
72. Scott LD, Hwang WT, Rogers AE, Nysse T, Dean GE, Dinges DF. The relationship between nurse work schedules, sleep duration and drowsy driving. Sleep. 2007;30(12):1801–7.
73. Dula DJ, Dula NL, Hamrick C, Woods C. The effect of working serial night shifts on the cognitive functioning of emergency physicians. Ann Emerg Med. 2001;38(2):152–5.
74. Wucklund E. A telemedicine program links ICU patients to clinicians down under. May 15, 2018. https://mhealthintelligence.com/news/a-telemedicine-program-links-icu-patients-to-clinicians-down-under. Accessed 6/7/2018.

75. Emory cares for ICU patients remotely, turning 'night into day' from Australia. May 9th, 2018. http://news.emory.edu/stories/2018/05/buchman-hiddleson_eicu_perth_australia/index.html. Accessed 7/11/2018.
76. Emory patients get care from Australia: Doctors, nurses on day shifts in Australia help Emory centers at night. Atlanta Journal Constitution http://epaper.ajc.com/popovers/dynamic_article_popover.aspx?appid=2870&artguid=36ea93e4-adf8-414c-8214-c81431ae59d1. Accessed 7/19/2018.
77. From Sydney, Australia, Emory Healthcare Leverages Tele-ICU to Address Specialist Shortages. https://www.healthcare-informatics.com/article/telemedicine/atlanta-s-emory-healthcare-turns-australia-address-specialist-shortages. Accessed 7/19/2018.
78. The Business Model Data Base. http://tbmdb.blogspot.com/2009/02/scalable-business-models.html. Accessed 7/16/2018.
79. Horizontal Scalability. http://searchcio.techtarget.com/definition/horizontal-scalability. Accessed 7/16/2018.
80. Vertical Scalability. http://searchcio.techtarget.com/definition/vertical-scalability. Accessed 7/16/2018.
81. Avera eCare Telemedicine. https://www.averaecare.org. Accessed 7/16/2018.
82. Intermountain creates a virtual hospital with telehealth tools and services. https://www.healthcareitnews.com/news/intermountain-creates-virtual-hospital-telehealth-tools-and-services. Accessed 8/24/2018.
83. Intermountain Healthcare Opens New Virtual Hospital. https://www.healthcare-informatics.com/news-item/telemedicine/intermountain-healthcare-opens-new-virtual-hospital. Accessed 8/24/2018.
84. Politico: A hospital without beds. https://www.politico.com/agenda/story/2017/11/08/virtual-hospital-mercy-st-louis-000573. Accessed 8/24/2918.
85. Mercy Opens World's First Virtual Care Center, Oct 6, 2015. https://www.mercy.net/newsroom/2015-10-06/mercy-opens-worlds-first-virtual-care-center/. Accessed 8/24/2018.
86. Advanced ICU Care. http://advancedicucare.com/. Accessed 7/16/2018.
87. Reynolds HN, Zubrow M, Sikka N, Alcorta R. Adult Emergency and Critical Care Telehealth, first edition of "Understanding Telehealth" , edited by Rheuban K and Puchinski E, McGraw Hill Education, Chapter 8, 89–112, January 2018.
88. History of the shock trauma center: a tribute to R Adams Cowley, M.D. https://www.umms.org/ummc/health-services/shock-trauma/about/history. Accessed 7/16/2018.
89. Project ECHO: a revolution in medical education and care delivery http://echo.unm.edu/. Accessed 8/23/2018.
90. Adopting the ECHO model (Extension for Community Healthcare Outcomes) https://www.stepsforward.org/modules/project-echo. Accessed 8/23/2018.

Chapter 2
Remote Proactive Physiologic Monitoring in the ICU

Venktesh R. Ramnath and Atul Malhotra

Key Points

- Intensivist-associated benefits in ICU outcomes are limited by predicted manpower shortages and increased critical care data, which led to enthusiasm for remote proactive physiologic monitoring (RPM)-based technology solutions, now a burgeoning market.
- The use of predictive analytics in critical care is at a tipping point as artificial intelligence, data science, and related disciplines make new clinical decision support (e.g., "Sepsis Sniffer") and the Internet of Things possible in the "smart ICU."
- Centralized and decentralized RPM tele-ICU vendors offer continuous, reactive, or scheduled care RPM models with differentiation based on cost, ease of implementation, and analytics capability to drive outcomes.
- Regardless of the RPM/tele-ICU platform chosen, impact upon remote and bedside provider workflows should be examined and collaborative teamwork emphasized.
- Administrators looking to use RPM and tele-ICU systems should seek to integrate them into a larger, institution-wide health IT vision and emphasize compatibility and interoperability between new and existing technology, operations, and workflows.

V. R. Ramnath (✉)
Critical Care Telemedicine Outreach, Division of Pulmonary, Critical Care, and Sleep Medicine, UC San Diego Health, San Diego, CA, USA
e-mail: vramnath@ucsd.edu

A. Malhotra
Division of Pulmonary, Critical Care, and Sleep Medicine, UC San Diego Health, San Diego, CA, USA
e-mail: amalhotra@ucsd.edu

M. A. Koenig (ed.), *Telemedicine in the ICU*,
https://doi.org/10.1007/978-3-030-11569-2_2

Critical Care in Crisis

- *Existing intensivist staffing strategy is inadequate*

Management of critically ill patients admitted to the intensive care unit (ICU) is at a crossroads. Though most studies indicate that ICUs staffed by intensivist physicians have improved ICU outcomes, including lower mortality [1, 2], most critical care in the USA is not delivered by intensivists [3]. One factor is the availability of intensivists, a problem that will likely worsen as the US population continues to age and demand for critical care expertise rises [4]. Further demands upon existing intensivist physicians are due to hospital expansion of ICU bed to hospital bed ratios as part of acute care services [5]. Together, these factors have created a "crisis" in the critical care workforce [6].

- *Rising critical care data compound the need for expertise*

Concurrent with shortcomings in access to critical care expertise, the types and amount of data that are available for the critical care physician to make care plans have escalated dramatically. This is due to a rapid advancement over the last decade in computer processing speeds and high-speed-internet-based technologies that have made the use of smartphones, cloud computing, and mobile data networks almost ubiquitous [7]. As a result, business practices of many nonmedical industries from retail to finance have become "disrupted" [8]. Following suit, the healthcare industry is now being increasingly influenced by rising availability, reliability, and quantities of digital data.

- *Critical care and digital data: the rise of remote proactive physiologic monitoring (RPM)*

Since ICU care involves multiple data sources and specialized personnel who may not be readily available in person, many have advocated for the use of remote proactive physiologic monitoring (RPM) technologies to address both access to expertise and provision of critical care decision support. As we will explain, RPM can be used to improve access to expertise in various ways, including direct audio-visual connections to remote intensivists via a video teleconference (VTC) platform, surveillance monitoring of physiologic changes, and decision support for clinicians by virtue of sophisticated analytic software and displays.

- *What exactly is RPM?*

RPM is defined as the collection (using digital technologies) of personal health data from a person in one location (e.g., ICU) and transfer of such information electronically to a different location where these data can be analyzed and used by healthcare providers to evaluate and create care recommendations [9–11]. As a whole, RPM incorporates various aspects of the "digital health" spectrum, which includes population health management, big data and analytics, telemedicine, consumer engagement, digital medical devices and apps, and personalized medicine [12]. Use of RPM in the ICU has been invoked as a possible solution to the intensivist workforce gap by improving patient triage to the ICU (e.g., Modified Early Warning System) [13] and through enhanced use of existing limited resources without increasing the supply of intensivists [14]. Furthermore, given that substantial healthcare costs are allocated to the ICU setting [15], new use of technology is expected to improve the overall value of ICU care.

Components of RPM include patient sensors, telecommunications platforms, data storage, analytics applications, and information displays with associated interventions (see Table 2.1). Sensors can acquire or receive information and can be obtained via invasive or noninvasive, digital or non-digital, manual or passive input,

Table 2.1 Types of RPM ICU components, types, and examples

Components	Types	Examples
Data capture	Invasive sensors Noninvasive sensors (e.g., wireless or wired devices and "wearables") Manual input by operator (via smartphone app, EMR, etc.) Social media feed VTC	Indwelling brain electrodes, blood sampling monitors [18] Therapeutic "wearable" devices (e.g., indwelling brain electrodes, hearing aids, insulin pumps, transcutaneous electrical nerve stimulation (TENS)) Diagnostic "wearable" devices (e.g., pulse oximeters, blood pressure monitors, wearable patches, ECG leads, activity trackers) "Eatable" sensors (e.g., pill sensors for gastrointestinal bleeding [19]) EMR notes Ultrasound probes
Data transmission	Wireless (WiFi) Wired Mobile network Satellite Bluetooth ZigBee Nearfield Infrared Ultrawide band	TCP/IP internet protocols Coder-Decoder (CODEC) compression software T-carrier lines 3G/4G/5G
Data storage (central)	EMR Cloud storage and services	Epic, Cerner, McKesson, Allscripts Amazon Web Services, Oracle, IBM, Google, Apple
Data analytics, artificial intelligence-based algorithms	Population health analysis Identification of opportunities for intervention (e.g., deviation from established norms)	APACHE, SAPS scoring Compliance and metric analysis
Data display and recommended treatment interventions	"Smart," logic-based clinical and operational decision support Dashboard-based alerts	Discharge Readiness Tool [20] "Sepsis Sniffer" [21] Irrelevant alarm reduction

APACHE Acute Physiology and Chronic Health Examination, *EMR* electronic medical record, *SAPS* Simplified Acute Physiology Score and/or real-time versus asynchronous means. For example, a device implanted in the brain can provide real-time data through an invasive electrode [16], while a wireless respiratory monitor may never be required to touch the patient's skin. Telecommunications can be through wired (e.g., T-carrier lines), wireless (WiFi), mobile network, satellite, infrared, ultrawide band, ZigBee, nearfield, or Bluetooth connections [17] and ensure Health Insurance Portability and Accountability Act (HIPAA) and other security compliance. Data storage must exist locally (within the device itself) as well as at the remote site where all device data are housed and ultimately examined for generation of treatment recommendations and statistical analyses (e.g., severity-adjusted acuity scores like Acute Physiology and Chronic Health Examination (APACHE)). Some digital devices, such as smartphones apps and wearable sensors, combine these capabilities and are able to monitor, record, transmit, and even provide treatment interventions.

- *Use cases of RPM in the ICU are promising but still early-stage*

How are these technologies used in the ICU? Many RPM technologies are still being tested in proof-of-concept and feasibility studies, but effective devices and strategies have emerged that use disease-specific approaches. Specific feasibility studies include the use of tele-electrocardiogram and tele-angiography [22, 23] in acute coronary syndrome, tele-echocardiography in congenital heart disease [23, 24], tele-delirium assessments via mobile devices [25], safety during transport of acutely ill [26], sleep disorder surveillance [27, 28], patient mobility [29], sedation levels [30], pressure ulcer monitoring [31–33], tele-electroencephalogram in epilepsy [34–38], and hyperbaric treatment [39]. RPM interventions have also applied to improving hand hygiene in the ICU [40].

When individual, disease-specific RPM technologies are grouped into collective strategies for delivering comprehensive ICU care, however, options narrow considerably. This finding is primarily due to the difficulties in integrating products that have been engineered and studied in diverse ways without overlapping or common standards, goals, or approaches. As a result, many disease-specific RPM technologies are wedded to particular technology ecosystems in which they were created. For example, there are differing quantities and types of mobile health apps that are specifically designed for Apple iOS or Android smartphone operating systems, but not both [41]. As a whole, integrated RPM platforms are still in a state of infancy.

RPM and Data Analytics in the ICU

- *RPM is a major step towards the Precision Medicine goal of personalized, data-driven critical care*

Interest in RPM took a large step forward with the introduction of the Precision Medicine Initiative of the National Institutes of Health [42, 43]. In early 2015,

President Obama laid the groundwork for a new approach to medicine and research in which care plans and treatment algorithms could be tailored to an individual person's unique makeup based on genetic, environmental, and lifestyle factors. In the President's words, "Doctors have always recognized that every patient is unique, and doctors have always tried to tailor their treatments as best they can to individuals. You can match a blood type – that was an important discovery. What if matching a cancer cure to our genetic code was just as easy, just as standard? What if figuring out the right dose of medicine was as simple as taking our temperature?" [43].

By using RPM and other digital health strategies, a new emphasis on creation of personalized care plans has now emerged in the ICU. Patient and context-relevant care plans can incorporate data from medical records and genomic, environmental, and even social media-based sources [44]. Along these lines, some have called for collecting digital patient health data to create a "digitized self" that could be shared with researchers and clinicians, who could then identify precise therapies [45]. Reflecting such enthusiasm, the global ICU RPM technology market is projected to grow with a compound annual growth rate at almost 20% from 2013 to 2024, with a projected overall value in North America of $2.5 billion [42].

- *RPM data and artificial intelligence in critical care: dawn of a new era in decision support*

Given the ongoing effects of Moore's Law upon processing power, RPM digital devices and enhanced cloud server storage capacities have allowed for exponentially growing repositories of health data, raising prospects for insights mined from such "big data." As a result, fields such as computer science, data science, and statistical analysis of large data sets have taken a special relevance in healthcare. In particular, artificial intelligence (AI) approaches such as deep learning and machine learning algorithms have shown much promise [16, 46–48], including better ICU patient acuity-based scoring and outcome predictions [20, 49], reduction of false arrhythmia alarms [50], predicting central-line bloodstream infections [51], and improved sepsis outcomes in the ICU [21, 52, 53].

One example is the Sepsis Sniffer [21], a detection and alert system that utilizes rules-based algorithms using EMR data to identify two key components of severe sepsis management: its presence and associated delays in recognition and treatment. The sepsis detection component of the algorithm uses multiple parameters gleaned from the EMR based on the physiology of sepsis (orders for body fluid cultures for suspicion of infection): white blood cell count, temperature, respiratory rate, and heart rate (markers of systemic inflammatory response syndrome (SIRS)); blood lactate levels and systolic blood pressure (signs of organ hypoperfusion-related dysfunction); and fluid-resistant low blood pressure readings and use of vasopressors documenting clinical shock. The delay in recognition and treatment component is based on lactate and central venous pressure (CVP) values only. Using both recursive data partitioning (a statistical modeling method) and an iterative process to refine the algorithm, the Sniffer had a sensitivity of 80% and specificity 96% for detection of severe sepsis. It was then used to demonstrate that 68% of patients had a delay in recognition of treatment component such as not having lactate and CVP measurements done in a timely manner. In addition, the Sniffer showed that the existence of low systolic blood pressure had the greatest predictive value for detecting severe sepsis [21].

Riding this momentum, we appear to be at a tipping point, given that 86% of hospitals now use some form of AI in their operations, with applications ranging from claims collection to clinical decision support [54]. In the ICU, the need for "smart" approaches to the rising data collection is inescapable.

- *RPM makes "The Internet of ICU Things" a realistic possibility*

The "Internet of Things" (IoT) is a description of how activities and objects of daily life continue to be transformed by the power of data from mobile computing technologies coupled with cloud-based storage servers, high-speed internet connectivity, and analytics platforms. Like "smart grids" that aim to improve utilization, efficiency, and reliability of electricity use [56], IoT now appears within reach in healthcare [57, 58], including the ICU, and depends on the use of RPM. Bhatia [55] introduced and implemented an ICU IoT framework that showed both high anomaly recognition and low false positive rate (~3%) compared to manual and audiovisual monitoring practices. The ICU IoT they propose includes the following features: data acquisition and synchronization, event classification and cloud server-based storage, information mining and analysis, and presentation of notifications to the physician provider (Fig. 2.1). Numerical, graphic, and textual data from patients are assigned attributes that are grouped into datasets and classified into "events" (such as physiologic values (e.g., vital signs), discrete therapies (e.g., medications and procedures), environmental factors (e.g., ambient noise and air quality), behavioral stigmata (e.g., stress), or diet features (e.g., type of nutrition). These events are then stored in cloud servers where they can be mined and analyzed, with eventual notification via alerts to the medical provider [59]. This IoT model is the natural extension of the informatics foundation well described by Halpern [17], in which he describes the steps toward creating the informatics backbone of the "smart ICU" through the use of the following: a wired and wireless device infrastructure, data connectivity hardware, automatic identification tags, adapters for interoperable data sharing, and ICU middleware (e.g., servers and applications) such as real-time locating systems, decision support, VTC, and smart displays (Fig. 2.2). With this scaffold in place, the various RPM technologies, IoT strategies, and AI-based algorithmic analyses (such as "just-in-time learning" [60]) can create an integrated technological approach that achieves the goals of Precision Medicine [61].

S.No.	Dataset	Attributes	Description	IoT Technology Used
(1)	Health Data	Heart rate, Blood pressure, Respiration rate, ECG	Data about health condition about patient under consideration	Smart wearable, Body sensors, Heart sensor, and ECG monitor
(2)	Medicinal Data	Strength, Type, Form, Proportion	Data about medication given to patient	RFID tag, Bedside sensor, and Camcorder
(3)	Environmental Data	Noise level, Light, Room temperature, Air-quality, Toxic waste	Data about ICU room environmental conditions	Room sensor, Chemical detector, Noise sensor, and Light sensor
(4)	Behavioural Data	Stress, Anxiety, Restlessness	Data regarding behavioural aspects of patient during ICU stay	Bio-Sensors, Smart wearable, and Monitor
(5)	Dietary Data	Nutritional value, Quantity, Nature	Data about eatables consumed by the patient	RFIDs, and Swallow sensor

Fig. 2.1 Classification of events in an "Internet of Things" ICU framework. (Adapted with permission from Bhatia et al. [55])

Step 1
Install robust wired and wireless infrastructure
↓
Step 2
Install tracking and data acquisition hardware
↓
Step 3
Attach Auto-Identification (Auto-ID) tags to all data sources
↓
Step 4
Attach adaptors and/or computers to medical device data output ports
↓
Step 5
Install middleware (servers/applications) on hospital and ICU networks

Fig. 2.2 Steps in creating an informatics foundation in the "smart" ICU. (From Halpern [17])

Current Comprehensive Tele-ICU Options

Although many RPM strategies to date have focused on feasibility and single applications, some integrated RPM platforms have demonstrated benefit in particular ICU populations under an umbrella term of "tele-ICU." These tele-ICU systems often integrate various different RPM components, such as real-time, high-definition VTC, EMR and imaging access, physiologic data acquired from sensors, secure data storage centers, and clinical decision support functionalities. In neurocritical care [62], iSyNCC provides patient monitoring and information and clinical decision support. There are other similar applications in neonatal care [63–66], pediatric care [65, 67], and cardiac care [23].

In general, tele-ICU systems for adult patients can be categorized as centralized or decentralized, employ open or closed architecture, and utilize either continuous, reactive, or scheduled care models [68, 69].

Centralized Monitoring Tele-ICU

- *CM systems provide a hub-and-spoke platform and continuous, reactive, and/or scheduled care models*

CM tele-ICU systems usually involve a hub-and-spoke structure in which RPM data (e.g., vital signs, EMR, picture archiving and communications system (PACS), VTC-based communication) are continually transmitted from all monitored ICU beds in the spoke ICU through high-fidelity, fixed T1-carrier connections to a dedicated team in the hub command center. The RPM data are constantly analyzed using sophisticated clinical information system (CIS) software to generate acuity scores, assess compliance with evidence-based care standards [70, 71], and create electronic displays. Using such information, the remote providers have the ability to make immediate and proactive interventions according to the recommendations of the analytic software. While reactive (i.e., upon request) or scheduled care models are possible, most CM systems employ a continuous care model in which the hub team constantly processes data inputs and intervenes in real-time. Actual or potential clinical problems can be visualized through acuity-based patient dashboards generated by the CM software, and the hub team can provide support via telephone and/or VTC for any questions from the on-site providers.

- *CM tele-ICU systems demonstrate improved outcomes through early recognition of critical disease and improved protocol compliance*

Use of CM systems has been associated with clinical outcome improvements, including enhanced sepsis management like the "Sepsis Sniffer" and "Sepsis Prompt" [21, 52, 72–75], adherence to lung protection goals [76, 77], prevention of ventilator-associated pneumonia [71], improved outcomes in ST-segment elevation myocardial infarction [78], and ventilator bundle compliance [79]. ICU survival benefits have also been observed [80, 81]. Furthermore, the wealth of actionable data from these CISs opens new opportunities in resource utilization, such as appropriately triaging patients into and out of the ICU [20, 82]. One such example is the Discharge Readiness Score (of the Philips eCareManager®) that utilizes calculated APACHE and/or Simplified Acute Physiology Score (SAPS) severity scores [20, 83], trends in clinical markers, benchmarks, and other data to indicate appropriate timing for discharge from the ICU care setting [20, 79]. In these ways, CM tele-ICU systems appear to be a major step toward the Precision Medicine goal of the "smart ICU."

- *CM tele-ICU vendors offer enterprise-level, end-to-end products*

CM tele-ICU systems are largely offered by vendors as a comprehensive, end-to-end enterprise-level package including hardware, software, and project management personnel to facilitate implementation. Some companies like Banner Health and Advanced ICU Care also offer telehealth providers for an installed CM tele-ICU system. Major vendors of CM tele-ICU products are global and include GE Healthcare (Chalfont St. Giles, UK) and Philips Healthcare (Andover, MA), which owns Philips-VISICU (Baltimore, MD). Smaller vendors include iMDsoft® (Dusseldorf, Germany) and INTeleICU (Chennai, India). Philips-VISICU offers an end-to-end solution including provision of hardware, software, and project management resources. Hardware is offered at cost from Philips itself or third-party vendors, while the software (eCareManager®) is a strictly proprietary product. iMDsoft® offers a software overlay that integrates with native EMRs to provide an early warning dashboard display using RPM data streams.

- *CM tele-ICU systems drawbacks: high cost, required resources, and time to implement*

One chief disadvantage of CM tele-ICU systems is cost, with initial startup estimates ranging from \$50,000 to \$100,000 per ICU patient bed [42, 84]. Another is time to full implementation, since enterprise solutions often require many months to prepare effectively and execute the launch. Therefore, committing to a CM tele-ICU platform requires significant investments in new hardware, software, and manpower, which can provide difficulties to smaller hospitals on a tight budget.

Decentralized Tele-ICU

- *DC systems emulate the bedside consultant experience through reactive or scheduled care models only*

DC tele-ICU systems most often involve a standalone platform in which a portable, mobile VTC device is used for direct bedside care through an open architecture design in which single or multiple providers can deliver care without being required to be in a single location. In this way, reactive or scheduled care models are primarily possible with DC systems as they mirror traditional clinical settings in which a clinician arrives at the bedside at the request of a referring provider (continuous care models require a separate system). The DC tele-consultant appears at the bedside on a VTC screen (i.e., positioned on a mobile robot or cart, desktop, or tablet), interviews the patient, and performs a physical examination with the help of an on-site medical provider (e.g., nurse). The tele-consultant reviews relevant patient health information in data repositories that are almost always separate from the VTC technology (e.g., EMR, PACS). In this way, the tele-consultant workflow is almost identical to a live consultant, except that the interview and exam are done remotely with the help of an on-site clinical provider. Clinical decision support, unlike CM tele-ICU systems, relies on existing IT systems that are traditionally EMR-based.

- *DC tele-ICU vendors offer many different hardware and software options*

DC tele-ICU system hardware device options include autonomous mobile robot units (e.g., InTouch Health (Santa Barbara, CA)), semiautonomous robot units (e.g., Double Robotics (Mountain View, CA), Suitable Technologies (Palo Alto, CA), Vgo (Cambridge, MA), VSee (Sunnyvale, CA)), cart-based units (e.g., Cisco (San Jose, CA), Lifesize (Austin, CA), Polycom (San Jose, CA)), and handheld tablets (e.g., Apple iPad®, Microsoft Surface Pro®). Separate software purchase is usually unnecessary, as most devices have their own embedded software allowing connections through available internet networks, but hospitals must ensure that high-speed internet connectivity (at least 1 MBPS) is available through either fixed ports in patient rooms or wireless access points to avoid signal interruptions. Patient examination "peripheral" devices include tele-stethoscopes, and ultrasound monitors can be helpful in direct patient evaluation. However, most DC-based patient examination primarily relies on the power of the VTC interface (particularly the resolution of camera zoom, which is often 10× to 12×) in conjunction with direct patient contact by on-site providers' "surrogate hands" [68].

- *DC tele-ICU systems are relatively inexpensive and flexible*

The main advantages to DC tele-ICU systems involve cost and flexibility. Device prices generally continue to decrease over time, given the low barriers to market entry of competitors and evolving manufacturing costs, and are device-specific. Tablets are generally \$500–\$2000 while mobile robot units are \$5000–\$10,000 and cart-based units range from \$10,000 to \$100,000 (based on available MSRP information). From a technical standpoint, introducing a DC device, which usually operates independently from other health IT infrastructure, can be relatively straightforward provided that high-speed internet connectivity is available. As a result, time to initial implementation can be minimal. Maintenance costs include hardware and software upgrades but are often included in purchase contracts.

- *DC tele-ICU drawback: lack of integrated IT/analytics platform to drive outcomes*

The main drawback of DC tele-ICU systems is the lack of an integrated CIS to allow seamless analytics-based intervention via a continuous care model. Instead, each remote provider must access RPM data separately via health IT platforms (e.g., EMR), which are often limited in functionality as they are frequently not engineered for population health-based analytics. While the ultimate efficacy upon clinical outcomes of DC systems is currently unclear (in comparison to CM tele-ICU systems which have been better studied [85]), it is also important to recognize that direct comparison studies between continuous and reactive care models have yet to be performed [86].

Bespoke (Hybrid) Models of Tele-ICU

Given the limitations of current vendor offerings in CM (i.e., cost of resources, time to execute) and DC (i.e., lack of CIS) tele-ICU systems, some have turned to create their own hybrid systems, often trying to incorporate advantages of both systems while minimizing respective downsides. For example, Navy Medical Center [87] created an early warning dashboard emulating a CM tele-ICU system with purchase of VTC equipment from third-party vendors and integrating them alongside other RPM devices with the legacy CliniComp EMR. Banner Health (Phoenix, AZ) created iCare™ that allows interoperability between devices across their multistate clinical network. iMDsoft® provides a software overlay product that allows legacy EMR systems to create customizable dashboards, while hospitals choose hardware options and provide their own internal IT support personnel. Disaster management models involving telemedicine often purport the importance of both CM and DC tele-ICU elements [88]. EMR vendors themselves (e.g., Epic (Verona, WI), Cerner (North Kansas City, MO)) are now developing their own tools to match the competition, like the APeX EMR used by the University of California at San Francisco that is capable of machine learning algorithms to improve sepsis outcomes [53]. Along these lines, larger academic medical institutions like UC San Diego Health are exploring mobile VTC solutions to complement and spur innovation in EMR capability. These developments have put pressure on the larger vendors of CM tele-ICU systems to provide "lighter" options to address the growing market niche for a more versatile, effective, and less costly solution.

Launching a Tele-ICU Program: Impact Upon Clinicians and Their Respective Workflows

In any tele-ICU system, clinical workflow and operations in both on-site and remote locations are important to understand to promote continuity of care. The following are some important points for clinicians to keep in mind in CM as well as DC tele-ICU systems:

Remote Tele-Clinicians

- Remember that credentialing/privileging requirements can be burdensome. This can be an overlooked point, but time, effort, and expense are required to complete and maintain hospital-based requirements at all potential care sites, especially if care crosses state borders [89].
- Understand the remote team structure. The number of individuals (nurses/intensivists/clerical staff) and reporting structure should be well defined and understood by all team members. CM usually involves multiple members, while DC can involve either single or multiple providers. Team-building activities are important to build morale and efficiency of the remote team.
- Expect to document tele-interventions and encounters. Most clinical interventions require EMR documentation in the medical record, which can be labor-intensive, particularly with higher numbers of beds monitored.
- Learn to utilize bedside providers as "surrogate hands" [68]. This is often challenging in both CM and DC systems. Expect a learning curve to proficiency, patience, and time spent to direct and obtain exam findings from a bedside in-person nurse. Proper training is crucial, especially for high stress situations such as cardiac resuscitation protocols and other urgent clinical deteriorations.
- Beware of alarm fatigue. Depending on the sophistication of embedded analytics and "smart" systems that can reduce clinically irrelevant alarms [50, 90], alert frequency can be substantial [71, 91] in CM and DC systems alike.

- Be familiar with expectations regarding coding and billing for services. While most users of tele-ICU systems currently do not submit bills for a variety of reasons [89], some do. DC models are more aligned with reimbursement if the geographic and other criteria are met [89].
- Participate in team-building exercises with on-site staff. Developing a "How can we help?" customer service-oriented approach is essential in both DC and CM systems. Create call schedules with continuity of providers so that familiarity between on-site and remote providers can grow.

On-site Clinicians

- Welcome tele-staff as part of the local care team. Tele-ICU staff are most often seen as extensions to local teams to provide extra resources in terms of specialist input for complex cases and a "second pair of hands" for routine surveillance and nurse charting [92–94].
- Expect changes in call coverage and local staffing structure. Given new access to critical care tele-specialists, availability of on-site physicians (especially at night) may be different [94]. Also, on-site staffing may include the introduction of advanced practice providers (i.e., nurse practitioners or physician assistants) to assist in bedside care needs.
- Review documentation from tele-ICU staff. On-site staff should expect to review notes made by remote tele-ICU staff frequently to be aware of any interventions, changes in care goals, and deviations from evidence-based standards that occurred.
- Learn how to be effective "surrogate hands." On-site providers will often be asked to develop and perform physical exam skills under the direct coaching of a remote physician and/or provider. Comfort and confidence come with practice.
- Be open to feedback and communication. Picking up the phone to ask for help and being receptive to feedback from "anonymous" providers can feel awkward at first but improves with time and familiarity. When on duty, using face-to-face visualization on the VTC whenever possible can help.

Considerations for administrative and clinical leaders to improve the relationship between on-site and remote providers:

- Identify physician, nursing [95], and other champions who have prior experience and enthusiasm for telemedicine and technology and provide tangible support for their efforts (e.g., funding, protected time).
- Create a plan for transparent communication [96, 97] and feedback through the pre-implementation, implementation, and post-implementation phases of roll-out. Clear designation of competencies [76] and roles of the remote and on-site providers can avoid "diffusion of responsibility" issues with multiple providers dedicated to the same task(s) that can lead to inadvertent neglect [98].

- Emphasize ongoing staff training. Increase familiarity with online data, alarms [99], and audiovisual connections for consultation and monitoring, with one-on-one and single patient experiences [100]. Consider use of virtual simulators [88, 101] and role-reversal exercises for both on-site and remote staff [97].
- Foster team and relationship building prospectively through encouragement of direct communication and visualization, continuity of staffing, arrangement of periodic in-person visits (on-site visits by remote staff as well as on-site provider visits to the remote staff location), and social engagements between all staff.

Making the Right Choice for Your Institution: Where Administrators Should Focus

Given the plethora of tele-ICU products, a thoughtful approach is important. The following key points should be considered:

1. Value proposition: What is the main driver behind taking on a change to the status quo and how urgent is the need? Examples include improving population-based ICU clinical outcomes [102], reducing patient transfers, mitigating burnout levels in on-site staff, improving ICU bed utilization [103], and closing ICU coverage gaps.
2. Operational assessment: How many ICU beds, units, hospitals, and hours of coverage (daytime/nighttime) are being considered? How many staff members are needed in the tele-ICU? CM tele-ICU systems often see financial economies of scale when more than 75 ICU beds are envisioned for coverage, while DC can be helpful in lower patient loads. Some vendors offer trial periods, subscription models, upgrade packages, and rentals in addition to direct purchase [96]. Credentialing-by-proxy [89] and tele-proctoring (for focused and ongoing professional practice evaluation requirements) should be considered. Remember that success of any tele-ICU system is contingent upon pre- and post-implementation periods as much as during the initial rollout itself.
3. Emphasize interoperability within the entire health IT ecosystem. Interoperability of RPM hardware and software is important in order to minimize technology and workflow silos. An initial technical point is to understand how extant WiFi, cellular, Bluetooth, mobile, and satellite network capability in and around the hospital(s) can and will impact RPM technologies of a planned tele-ICU system. Next, one should examine the impact of interoperability upon technology workflows. For example, DC tele-ICU systems usually offer standalone VTC services and, from an analytics standpoint, are largely independent of native EMR systems and thereby generally cannot harness the power of integrated CIS metrics that can improve outcomes. On the other hand, CM tele-ICU systems offer CIS-based interventions but also heavily depend on compatibility between devices and data streams for optimal results.

- *Synchronize and coordinate hospital-wide RPM approaches and departmental IT systems as much as possible to optimize overall system efficiency.*

Some specific considerations regarding interoperability should be highlighted. First, continuous care models using CIS (whether as part of a CM system or an adjunct to DC system) require full integration between legacy IT systems and analytic software to realize the full potential [58]. Reduced or partial integration hamstrings functionality and can detract from utilization by providers with strong consequences on overall efficacy [104]. Second, tele-ICU systems should synchronize with other similar technology-driven efforts elsewhere in the hospital to minimize overall costs and enhance continuity of analytics-driven care to maximize system-wide gains. The EarlySense system in the Veterans Administration is a low-acuity early warning system that involves sensors placed in patients' beds, bedside monitors, central display station, and proprietary analytic tools to prevent ICU admissions [105]. Other examples include the use of tele-ICU-like RPM systems for rapid response team support [106], progressive care units [107], and even general medical/surgical ward units [108]. Third, tele-ICU technology should include capacity to interface easily with nonclinical technology systems in order to reduce data stream conflicts and broaden the data spectrum available for analysis. Indeed, health data sharing across disparate devices, which is promoted by the Integrating the Healthcare Environment initiative (www.ihe.net), has yielded notable benefits. For example, the University of Utah gained valuable insight when using computer system to analyze data from various sources (e.g., ICU supplies, laboratory ordering, imaging and other diagnostic tests, medication orders) eventually finding that surgical ICU costs amounted to $1.43 per minute [109]. Cismondi found that AI-based modeling could reduce unnecessary lab tests in the ICU by around 50% [110]. With such clarity, "smart" use of existing resources is possible, akin to "just-in-time" approaches seen in the supply chain management in the manufacturing industry since the 1970s [111].

- *Encourage interoperability with regional and national networks.*

Similarly, promoting interoperability beyond the hospital (i.e., intra-institution, inter-hospital, intra-network (regional, national)) contexts is important, to extend gains based on facilitated information sharing across a wider set of patients. For institutions seeking to grow and leverage population health-based gains, seamless information sharing between all the member institutions is essential, with the Veterans Administration leading new efforts through promotion of the Open Application Programming Interface Pledge [112]. By engaging in such public-private partnerships, new innovative ideas are likely to surface as experiences and approaches are shared with others in the regional and national health system facing similar challenges.

- *Anticipate any new technology to be launched in the medium (1–5-year) time frame.*

Finally, it may be worthwhile to examine if any new or expanded technologies are envisioned in the near future (1–5-year time frame). Examples might include upgrading or switching an EMR platform, launching a new secure messaging application [113], purchasing a new set of ventilators or monitors, changing data server hosting, or studying a new technology (e.g., blockchain, augmented/virtual/mixed reality). If so, attention should be made to consider interoperability concerns in the short, medium, and long term.

4. Prioritize compatibility of tele-ICU systems with existing clinical workflows, operations, and technology.

Technology does not exist in a vacuum. In both CM and DC tele-ICU systems, the interoperability of RPM products and data sharing platforms must be coordinated with clinician interventions to maximize overall benefits. Studies continue to show that the more the tele-ICU system is used, the more the benefits may accrue [71, 81], especially if a direct intervention or logistic center is involved [114, 115]. Therefore, it is important to focus upon the usability and compatibility of technology with existing clinical (and other) workflows and communication between providers [116]. Focus groups involving all stakeholders to a planned tele-ICU system should take place to understand all the current and potential pain points. This would include not just physicians (especially those who regularly admit to the ICU, such as surgeons, hospitalists, critical care intensivists, and cardiologists) and nurses [95], who would be the highest users of the tele-ICU service, but also ancillary staff such as pharmacists as well as administrators.

- *Who are the potential proponents and detractors of a tele-ICU program?*

In addition, scrutiny must be placed on who will be directly or indirectly affected by launching a tele-ICU program. Who will lose or dissuade others from using tele-ICU and who will gain or promote its use? This is a key consideration, since the success of the tele-ICU program will depend on the strength and balance of local champions and detractors [71, 95, 117]. Some key issues to consider from enacting a tele-ICU system include the local staff response to remote providers and the effect upon staff in non-ICU wards, who may now need to handle higher acuity patients [118].

Tele-ICU implementation should also synchronize existing contract-based services to minimize friction during transition. For example, if the RPM system will replace or impact a specific service line (e.g., intensivist staffing), contractual adjustments should be anticipated in advance, particularly with external provider groups. By recognizing that business transparency is a major market challenge in healthcare, administrators should avoid using multiple different and simultaneously operating IT platforms in order to reduce redundancy, confusion, and cross-competition for resources [57]. Finally, the public policy landscape should be compatible with the tele-ICU plan, given implications on licensing and restrictions on the use of telemedicine, including billing practices depending on state [89].

5. Reflect on longer-range strategic vision: What role does technology play? Remember overall tele-ICU and health IT trends.

From a global market perspective, tele-ICU systems are still in their infancy [42]. Given the current interdependence of technology with human resources, there still remains some uncertainty about the true effectiveness of tele-ICU alone, since they are considered "just one aspect of the health information technology bundle." [96]. To date, CM tele-ICU systems demonstrate unclear cost-effectiveness [119], though financial gains may increase if technology is complemented by a decision support model in which RPM information was used to triage patients as well as deliver care [115]. In other words, technology alone is not enough.

Overall health IT trends are pointing toward increased options in healthcare data storage and analysis. Hospitals, which have traditionally been the location for patient data server hosting and other IT services, are now moving to outsource such activities to third parties in order to save costs and improve operational efficiency by streamlining workflows to core competencies [57]. Current market trends in the tele-ICU technology product space favor growth in software over hardware [42, 57] which suggests that the greatest gains will be seen by using software analytics that leverage existing hardware to optimize economies of scale. Many cloud computing vendors reliably meet governmental regulations and data privacy and security requirements, thereby allowing increased market entry of offerings such as software as a service (SAAS), platform as a service (PAAS), and software as a medical device (SaMD) products for health data analysis. The decisions of various large tech companies (e.g., Apple, Amazon, IBM, Google) to enter the health analytics space further substantiate this trend [47, 120]. As noted earlier, EMR vendors such as Epic are also developing their own internal tele-ICU dashboards and electronic triage tools. For these reasons, we are in the midst of a sea change in ICU health IT and data analytics.

Recognizing this trend can aid decision-making about tele-ICU investment and where the longer-term return on investment lies. For example, some institutions may find it better to devise a more custom-fit solution by partnering with a cloud storage and data analytics company or invest in a robust EMR platform that has embedded ICU analytics capabilities, in conjunction with a DC VTC interface for the face-to-face component. Others may find higher value in selecting an established CM tele-ICU vendor product if many hospitals in a given network have aligned objectives and health IT structures that would make such a transition more straightforward.

Common Pitfalls for Physician Leaders and Administrators

1. Avoid making decisions based on a limited perspective. When choosing a DC or CM system, use a wide lens when considering system-based health IT, clinical operations, and market trends.
2. Do not underestimate how much team-building and trust-sharing is required to launch and sustain a successful tele-ICU program. Remember to incent and

support tele-ICU champions, since an effective champion will weather criticism from peers and promote adoption, help anticipate and troubleshoot problems, and augment overall program sustainability.
3. Don't forget interoperability *and* compatibility. This is the sweet spot for choosing something that works today, tomorrow, and beyond.
4. Think of your tele-ICU as a startup business. There are no "failures" in entrepreneurship. Too often, valuable projects lose support because hard targets are not met. Learn from the mistakes made. As the startup adage goes, "fail frequently and quickly" in order to home in on more sustainable successes for the long term.

Summary

Use of RPM in an ICU setting, whether it be a comprehensive tele-ICU solution or disease-specific approaches, is here to stay. We have discussed the importance of the various RPM strategies and how integration, interoperability, and compatibility from various standpoints lie at the heart of a successful move forward toward the development of a "smart" ICU and IoT. As with all healthcare endeavors, the people involved – in the case of the tele-ICU, remote and on-site providers – are a central component, and fostering this relationship is vital. As we move further into the twenty-first century, the capability of technology-driven clinical decision-making will likely increase exponentially with the power of AI, data science, and other tools. Even in such scenarios, however, people will need to work together in creative and mutually supportive ways to achieve the most that technology has to offer.

References

1. Wilcox ME, Chong CAKY, Niven DJ, Rubenfeld GD, Rowan KM, Wunsch H, et al. Do intensivist staffing patterns influence hospital mortality following ICU admission? A systematic review and meta-analyses. Crit Care Med. 2013;41(10):2253–74.
2. Gajic O, Afessa B. Physician staffing models and patient safety in the ICU. Chest. 2009;135(4):1038–44.
3. Angus DC, Shorr AF, White A, Dremsizov TT, Schmitz RJ, Kelley MA, et al. Critical care delivery in the United States: distribution of services and compliance with Leapfrog recommendations. Crit Care Med. 2006;34(4):1016–24.
4. Krell K. Critical care workforce. Crit Care Med. 2008;36(4):1350–3.
5. Vincent J-L. Critical care--where have we been and where are we going? Crit Care Lond Engl. 2013;17(Suppl 1):S2.
6. Kelley MA, Angus D, Chalfin DB, Crandall ED, Ingbar D, Johanson W, et al. The critical care crisis in the United States: a report from the profession. Chest. 2004;125(4):1514–7.
7. Friedman TL. Thank you for being late: an optimist's guide to thriving in the age of accelerations. 1st ed. New York: Farrar, Straus and Giroux; 2016. 486 p.
8. Grossman R. The industries that are being disrupted the most by digital [Internet]. Harv Bus Rev. 2016 [cited 2018 Mar 7]. Available from: https://hbr.org/2016/03/the-industries-that-are-being-disrupted-the-most-by-digital.

9. What is Telehealth? | Center for Connected Health Policy [Internet]. [cited 2018 Mar 6]. Available from: http://www.cchpca.org/what-is-telehealth.
10. Vegesna A, Tran M, Angelaccio M, Arcona S. Remote patient monitoring via non-invasive digital technologies: a systematic review. Telemed J E Health. 2017;23(1):3–17.
11. Telehealth Programs | Official web site of the U.S. Health Resources & Services Administration [Internet]. [cited 2018 Mar 6]. Available from: https://www.hrsa.gov/rural-health/telehealth/index.html.
12. Digital Health Funding: 2014 Year in Review [Internet]. Rock Health. [cited 2018 Mar 7]. Available from: https://rockhealth.com/reports/digital-health-funding/.
13. Gardner-Thorpe J, Love N, Wrightson J, Walsh S, Keeling N. The value of Modified Early Warning Score (MEWS) in surgical in-patients: a prospective observational study. Ann R Coll Surg Engl. 2006;88(6):571–5.
14. Kahn JM, Rubenfeld GD. The Myth of the workforce crisis. Why the United States does not need more intensivist physicians. Am J Respir Crit Care Med. 2015;191(2):128–34.
15. Halpern NA, Pastores SM. Critical care medicine in the United States 2000-2005: an analysis of bed numbers, occupancy rates, payer mix, and costs. Crit Care Med. 2010;38(1):65–71.
16. How brains and machines can be made to work together | The Economist [Internet]. [cited 2018 Mar 6]. Available from: https://www.economist.com/news/technology-quarterly/21733196-brain-computer-interfaces-sound-stuff-science-fiction-andrew-palmer.
17. Halpern NA. Innovative designs for the smart ICU. Chest. 2014;145(4):903–12.
18. Frost MC, Meyerhoff ME. Real-time monitoring of critical care analytes in the bloodstream with chemical sensors: progress and challenges. Annu Rev Anal Chem (Palo Alto Calif). 2015;8:171–92.
19. Schostek S, Zimmermann M, Keller J, Fode M, Melbert M, Schurr MO, et al. Telemetric real-time sensor for the detection of acute upper gastrointestinal bleeding. Biosens Bioelectron. 2016;78:524–9.
20. Badawi O, Liu X, Hassan E, Amelung PJ, Swami S. Evaluation of ICU risk models adapted for use as continuous markers of severity of illness Throughout the ICU stay. Crit Care Med. 2018;46(3):361–7.
21. Harrison AM, Thongprayoon C, Kashyap R, Chute CG, Gajic O, Pickering BW, et al. Developing the surveillance algorithm for detection of failure to recognize and treat severe sepsis. Mayo Clin Proc. 2015;90(2):166–75.
22. Bilgi M, Erol T, Güllü H, Sezgin AT, Hamad S, Bilgel ZG, et al. Teleconsultation of coronary angiograms using smartphones and an audio/video conferencing application. Technol Health Care. 2013;21(4):407–14.
23. Raikhelkar J, Raikhelkar JK. The impact of telemedicine in cardiac critical care. Crit Care Clin. 2015;31(2):305–17.
24. George KJ, Walsh-Irwin C, Queen C, Heuvel KV, Hawkins C, Roberts S. Development of evidence-based remote telemetry policy guidelines for a multifacility hospital system. Dimens Crit Care Nurs DCCN. 2015;34(1):10–8.
25. Ji M, Wu Y, Chang P, Yang X, Yang F, Xu S. Development and usability evaluation of the mobile delirium assessment app based on confusion assessment method for intensive care unit (CAM-ICU). Stud Health Technol Inform. 2015;216:899.
26. Correa BSPM, Gonçalves B, Teixeira IM, Gomes ATA, Ziviani A. AToMS: a ubiquitous teleconsultation system for supporting AMI patients with prehospital thrombolysis. Int J Telemed Appl. 2011;2011:1–12.
27. Vacas S, McInrue E, Gropper MA, Maze M, Zak R, Lim E, et al. The feasibility and utility of continuous sleep monitoring in critically ill patients using a portable electroencephalography monitor. Anesth Analg. 2016;123(1):206–12.
28. Knauert MP, Yaggi HK, Redeker NS, Murphy TE, Araujo KL, Pisani MA. Feasibility study of unattended polysomnography in medical intensive care unit patients. Heart Lung J Crit Care. 2014;43(5):445–52.
29. Ma AJ, Rawat N, Reiter A, Shrock C, Zhan A, Stone A, et al. Measuring patient mobility in the ICU using a novel noninvasive sensor. Crit Care Med. 2017;45(4):630–6.

30. Raj R, Ussavarungsi K, Nugent K. Accelerometer-based devices can be used to monitor sedation/agitation in the intensive care unit. J Crit Care. 2014;29(5):748–52.
31. Behrendt R, Ghaznavi AM, Mahan M, Craft S, Siddiqui A. Continuous bedside pressure mapping and rates of hospital-associated pressure ulcers in a medical intensive care unit. Am J Crit Care. 2014;23(2):127–33.
32. Pickham D, Ballew B, Ebong K, Shinn J, Lough ME, Mayer B. Evaluating optimal patient-turning procedures for reducing hospital-acquired pressure ulcers (LS-HAPU): study protocol for a randomized controlled trial. Trials. 2016;17:190.
33. Pickham D, Berte N, Pihulic M, Valdez A, Mayer B, Desai M. Effect of a wearable patient sensor on care delivery for preventing pressure injuries in acutely ill adults: a pragmatic randomized clinical trial (LS-HAPI study). Int J Nurs Stud. 2017;80:12–9.
34. Bosco E, Marton E, Feletti A, Scarpa B, Longatti P, Zanatta P, et al. Dynamic monitors of brain function: a new target in neurointensive care unit. Crit Care. 2011;15(4):R170.
35. Bai Y, Sow D, Vespa P, Hu X. Real-time processing of continuous physiological signals in a neurocritical care unit on a stream data analytics platform. In: Ang B-T, editor. Intracranial pressure and brain monitoring XV [Internet]. Cham: Springer International Publishing; 2016 [cited 2018 Mar 6]. p. 75–80. Available from: http://link.springer.com/10.1007/978-3-319-22533-3_15.
36. Herta J, Koren J, Fürbass F, Zöchmeister A, Hartmann M, Hosmann A, et al. Applicability of NeuroTrend as a bedside monitor in the neuro ICU. Clin Neurophysiol. 2017;128(6):1000–7.
37. Riviello JJ. Digital trend analysis in the pediatric and neonatal intensive care units. J Clin Neurophysiol. 2013;30(2):143–55.
38. Global Wearable Medical Devices Market 2017-2021 [Internet]. Infiniti Research Limited; Available from: www.technavio.com.
39. Kronlund P, Lind F, Olsson D. Hyperbaric critical care patient data management system. Diving Hyperb Med. 2012;42(2):85–7.
40. Armellino D, Trivedi M, Law I, Singh N, Schilling ME, Hussain E, et al. Replicating changes in hand hygiene in a surgical intensive care unit with remote video auditing and feedback. Am J Infect Control. 2013;41(10):925–7.
41. Apple still leads Android in total number of medical apps [Internet]. iMedicalApps. 2013 [cited 2018 Mar 6]. Available from: https://www.imedicalapps.com/2013/07/apple-android-medical-app/.
42. Tele-ICU Market Analysis And Segment Forecasts To 2024. Grand View Research, Inc.;
43. Precision Medicine Initiative | The White House [Internet]. [cited 2018 Mar 6]. Available from: https://obamawhitehouse.archives.gov/node/333101.
44. Ghassemi M, Celi L, Stone DJ. State of the art review: the data revolution in critical care. Crit Care. 2015;19(1):118.
45. Topol EJ. The creative destruction of medicine: how the digital revolution will create better health care. 1st pbk ed. New York: Basic Books; 2013. 319 p.
46. Demystifying AI and machine learning in healthcare [Internet]. Rock Health. [cited 2018 Mar 6]. Available from: https://rockhealth.com/reports/demystifying-ai-and-machine-learning-in-healthcare/
47. Rajkomar A, Oren E, Chen K, Dai AM, Hajaj N, Liu PJ, et al. Scalable and accurate deep learning for electronic health records. ArXiv Prepr ArXiv180107860. 2018.
48. Pinsky MR, Dubrawski A. Gleaning knowledge from data in the intensive care unit. Am J Respir Crit Care Med. 2014;190(6):606–10.
49. Jalali A, Bender D, Rehman M, Nadkanri V, Nataraj C. Advanced analytics for outcome prediction in intensive care units. In: Engineering in Medicine and Biology Society (EMBC), 2016 IEEE 38th Annual International Conference of the. IEEE; 2016. p. 2520–2524.
50. Ansari S, Belle A, Ghanbari H, Salamango M, Najarian K. Suppression of false arrhythmia alarms in the ICU: a machine learning approach. Physiol Meas. 2016;37(8):1186–203.
51. Parreco JP, Hidalgo AE, Badilla AD, Ilyas O, Rattan R. Predicting central line-associated bloodstream infections and mortality using supervised machine learning. J Crit Care. 2018;45:156–62.

52. Nemati S, Holder A, Razmi F, Stanley MD, Clifford GD, Buchman TG. An interpretable machine learning model for accurate prediction of sepsis in the ICU. Crit Care Med. 2018;46(4):547–53.
53. Shimabukuro DW, Barton CW, Feldman MD, Mataraso SJ, Das R. Effect of a machine learning-based severe sepsis prediction algorithm on patient survival and hospital length of stay: a randomised clinical trial. BMJ Open Respir Res. 2017;4(1):e000234.
54. Artificial intelligence and machine learning took hold in healthcare during 2017 [Internet]. Healthcare IT News. 2017 [cited 2018 Mar 7]. Available from: http://www.healthcareitnews.com/news/artificial-intelligence-and-machine-learning-took-hold-healthcare-during-2017.
55. Bhatia M, Sood SK. Temporal informative analysis in Smart-ICU monitoring: M-HealthCare perspective. J Med Syst [Internet]. 2016 Aug [cited 2018 Mar 6];40(8). Available from: http://link.springer.com/10.1007/s10916-016-0547-9.
56. Building the smart grid | The Economist [Internet]. [cited 2018 Mar 6]. Available from: https://www.economist.com/node/13725843.
57. Global Healthcare IT Market 2016-2020 [Internet]. Infiniti Research Limited; Available from: www.technavio.com.
58. Global Telemonitoring Systems Market 2017-2021 [Internet]. Infiniti Research Limited; Available from: www.technavio.com.
59. Srinivas P, Reddy MC, Faiola A. Better managing technology-mediated interruptions in the ICU: examining the role of patient information for improving text message notifications. AMIA Annu Symp Proc. 2016;2016:1159–68.
60. Li X, Wang Y. Adaptive online monitoring for ICU patients by combining just-in-time learning and principal component analysis. J Clin Monit Comput. 2016;30(6):807–20.
61. Belard A, Buchman T, Forsberg J, Potter BK, Dente CJ, Kirk A, et al. Precision diagnosis: a view of the clinical decision support systems (CDSS) landscape through the lens of critical care. J Clin Monit Comput. 2017;31(2):261–71.
62. Feng M, Zhang Z, Zhang F, Ge Y, Loy LY, Vellaisamy K, et al. iSyNCC: an intelligent system for patient monitoring & clinical decision support in Neuro-Critical-Care. Conf Proc IEEE Eng Med Biol Soc. 2011;2011:6426–9.
63. Singh H, Yadav G, Mallaiah R, Joshi P, Joshi V, Kaur R, et al. iNICU - integrated neonatal care unit: capturing neonatal journey in an intelligent data way. J Med Syst. 2017;41(8):132.
64. Makkar A, McCoy M, Hallford G, Escobedo M, Szyld E. A hybrid form of telemedicine: a unique way to extend intensive care service to neonates in medically underserved areas. Telemed J E Health. 2018;24(9):717–21.
65. Ellenby MS, Marcin JP. The role of telemedicine in pediatric critical care. Crit Care Clin. 2015;31(2):275–90.
66. Garingo A, Friedlich P, Chavez T, Tesoriero L, Patil S, Jackson P, et al. "Tele-rounding" with a remotely controlled mobile robot in the neonatal intensive care unit. J Telemed Telecare. 2016;22(2):132–8.
67. Hernandez M, Hojman N, Sadorra C, Dharmar M, Nesbitt TS, Litman R, et al. Pediatric critical care telemedicine program: a single institution review. Telemed J E Health. 2016;22(1):51–5.
68. Reynolds HN, Rogove H, Bander J, McCambridge M, Cowboy E, Niemeier M. A working lexicon for the tele-intensive care unit: we need to define tele-intensive care unit to grow and understand it. Telemed J E Health. 2011;17(10):773–83.
69. Reynolds HN, Bander JJ. Options for tele-intensive care unit design: centralized versus decentralized and other considerations. Crit Care Clin. 2015;31(2):335–50.
70. Kahn JM, Gunn SR, Lorenz HL, Alvarez J, Angus DC. Impact of nurse-led remote screening and prompting for evidence-based practices in the ICU*. Crit Care Med. 2014;42(4):896–904.
71. Khunlertkit A, Carayon P. Contributions of tele–intensive care unit (Tele-ICU) technology to quality of care and patient safety. J Crit Care. 2013;28(3):315.e1–315.e12.
72. Rincon TA, Manos EL, Pierce JD. Telehealth intensive care unit nurse surveillance of sepsis. Comput Inform Nurs CIN. 2017;35(9):459–64.

73. Badawi O, Hassan E. Telemedicine and the patient with sepsis. Crit Care Clin. 2015;31(2):291–304.
74. Rincon TA, Bourke G, Seiver A. Standardizing sepsis screening and management via a tele-ICU program improves patient care. Telemed J E Health. 2011;17(7):560–4.
75. Croft CA, Moore FA, Efron PA, Marker PS, Gabrielli A, Westhoff LS, et al. Computer versus paper system for recognition and management of sepsis in surgical intensive care. J Trauma Acute Care Surg. 2014;76(2):311–7; discussion 318-319.
76. Schleifer SJ, Carroll K, Moseley MJ. Developing criterion-based competencies for tele–intensive care unit. Dimens Crit Care Nurs. 2014;33(3):116–20.
77. Richter A. Use of tele-ICU to improve adherence to ventilator tidal volume goals. Crit Care Med. 2016;44:372.
78. Gupta S, Dewan S, Kaushal A, Seth A, Narula J, Varma A. eICU reduces mortality in STEMI patients in resource-limited areas. Glob Heart. 2014;9(4):425–7.
79. Kalb TH. Increasing quality through telemedicine in the intensive care unit. Crit Care Clin. 2015;31(2):257–73.
80. Kahn JM, Le TQ, Barnato AE, Hravnak M, Kuza CC, Pike F, et al. ICU telemedicine and critical care mortality: a national effectiveness study. Med Care. 2016;54(3):319–25.
81. Lilly CM, McLaughlin JM, Zhao H, Baker SP, Cody S, Irwin RS. A multicenter study of ICU telemedicine reengineering of adult critical care. Chest. 2014;145(3):500–7.
82. Blackburn HN, Clark MT, Moorman JR, Lake DE, Calland JF. Identifying the low risk patient in surgical intensive and intermediate care units using continuous monitoring. Surgery. 2018;163(4):811–8.
83. Cubrilo-Turek M, Babic Z, Pilas V, Soric N. Comparison of SAPS and APACHE II scores in patients admitted to intensive care unit. Croat J Gastroenterol Hepatol. 1996;4:39–42.
84. Kumar S, Merchant S, Reynolds R. Tele-ICU: efficacy and cost-effectiveness of remotely managing critical care. Perspect Health Inf Manag. 2013;10:1f.
85. Ramnath VR, Khazeni N. Centralized monitoring and virtual consultant models of tele-ICU care: a side-by-side review. Telemed J E-Health. 2014;20(10):962–71.
86. Venkataraman R, Ramakrishnan N. Outcomes related to telemedicine in the intensive care unit. Crit Care Clin. 2015;31(2):225–37.
87. Kavanaugh MJ, So JD, Park PJ, Davis KL. Validation of the intensive care unit early warning dashboard: quality improvement utilizing a retrospective case–control evaluation. Telemed J E Health. 2017;23(2):88–95.
88. Rolston DM, Meltzer JS. Telemedicine in the intensive care unit - its role in emergencies and disaster management. Crit Care Clin. 2015;31(2):239–55.
89. Rogove H, Stetina K. Practice challenges of intensive care unit telemedicine. Crit Care Clin. 2015;31(2):319–34.
90. Schmid F, Goepfert MS, Reuter DA. Patient monitoring alarms in the ICU and in the operating room. Crit Care. 2013;17(2):216.
91. Winters BD, Cvach MM, Bonafide CP, Hu X, Konkani A, O'Connor MF, et al. Technological distractions (Part 2): a summary of approaches to manage clinical alarms with intent to reduce alarm fatigue. Crit Care Med. 2018;46(1):130–7.
92. Thomas JT, Moeckli J, Mengeling MA, Goedken CC, Bunch J, Cram P, et al. Bedside critical care staff use of intensive care unit telemedicine: comparisons by intensive care unit complexity. Telemed J E Health [Internet]. 2017 Feb 16 [cited 2018 Mar 6]; Available from: http://online.liebertpub.com/doi/10.1089/tmj.2016.0243
93. Hoonakker PLT, Carayon P, McGuire K, Khunlertkit A, Wiegmann DA, Alyousef B, et al. Motivation and job satisfaction of Tele-ICU nurses. J Crit Care. 2013;28(3):315.e13–21.
94. Goedken CC, Moeckli J, Cram PM, Reisinger HS. Introduction of Tele-ICU in rural hospitals: changing organisational culture to harness benefits. Intensive Crit Care Nurs. 2017;40:51–6.
95. Hoonakker PLT, Pecanac KE, Brown RL, Carayon P. Virtual collaboration, satisfaction, and trust between nurses in the tele-ICU and ICUs: Results of a multilevel analysis. J Crit Care. 2017;37:224–9.

96. Kruklitis RJ, Tracy JA, McCambridge MM. Clinical and financial considerations for implementing an ICU telemedicine program. Chest. 2014;145(6):1392–6.
97. Wilkes MS, Marcin JP, Ritter LA, Pruitt S. Organizational and teamwork factors of tele-intensive care units. Am J Crit Care. 2016;25(5):431–9.
98. Dayton E, Henriksen K. Communication failure: basic components, contributing factors, and the call for structure. Jt Comm J Qual Patient Saf. 2007;33(1):34–47.
99. Brantley A, Collins-Brown S, Kirkland J, Knapp M, Pressley J, Higgins M, et al. Clinical trial of an educational program to decrease monitor alarms in a medical intensive care unit. AACN Adv Crit Care. 2016;27(3):283–9.
100. Larinkari S, Liisanantti JH, Ala-Lääkkölä T, Meriläinen M, Kyngäs H, Ala-Kokko T. Identification of tele-ICU system requirements using a content validity assessment. Int J Med Inform. 2016;86:30–6.
101. Venditti A, Edelstein T, Brock AJ. Transformation of ICU and tele-ICU annual competencies. Nurs Manag (Harrow). 2015;46(10):8–13.
102. Kopec I. Improving population health of acute patients through Tele-ICU. Crit Care Med. 2016;44:363.
103. Wunsch H, Wagner J, Herlim M, Chong DH, Kramer AA, Halpern SD. ICU occupancy and mechanical ventilator use in the United States. Crit Care Med. 2013;41(12):2712–9.
104. Berenson RA, Grossman JM, November EA. Does telemonitoring of patients--the eICU--improve intensive care? Health Aff Proj Hope. 2009;28(5):w937–47.
105. Helfand M, Christensen V, Anderson J. Technology Assessment: Early Sense for Monitoring Vital Signs in Hospitalized Patients. Evidence-based Synthesis Program (ESP) Coordinating Center, Portland VA Healthcare System, Portland, OR for Department of Veterans Affairs, Veterans Health Administration, Quality Enhancement Research Initiative, Health Services Research & Development Service, Washington, DC 20420.; 2016.
106. Pappas PA, Tirelli L, Shaffer J, Gettings S. Projecting critical care beyond the ICU: an analysis of tele-ICU support for rapid response teams. Telemed J E Health. 2016;22(6):529–33.
107. Armaignac DL, Saxena A, Rubens M, Valle CA, Williams L-MS, Veledar E, et al. Impact of telemedicine on mortality, length of stay, and cost among patients in progressive care units: experience from a large healthcare system. Crit Care Med. 2018;46:728–35.
108. Slight SP, Franz C, Olugbile M, Brown HV, Bates DW, Zimlichman E. The return on investment of implementing a continuous monitoring system in general medical-surgical units. Crit Care Med. 2014;42(8):1862–8.
109. What are a Hospital's Costs? Utah system is trying to learn – The New York Times [Internet]. [cited 2018 Mar 6]. Available from: https://www.nytimes.com/2015/09/08/health/what-are-a-hospitals-costs-utah-system-is-trying-to-learn.html
110. Cismondi F, Celi LA, Fialho AS, Vieira SM, Reti SR, Sousa JMC, et al. Reducing unnecessary lab testing in the ICU with artificial intelligence. Int J Med Inform. 2013;82(5):345–58.
111. Just-in-time | The Economist [Internet]. [cited 2018 Mar 6]. Available from: https://www.economist.com/node/13976392
112. Affairs O of P and I. VA Secretary Announces VA Open Application Programming Interface Pledge [Internet]. [cited 2018 Mar 22]. Available from: https://www.va.gov/opa/pressrel/pressrelease.cfm?id=4022
113. Pimintel DM, Wei SH, Odor A. A software communication tool for the tele-ICU. AMIA Annu Symp Proc. 2013;2013:1139–48.
114. Hawkins HA, Lilly CM, Kaster DA, Groves RH, Khurana H. ICU telemedicine comanagement methods and length of stay. Chest. 2016;150(2):314–9.
115. Lilly CM, Motzkus C, Rincon T, Cody SE, Landry K, Irwin RS. ICU telemedicine program financial outcomes. Chest. 2017;151(2):286–97.
116. Nguyen C, McElroy LM, Abecassis MM, Holl JL, Ladner DP. The use of technology for urgent clinician to clinician communications: a systematic review of the literature. Int J Med Inform. 2015;84(2):101–10.

117. Moeckli J, Cram P, Cunningham C, Reisinger HS. Staff acceptance of a telemedicine intensive care unit program: a qualitative study. J Crit Care. 2013;28(6):890–901.
118. Ward MM, Ullrich F, Potter AJ, MacKinney AC, Kappel S, Mueller KJ. Factors affecting staff perceptions of tele-ICU service in rural hospitals. Telemed J E Health. 2015;21(6):459–66.
119. Ries M. Evaluating tele-ICU cost—an imperfect science. Crit Care Med. 2016;44(2):441–2.
120. Big Data in Healthcare 2017 [Internet]. Kalorama Information; 2017. Available from: www.kaloramainformation.com

Chapter 3
Reimbursement and Payment Models for Tele-ICU

Herbert J. Rogove and Jordana Bernard

Telemedicine has reached the inflection point where acceptance and utilization have accelerated its growth from the early adopter to the early majority stage. From Geoffrey A. Moore's classic book about the stages of technology acceptance, it is clear that telemedicine has crossed the chasm [1].

With the advancement of a clinical delivery system such as the tele-ICU platform, questions abound. In particular, since 2017, new billing codes have been published by the Centers for Medicare and Medicaid Services (CMS). For years the Medicare Payment Advisory Commission (MedPAC), which considers and comments upon new billing codes, had not recognized nor recommended a billing code for tele-ICU until recently. The purpose of this chapter is to provide a step-by-step approach to billing in the context of third-party payers.

Similar to the clinical practice of caring for the critically ill, a logical and systematic approach to coding and billing should occur first and foremost. Fundamental questions should include: what type of insurance does the patient have, do telehealth parity laws exist within the state where the patient is located, is the patient in an eligible geographic region, and does the cost of billing justify the reimbursement? These and many other questions will be addressed in this chapter starting with an understanding of the primary payers and existing legislation.

H. J. Rogove (✉)
Residential Connected Health, New York, NY, USA

J. Bernard
Policy and Public Affairs for InTouch Health, Santa Barbara, CA, USA

M. A. Koenig (ed.), *Telemedicine in the ICU*,
https://doi.org/10.1007/978-3-030-11569-2_3

The Payers

Reimbursement for telemedicine for Medicare, Medicaid, and the private payers will be reviewed. The Veterans Administration (VA) will not be considered other than the fact that the VA has developed a very advanced telehealth presence and demonstrates how the barrier of interstate licensing is removed from the practice of telemedicine.

Medicare

Telehealth reimbursement emerged when the Balanced Budget Act of 1997 (BBA) mandated Medicare coverage of telehealth care and funded federal telemedicine demonstration projects throughout the country [2]. Although it was passed in 1997, payment was not required to begin until 1999 [2]. The law sets up some significant policy barriers facing telehealth providers seeking reimbursement from Medicare including the need for a Medicare physician to be with the patient at the time of the video consultation, and the fees had to be shared between the consulting and referring physician.

In 2000, the Benefits Improvement and Protection Act (BIPA) was passed and expanded Medicare's coverage of telehealth [2]. The BIPA law included the following changes:

1. Defining telehealth visits as occurring between an originating site and distant site
2. Extending coverage for federal demonstration projects and non-metropolitan statistical areas
3. Eliminating the fee-sharing requirement by allowing the distant-site practitioner to get the current fee amount for the service provided and the originating site to get a facility fee
4. Eliminating the need for a tele-presenter
5. Expanding telehealth services to include direct patient care, physician consultations, and office psychiatry services
6. Permitting the use of store-and-forward applications for Alaska and Hawaii federal telemedicine demonstration projects
7. Specification of the type of provider who may be reimbursed by Medicare for services provided via telehealth

The Medicare Improvements for Patients and Providers Act of 2008 (MIPPA) added the following types of facilities to their eligible originating sites [2]:

1. Hospital-based or critical access hospital-based renal dialysis centers
2. Skilled nursing facilities
3. Community mental health centers

The Bipartisan Budget Act of 2018 (BBA) expanded the coverage of telehealth services under the physician fee schedule to include the treatment of acute strokes in urban areas. BBA also expanded flexibility for Medicare Advantage plans to add additional costs of telehealth services in their annual plan bid amounts. Finally, the act permitted accountable care organizations that accept the financial risk to bill Medicare for telehealth services originating from the patient's residence and urban areas [3].

Accelerated adoption of telehealth and the introduction of approved CMS codes have seen the approval of 95 codes in 2018 up 7 from 2017. Critical care telehealth codes were first introduced in January 2017 [4].

A persistent reimbursement barrier relates to the qualifications of originating sites discussed below. With the passage of coverage laws for acute stroke patients not restricted by the originating sites geographical limitations, payment for telestroke care in urban areas will begin in January 2019.

For those patients who have Medicare Advantage (MA), these patients are covered for telehealth similar to the fee-for-service (FFS) in traditional Medicare. In fact, MA patients may have coverage beyond FFS. Recent telehealth legislation supports more avenues to receive payment for telehealth care [5].

The critical steps for ensuring patient and provider qualifications for coding and billing for Medicare tele-ICU services include the following:

1. *Originating Sites*
   The first step in consideration of billing for a tele-ICU visit is to verify the eligibility of the Medicare beneficiary. Eligibility means that the patient is in a facility that meets the definition of an originating site. CMS has defined these sites as either in a county outside of a metropolitan statistical area (MSA) or in a health professional shortage area (HPSA). Who determines if a site is in one of these areas? It is the Health Resources and Services Administration (HRSA) which advises CMS for HPSA classification. The US Census Bureau determines the MSA or non-MSA areas. To check on eligibility, go to the HRSA Data Warehouse [6]. The current list of originating sites and facility fees are in Tables 3.1 and 3.2 [7].

Table 3.1 Authorized originating sites [6]

Offices of physicians and providers
Hospitals
Critical Access Hospitals (CAHs)
Rural Health Clinics
Federally Qualified Health Centers
Hospital-based or CAH-based renal dialysis centers (including satellites)
Skilled nursing facilities (SNFs)
Community mental health centers (CMHCs)

Note: Independent renal dialysis facilities are not eligible originating sites

Table 3.2 Originating site fee [7]

2002 (baseline)	$20.00
2015	$24.83
2016	$25.10
2017	$25.40
2018	$25.76

Table 3.3 Distant-site practitioners [4]

Physicians
Nurse practitioners (NP)
Physician assistants (PA)
Nurse-midwives
Clinical nurse specialists (CNSs)
Certified registered nurse anesthetists
Clinical psychologists (CP) and clinical social workers (CSW)
Registered dietitians or nutrition professionals

Additionally, originating sites can only be physician offices, hospitals, critical access hospitals (CAH), rural health centers, skilled nursing facilities (SNF), federally qualified health centers (FQHC), community mental health centers, or hospital-based dialysis facilities. In January 2019, mobile stroke units and the patient's home will be added to this list for specific services such as telestroke and home dialysis evaluation.

One exception to the above criteria is the federal telemedicine demonstration projects approved by the Secretary of Health and Human Services. This rare exception removes the geographic restrictions described above.

For hospital inpatients, payment for the originating site facility fee must be made outside the diagnosis-related group (DRG) payment, since this is a Part B benefit, similar to other services paid separately from the DRG payment [8].

It is essential to check on the eligibility of a site as these may change by an annual adjustment based on the preceding year ending on December 31.

2. *Distant-Site Practitioners*
For the healthcare practitioner who is providing the tele-ICU service to the originating site, the same criteria for billing exist as in-person critical care. Not only are intensivists and other physicians eligible but also nurse practitioners (NPs), physician assistants (PAs), clinical nurse specialists (CNSs), and registered dietitians. A full list of distant-site practitioners is in Table 3.3 [4].
3. *Tele-ICU Services Defined*
CMS defines telehealth as a real-time interactive audiovisual communication between the healthcare professional from the distant site and the patient at the originating site [4]. It explicitly does not include asynchronous or store-and-forward telehealth with the exception of federally qualified telemedicine demonstration projects in Alaska and Hawaii.
4. *Claims*
Submission of claims to the state-specific Medicare Administrative Contractor (MAC) is similar to the process for an in-person intensivist or qualified

practitioner. While the claim forms are the same, there are Current Procedural Terminology (CPT) and Healthcare Common Procedure Coding Systems (HCPCS) codes that may be different and require detailed attention and understanding. While many of the codes are similar, the distinction is the CPT codes which were developed by the American Medical Association (AMA), and the HCPCS codes were developed by the Centers for Medicare and Medicaid (CMS) both for the same reason, for reporting medical procedures and services.

As of January 2017, new critical care codes were introduced. The new HCPCS code G0508 is for the initial physician-to-patient encounter that typically defines a 60-minute communication with patient and providers utilizing a telehealth platform. For a subsequent visit, typically 50 minutes in duration, the HCPCS code G0509 is used. Interestingly, these codes are considered telehealth consultations when ironically the in-person consultation codes were eliminated in 2010 by the CMS [4]. Table 3.4 lists all the most frequently used reimbursement codes and national averages for reimbursement for the year 2018 [9].

As ICU patients reach a point when they are not critically ill and do not qualify for a critical care code, in-person intensivists use the subsequent hospital care codes 99231-33. One must be cognizant when billing for tele-ICU patients that these codes may only be utilized every 3 days. It seems that the better alternative, at this time, is to utilize HCPCS G0406-08 which is a follow-up for inpatient telehealth consultation furnished to beneficiaries in hospitals or SNFs. After communication with Noridian Healthcare Solutions (NHS), one of the MACs, there may be lack of clarity about the correct coding for tele-ICU care as the

Table 3.4 Tele-ICU reimbursement (national averages) [9]

Code	Description	Fee schedule for CY 2018
G0508	Telehealth consultation, critical care, initial, physicians typically spend 60 minutes communicating with the patient and providers via telehealth	$204.12
G0509	Telehealth consultation, critical care, subsequent, physicians typically spend 50 minutes communicating with the patient and providers via telehealth	$197.28
G0406	Follow-up inpatient consultation, limited, physicians typically spend 15 minutes communicating with the patient via telehealth	$39.24
G0407	Follow-up inpatient consultation, intermediate, physicians typically spend 25 minutes communicating with the patient via telehealth	$73.44
G0408	Follow-up inpatient consultation, complex, physicians typically spend 35 minutes communicating with the patient via telehealth	$105.48
99231	Subsequent hospital care services (focused), with limitation of one telehealth visit every 3 days	$39.96
99232	Subsequent hospital care services (expanded), with limitation of one telehealth visit every 3 days	$74.16
99233	Subsequent hospital care services (detailed), with limitation of one telehealth visit every 3 days	$106.20
Q3014	Telehealth originating site facility fee	$25.76

patient improves from their critical status. NHS has referred the authors to the AMA website [10, 11] to review the CPT codes and descriptors and allow CMS to realign use of the new telehealth codes with the actual tele-ICU patient care model. It is the authors' understanding, based upon current descriptions of care, that the majority of subsequent inpatient hospital care services require in-person visits to facilitate the comprehensive, coordinated, and personal care that medically unstable, acutely ill patients require on an ongoing basis. Also, one must understand whether there is a limitation to the use of the G0406-08 codes if the teleintensivist has entered into a more direct management capacity rather than a consultative role. Perhaps since the tele-ICU codes are recent and the current volume may not yet be high enough for adequate interpretation, CMS may provide coding clarity for teleintensivists in the future.

Also, before the implementation of a tele-ICU program, consideration should be given about whether the billing entity represents intensivists from the same group that is providing in-person care or an independent Physician Service Organization (PSO) intensivist group, with a different National Provider Identification (NPI) number. The PSO may be providing tele-ICU care for gap or supplemental coverage for the in-person intensivist group. Based upon the new tele-ICU code, one needs to understand if a bedside intensivist bills 99291, can the teleintensivist later bill G0509 (second 50 minutes of critical care) if the patient is in need of critical care management when they cover for the in-person intensivist? The inverse applies in the case in which the teleintensivist provides the initial encounter and the bedside intensivist later sees the patient in need of additional critical care. What complicates this scenario is if the bedside and teleintensivist groups are separate entities. In this situation, each has a different NPI provider number. At this time the authors were unable to acquire an appropriate clarification from CMS, so this remains an area of uncertainty.

Modifiers are a necessity to include with coding as they inform CMS that the physician encounter is a telehealth visit from a distant site. As of January 1, 2017, place of service (POS)-2 must be included for Medicare claims [12]. The POS-02 code has replaced the GT modifier in most circumstances. The only use of the GT modifier became effective on January 2018 for distant-site physicians billing for the CAH Optional Payment Method. The Optional Payment Method means the physician reassigns his or her billing rights to the hospital and therefore cannot bill for professional services. The CAH bills on behalf of the teleintensivist, and the payment is 80% of the Medicare Physician Fee Schedule (PFS).

The pitfalls for billing for tele-ICU services are not unlike in-person intensivists. Meticulous documentation of the patient and practitioner encounter is vital and includes the reason for the consultation. Critical is the inclusion of the POS-02 code for all Medicare claims. Be mindful that multiple days or weeks in the ICU may demonstrate that the first days are consistent with the critical nature of the patient's condition. However, as the patient stabilizes or shows signs of recovery and is headed for ICU discharge, the failure to submit the appropriate level of care such as a follow-up consultation or subsequent hospital visit rather than a critical care code may raise a red flag resulting in an audit. It is essential to abide by legal and ethical standards for billing tele-ICU visits since these new codes are likely to draw heightened scrutiny from regulatory bodies.

5. *Alternative Payment Models (APMs)*
The one area of joint agreement between Medicare, Medicaid, and the private payers is the need to replace the fee-for-service volume-based model with a value-based system.

It is under alternative payment models (APMs) that telehealth has the opportunity to prove itself as a means to be a quality-driven, value-enhanced system of healthcare delivery. Tele-ICU care is undoubtedly a prime example of meeting the needs especially in light of the increasing shortage of intensivists.

APMs will disrupt fee-for-service by combining quality and cost targets into the determination of reimbursement [13]. Examples are accountable care organizations (ACOs) where annual cost quality targets are expected and bundled payment quality and cost targets are determined at 30-, 60-, or 90-day care periods.

It is with APMs that high-cost care, such as in the ICU, offers the most opportunities to improve value. For example, with both in-person and tele-ICU care, compliance with guidelines will potentially lead to decreasing inappropriate tests, accelerated ventilator weaning, and the early sepsis treatment bundle among other quality metrics and bundles associated with critical care.

Medicare Shared Savings Programs (MSSP), part of the Affordable Care Act, introduced the concept of ACOs and have expanded to include similar models that can be incorporated into telehealth programs.

Next Generation ACOs, which assume financial risk, have a telehealth waiver which eliminates the rural geographic restrictions of the originating sites, including a patient's home and for the use of asynchronous telehealth such as teledermatology and teleophthalmology [14]. Billing for these services is the same as billing for any Medicare service and can be found under the Medicare claims processing manual section on payment for telehealth services [15]. Now, these ACOs may be able to bill in urban settings.

Medicare Advantage Value-Based Insurance Design (VBID) as of January 2017 has allowed seven states to test enrollee cost sharing and design for high-value clinical services that have the highest potential to positively impact an enrollee's health [16]. As of 2018, the number of states will have increased to ten. MA patients already have more flexible telehealth coverage than traditional Medicare patients. With the introduction of remote patient monitoring under VBID, one could predict growth of follow-up for ICU patients especially those who suffer from post-ICU syndrome. Seeing these patients would afford the opportunity for intensivist interaction at the patient's home rather than having the patient travel to a clinic. The cost savings for both the patient and the in-person clinic (e.g., a decrease in time, support staff, and rent) would be significant.

A broader question to consider is how can FFS be transitioned into a valued-based system? Some will argue that such a system may still contain an element of FFS. A value-based system may take portions of FFS and combine bundled payments, capitation, and increased financial risk sharing [17].

For a tele-ICU program, financial risk sharing can be accomplished through the contract between the hospital and teleintensivist group. A threshold percent of an achieved metric will determine if the physician receives a bonus or a penalty. Examples including response time for calls utilizing the Leapfrog teleintensivist response of 5 minutes 95% or more of the time, bundle compliance, utilization of a checklist, compliance with the Surviving Sepsis Guidelines, and a satisfaction survey may all be utilized as contractual incentivize metrics. Telemedicine and other forms of remote communication have improved outcomes for many types of patients, including those in remote ICUs in both metropolitan and rural areas and thus should be reimbursed [18].

The authors' experience would suggest that the intensivist group in conjunction with the payer or hospital agrees upon the method in which the shared savings will be determined. Mutually agreed-upon value metrics must be clearly articulated. It is imperative before the start of a tele-ICU program to be sure the payer or hospital can access and provide the needed data. The teleintensivist group must be in a position where data exchange is bidirectional and in a predetermined time frame. Having the performance data along with the targets should be available for physician review so that any adjustments in the clinical program can be made. Refinement of any process requires the constant monitoring of data and the ability to be facile in making any needed changes. Finally, the providers should always do their financial risk assessment to look at any potential downside that might have an adverse monetary impact. There are many unforeseen variables in the care of the critically ill, so an eyes wide open approach is encouraged.

The Society of Critical Care Medicine called together a task force of academic leaders in critical care medicine in 2016 to develop a strategy for value-based care [19]. The task force concluded that organizations should be integrated both horizontally and vertically, align strategy and operations with the parent health system, and include a solid understanding of finance and risk to position for success in a value-based world [19].

Medicaid

At the state level, Medicaid is not restricted by the federal rules for telemedicine under Medicare. In fact, CMS allows each state to set its own Medicaid reimbursement policies for telemedicine as long as the rules satisfy federal requirements of "efficiency, economy, and quality of care" [20].

Because states have the flexibility to determine their coverage and payment policies, no two state's policies are alike, resulting in wide variations across all 50 states and the District of Columbia. However, similar to Medicare's rules for payment, the following factors may play a role when determining whether a telemedicine service will be covered and reimbursed under Medicaid: the type of service being delivered

Table 3.5 California Medicaid Telehealth Policies (May 2018) [23, 24]

Does not limit the type of setting or the type of practitioner
Requires consent and now verbal consent has replaced written consent
Reimburses for professional services delivered from the distant site at a rate equal to in-person care when services use (1) interactive, two-way audio-video communications and (2) the appropriate HCPCS codes G0508 or G0509 with GT or 95 modifiers.
Reimburses the originating site (patient location) facility fee when billed with code Q3014
Reimburses the transmission cost for services delivered via audio-video communications when billed with code T1014 (up to 90 minutes per patient, per day, per provider)

by telemedicine, the type of healthcare practitioner at the distant site, the setting and location of the patient at the time services are delivered, and the technological modality used to deliver services. States may also determine how much to reimburse for professional services, whether to reimburse for a separate facility fee to the originating site or additional costs associated with telemedicine visits such as transmission charges and technical support [21].

To determine if there is reimbursement for tele-ICU services in the state of practice, go to the online Medicaid provider/claims manual to see if the critical care codes for services delivered by telehealth are listed as eligible for payment. Also, state Medicaid policies will indicate which modifiers and place of service codes must be used when submitting claims for professional services. See Table 3.5 for an example of a state-based Medicaid policy for tele-ICU services in California [22, 23].

With a rapidly evolving policy environment, it can be challenging to stay apprised of regulatory changes that may impact the billing rules and requirements for the telemedicine services delivered. Current information on telemedicine reimbursement laws and policies for all 50 states and the District of Columbia can be found at the Center for Connected Health Policy, the National Telehealth Policy Resource Center [24], and the American Telemedicine Association [25].

Private Payers

Interest in telehealth has been growing among commercial insurers over the last several years. The reimbursement structure for telemedicine under commercial plans also varies widely between payers and state laws. However, many commercial plans cover and pay for telemedicine services to some extent [5]. For example, Anthem Blue Cross Blue Shield of California's telemedicine policy follows the coverage rules and fee schedule set by Medicaid under the California state statute. When California Medicaid (Medi-Cal) is "silent" about reimbursement for a specific service, then Anthem follows Medicare rules and pays when the service is listed as a Medicare-approved telemedicine service.

Some states have enacted payer parity laws to address private insurance coverage for telemedicine services. These laws are often referred to as "telehealth parity" laws. As of May 2018, 38 states and the District of Columbia have enacted

Table 3.6 States with telehealth parity laws (as of May 2018) [25, 26]

Alaska[a]	Georgia	Maryland	New Hampshire	Tennessee
Arizona	Hawaii	Michigan	New Jersey	Texas
Arkansas	Indiana	Minnesota	New Mexico	Utah[a]
California	Iowa	Mississippi	New York	Vermont
Colorado	Kansas	Missouri	North Dakota	Virginia
Connecticut	Kentucky	Montana	Oklahoma	Washington
Delaware	Louisiana	Nebraska	Oregon	
District of Columbia	Maine	Nevada	Rhode Island	

[a]Partial parity law

telehealth payer "parity" or "partial parity" legislation. See Table 3.6 for a listing of these states.

There are significant variations among state parity laws, but generally, parity legislation addresses coverage and access to telemedicine services [26]. Telemedicine coverage laws require commercial payers to cover services delivered by telemedicine to the same extent the plan already covers in-person services [27].

In addition to addressing coverage for telemedicine services, some state parity laws also address payment parity. Full payment parity legislation enables the practitioner to be reimbursed for telemedicine services equal to the rate had the service been provided to the patient in the traditional in-person setting. Partial payment parity laws only require payers to cover a narrowly defined area, such as mental health, on the same basis as in-person care. Here are two excerpts from telehealth commercial payer laws to illustrate different ways states have addressed coverage and payment policies in their statute:

Delaware (18 Del Code, Title 1, Chapter 33, Sec. § 3370)

This law has explicit language ensuring full payment parity for telemedicine services delivered in the state:

> An insurer, corporation, or health maintenance organization shall reimburse the treating provider or the consulting provider for the diagnosis, consultation, or treatment of the insured delivered through telemedicine services on the <u>same basis and at least at the rate</u> that the insurer, corporation, or health maintenance organization is responsible for coverage for the provision of the same service through in-person consultation or contact [28].

Mississippi (Miss Code Ann. § 83-9-351, 83-9-353)

This law could be interpreted as payment parity; however, the language is not explicit.

> All health insurance plans in this state must provide coverage for telemedicine services to the same extent that the services would be covered if they were provided through in-person consultation [29].

Similar to Medicaid, one must check with the private payer or locate the payer's online claims manual in the state of practice to determine if the critical care codes for services delivered by telehealth are eligible for payment. In some cases, payer policies regarding coding and modifiers for telehealth services may be different than Medicare.

Finally, in 2017 the AMA introduced a new modifier for telehealth services to patients who have private insurance, not Medicare [30]. Modifier 95 was defined as synchronous telemedicine services rendered via a real-time interactive audio and video telecommunications system. The modifier can be added to E&M codes such as 99231-33 for subsequent visits for a consultation. A clinical example would be a 45-year-old woman with pneumonia and acute respiratory failure who was extubated 3 days ago and is now stable, so her private insurer was billed 99231-95 for the tele-ICU follow-up consultation visit.

State-Based Alternative Payment Models (APMs)

Commercial payer policies including telehealth often follow the lead of CMS by implementing APMs or value-based care models such as ACOs and bundled payments. A majority of payers have stated strategies and goals toward value-based reimbursement models as a means to improve care coordination and patient outcomes and reduce healthcare spending [31].

What Else Do Intensivists Need to Know?

As of February 2018, the physician or practitioner who furnishes the emergency department or initial inpatient consultation via telehealth cannot be the physician of record or the attending physician, and the emergency department or initial inpatient telehealth consultation would be distinct from the care provided by the physician of record or the attending physician [15]. Thus, the patient cannot be admitted to the teleintensivists service. In most facilities, it will be the hospitalist who is the physician of record. When no hospitalist is present, then it would be the customary in-person admitting service to which the patient is assigned.

Utilization of a tele-ICU critical care code seems directed to programs that provide daily rounds on a continual basis which is consistent with a decentralized form of telehealth. The sum total of direct patient care must be the defined as 60 minutes to be eligible for coding G0508. It would seem that, in a centralized model such as the Philips eICU which provides more of an episodic form of care, the G0508 code would rarely if ever be utilized.

Documentation requirements should be no different than in-person ICU care. This most certainly includes the documentation of the reason for the consultation. To avoid claims rejection, all of the requirements of the critical care and E&M codes must be met. Also, adding the POS-02 code if Medicare or Medicaid and modifier-95 if a commercial payer is essential.

Technology requirements should include a platform that maintains a flawless record of connectivity. The vendor should maintain a help desk that is real-time and available 24/7/365. Anything less is unacceptable when providing patient care in an ICU setting. Quality metrics such as uptime and percent of failed consults due to technical issues should be tracked to ensure the highest level of connectivity is maintained.

Privacy for patient information means meeting HIPAA requirements and is no different when employing telehealth. It is important to consider that employment of telehealth technology is in itself no guarantee of patient privacy. Utilization of an encryption process alone does not provide adequate security, so a deep understanding of how a vendor provides security is imperative. If a vendor is Health Information Trust Alliance (HITRUST) accredited, then the security of health information meets the highest of standards [32].

Another pitfall for teleintensivist billing would include the recent findings by the Office of Inspector General (OIG) during a recent audit of 2014 and 2015 claims [33]. What prompted the audit was the significant increase in claims between 2001 and 2015 plus the number of physician claims where there was no claim from the originating site as reported in a 2009 Medicare Payment Advisory Commission study. The OIG found that 31% of the physician claims reviewed did not meet Medicare requirements. The specifics were beneficiaries who were at non-rural sites, providers who were ineligible, beneficiaries who were at unallowable originating sites, services that were by unallowable means of communication, non-covered services, and a physician located outside of the United States [34].

Finally, for teleintensivists and others who wish to see how relative value units (RVUs) impact reimbursement, it is necessary to compare the onsite and telehealth work or wRVU. Most physicians are aware that there are three components that comprise the RVU. These are the physician work, the practice overhead, and the malpractice coverage. The latter two are dependent upon geographic location of the physician thus leaving the wRVU as a constant number across all specialties and geographic physician locations. The wRVU for the onsite physician utilizing the 99291 code is 4.5 per unit, whereas, for the teleintensivist, the wRVU for the G0508 telemedicine critical care code is 4.0 [35]. One can only surmise at this time that CMS has determined that they value the work of the onsite intensivist as greater than the teleintensivist. For additional critical care time, the 99292 wRVU is 2.25 per unit, and the G0509 is 3.86 [35]. The authors were unable to uncover the rationale for the determination of the teleintensivist wRVU, but perhaps the 99292 being a 30-minute period of time compared to the 50 minutes required for the G0509 explains the difference in values.

What Do Administrators Need to Know?

Hospital administrators, by nature of providing leadership in a challenging healthcare environment, typically ask about costs first. This mindset was accepted standard practice until recently. As the early adopters have seen and understood how telehealth has augmented in-person care and helped to expand catchment areas, telemedicine programs are more mainstream now than ever before. The fundamental question should not only be centered around return on investment but should be focused on what a health system or hospital will lose if they have no telehealth offering. Continuity of care from inpatient to clinic to patient home utilizing telemedicine will become the core of hospitals and health systems that are recognized leaders who have optimized their chances to survive the economic realities of healthcare.

Spoke or originating site hospitals, particularly in rural locations, will score heavily in their community if patients can be cared for in their local ICU. Utilizing teleintensivists first to triage and determine whether a higher level of care is required is an important starting point. Maintaining them near home will be well received and appreciated by the patient and their family who may not have the time or finances to visit their loved ones at major medical centers hours away.

A second factor for originating sites is that they can bill a facility fee if they meet payer requirements. The fee may be increased annually and based upon the Medicare Economic Index (MEI). For Medicare patients, the fee is separately billed under Part B. The fees are updated annually and can be found in the Medicare Physician Fee Final Rule published in November of the year before its implementation [7]. HCPCS code Q3014 should always be utilized on claims for the originating site facility fee.

Administrators should be aware of the distinction of billing between originating and distant sites. The originating site where the patient is located can, of course, bill the site fee, and the distant site can bill on behalf of the teleintensivist for the physician component. The importance is to avoid duplicate billing.

One of the significant issues healthcare organizations face is the financial agreement between the sites. Often, the distant site (e.g., academic or tertiary medical center) must decide if there will be a charge to the originating site for the tele-ICU services. Some distant sites will not charge as there are often transfers to their site for procedures or higher levels of care. Receiving patients that require procedures and a higher level of care may offset the startup and maintenance costs. Sometimes a third party or PSO provides care as there may not be enough physicians at the distant site to cover critical care needs. Finally, sometimes there will be a hybrid model of both a distant-site teleintensivist and PSO physicians (representing the distant site) to provide the needed care at the originating site. The financial model should be worked out before a program's implementation. Items for discussion should include the fees for physician services. Currently, because of Medicare geographic restrictions, billing may not be allowable so physician charges to the originating site will either be a per diem fee, a per consult fee, or a combination of charges. As FFS transitions into value-based care, as discussed above, risk sharing will be part of these contracts.

Financial Considerations to Provide Services to Other Healthcare Organizations

In today's world, an intensivist, who in most cases is pulmonary–critical care trained, may have additional responsibilities including sleep medicine, outpatient clinic, and procedure commitments. In addition to clinical duties, such as ICU rounds, there are often added responsibilities for teaching, research, and administrative assignments. Now, added to this long list is telemedicine. It is easy to understand that even with well-staffed physician groups at academic and nonacademic hospitals, coverage for tele-ICU services may need an external workforce to augment tele-ICU coverage to other hospitals or healthcare organizations. There are critical financial considerations with whatever staff model fulfills the need. Here are some considerations:

- As introduced above, will the service provided be an offering that may benefit the distant healthcare system from patient referrals and the originating site by keeping their patients? The financial discussion centers around whether the service will be no charge, breakeven, or profitable for the distant site. One can argue this should be an included service with no additional charges. Others may charge a fee only based upon the actual cost of providing the service. One never wants to operate with a negative balance sheet nor miss the opportunity to offset costs by receiving reimbursement from third-party payers. Whatever financial direction is chosen, a detailed monetary analysis to ensure that the distant site does not suffer a noteworthy fiscal drain on their operations is paramount.
- Submitting claims to third-party payers is discussed above, but an understanding of limitations based on geographical restrictions is vital for tele-ICU program development.
- If a PSO is involved, then one is usually working with a for-profit organization which calculates the cost per day and the number of beds being covered. The pricing can be based upon 24/7/365 or gap coverage dependent upon the number of hours of coverage provided. Factored into the physician reimbursement, the PSO also has the burden of malpractice coverage, state licensure, and credentialing. Also included for the administrative costs of the PSO are accreditation, scheduling, invoicing, claims submission of billing, and the personnel for a quality improvement program to develop the strategy and implementation of the agreed-upon metrics.
- The receiving or distant-site hospital should consider not only the metrics of decreasing length of stay and survival statistics but also the gain in number of patients who no longer need to be transferred. This is an important metric that should be considered in the ROI of a tele-ICU program.
- Discussion of quality metrics should be part of the PSO-hospital (or healthcare organization) contract, and details should be considered before program implementation. This aspect of the contract is vital as the evolution of value-based outcomes will contain financial rewards or penalties. Focusing on cost, access, outcomes, and experience reflects four areas of importance in determining a successful tele-ICU program.

The critical care community is tasked with the onerous responsibility of collectively understanding the real costs and savings associated with tele-ICU programs. This responsibility is a shared responsibility for the hospitals requesting this service as well as for the providers.

Conclusion

The telehealth reimbursement policy environment is rapidly changing and moving in a positive direction. Today Medicare, Medicaid, and private payers offer reimbursement for tele-ICU based upon the location, but up-front planning is key to putting in place billing processes that capture available payment opportunities and comply with applicable federal and state rules and regulations for telehealth.

Part of the Bipartisan Budget Act of 2018 includes payment in 2019 of telehealth care for acute stroke patients in metropolitan as well as rural locations. This legislation will hopefully be the catalyst for expanded reimbursement for other telehealth services for patients in metropolitan areas, which currently comprise 77% of Medicare FFS beneficiaries [5].

Strict attention to the rules and details when submitting charges is imperative. Submitting claims for telehealth services is more complicated than bedside encounters as CMS regulations require place of service codes and currently limit visits to two-way interactive video visits in non-Metropolitan areas. There are differences between coding for Medicare, Medicaid, and private payers which all teleintensivists must account for in billing for their services. Being prepared for this new world order of expanding use and incorporation of tele-ICU care will necessitate a thorough understanding of the financial implications before the implementation of a program.

Acknowledgment The authors wish to thank Nathaniel Lacktman, Esq. for his guidance in connecting the authors with the appropriate CMS resources and Shelly Clark, RN, BSN.

References

1. Moore GA. Crossing the Chasm. 3rd ed. New York: Harper Business; 2014.
2. Medicare's Telemedicine/Telehealth Payment Policies – Telehealth Resource Center [Internet]. Telehealth Resource Center. 2018 [cited 11 March 2018]. Available from: http://bit.ly/2pbVlOU
3. Bipartisan Budget Act of 2018 [Internet]. Bipartisan Budget Act of 2018, Title III, Subtitle C, Section 50323. 2018 [cited 2018Apr26]. Available from: http://bit.ly/2JS35P1
4. MLN Booklet Telehealth Services [Internet]. cms.gov. 2018 [cited 2018Feb26]. Available from: https://www.cms.gov/Outreach-and-Education/Medicare-Learning-Network-MLN/MLNProducts/Downloads/TelehealthSrvcsfctsht.pdf
5. Medpac.gov. 2018, Chapter 16, page 483 and footnote 16 page 503 [cited 26 April 2018]. Available from: http://bit.ly/2Jwzz0b
6. HRSA – Medicare Telehealth Payment Eligibility Analyzer [Internet]. Datawarehouse.hrsa.gov. 2018 [cited 27 April 2018]. Available from: https://datawarehouse.hrsa.gov/tools/analyzers/geo/Telehealth.aspx
7. Telehealth Originating Site [Internet]. Noridian Healthcare Solutions. 2018 [cited 14 April 2018]. Available from: http://bit.ly/2JK0iqK
8. Novitas Telehealth Services[Internet]. Novitas Solutions. 2018 [cited 18 May 2018]. Available http://bit.ly/2IW3L8d

9. Cms.gov. 2018 [cited 15 April 2018]. Available from: https://www.cms.gov/Outreach-and-Education/Medicare-Learning-Network-MLN/MLNMattersArticles/downloads/MM6705.pdf
10. Coding & Billing Resources/AMA [Internet]. AMA-assn.org. 2018 [cited 18 April 2018]. Available from: https://www.ama-assn.org/practice-management/find-coding-resources
11. Noridian Health Solutions, Tana Williams, personal communication 5/11/18.
12. Place of Service Code Set – Centers for Medicare & Medicaid Services [Internet]. Cms.gov. 2018 [cited 18 May 2018]. Available from: https://www.cms.gov/Medicare/Coding/place-of-service-codes/Place_of_Service_Code_Set.html
13. Joynt Maddox K. Financial incentives and vulnerable populations — will alternative payment models help or hurt? N Engl J Med. 2018;378(11):977–9.
14. Next Generation ACOs [Internet]. 2018 [cited 7 May 2018]. Available from: https://innovation.cms.gov/Files/x/nextgenaco-telehealthwaiver.pdf
15. Medicare Claims Processing for Telehealth [Internet]. cms.gov; 2017 [cited 2018Apr12]. Section 190.3.2. Available from: https://www.cms.gov/Regulations-and-Guidance/Guidance/Manuals/downloads/clm104c12.pdf
16. Medicare Advantage Value-Based Insurance Design Model [Internet]. Innovation Models | Center for Medicare & Medicaid Innovation. [cited 2018Apr10]. Available from: https://innovation.cms.gov/initiatives/vbid/
17. Schroeder SA, Frist W. Phasing out fee-for-service payment. N Engl J Med. 2013;368(21):2029–32.
18. Cummings J, Krsek C, Vermoch K, Matuszewski K. Intensive care unit telemedicine: review and consensus recommendations. Am J Med Qual. 2007;22(4):239–50.
19. Leung S, Gregg SR, Coopersmith CM, Layon AJ, Oropello J, Brown DR, et al. Critical care organizations. Crit Care Med. 2018;46(1):1–11.
20. Telemedicine | Medicaid.gov [Internet]. Medicaid.gov. 2018 [cited 9 May 2018]. Available from: https://www.medicaid.gov/medicaid/benefits/telemed/index.html
21. State Telehealth Laws and Medicaid Program Policies. 2018 [cited 16 May 2018]. Available from: http://www.cchpca.org/sites/default/files/resources/50%20STATE%20FULL%20PDF%20SPRING%202018%20-%20PASSWORD.pdf
22. Medi-Cal: Provider Manuals [Internet]. Files.medi-cal.ca.gov. 2018 [cited 10 May 2018]. Available from: http://files.medi-cal.ca.gov/pubsdoco/manuals_menu.asp
23. Telehealth FAQ [Internet]. Dhcs.ca.gov. 2018 [cited 10 May 2018]. Available from: http://www.dhcs.ca.gov/provgovpart/Pages/TelehealthFAQ.aspx
24. Center for Connected Health. Cchpca.org. 2018 [cited 9 May 2018]. Available from: http://www.cchpca.org/sites/default/files/resources/50%20STATE%20FULL%20PDF%20SPRING%202018%20-%20PASSWORD.pdf
25. State Policy Resource Center – ATA Main [Internet]. Americantelemed.org. 2018 [cited 9 May 2018]. Available from: http://www.americantelemed.org/policy-page/state-policy-resource-center
26. Telehealth Private Payer Laws: Impact and Issues. Cchpca.org. 2018 [cited 9 May 2018]. Available from: http://www.cchpca.org/sites/default/files/resources/CCHP_%20Milbank-Telehealth-Report-FINAL.pdf
27. Breuer J, Broughton S, Frey A, Hansen J, Lacktman N, Rao V. Telehealth law handbook: a practical guide to virtual care. 1st ed. Washington, DC: American Health Lawyers Association; 2018.
28. Delaware TITLE 18 – CHAPTER 33. HEALTH INSURANCE CONTRACTS – Subchapter I. General Provisions [Internet]. Delcode.delaware.gov. 2018 [cited 9 May 2018]. Available from: http://delcode.delaware.gov/title18/c033/sc01/index.shtml
29. 2016 Mississippi Code: Title 83 – Insurance: Chapter 9 – Accident, Health and Medicare Supplement Insurance: Coverage for Telemedicine Services (§§ 83-9-351 - 83-9-353): § 83-9-353. Coverage and reimbursement for store-and-forward telemedicine services and remote patient monitoring services; definitions [Internet].
30. Justia Law. 2018 [cited 9 May 2018]. Available from: https://law.justia.com/codes/mississippi/2016/title-83/chapter-9/coverage-for-telemedicine-services/section-83-9-353

31. Modifier 95 [Internet]. Aapc.com. 2018 [cited 21 May 2018]. Available from: https://www.aapc.com/memberarea/forums/144185-modifier-95-a.html
32. Private Payers Follow CMS Lead, Adopt Value-Based Care Payment [Internet]. Health Payer Intelligence. 2018 [cited 16 May 2018]. Available from: https://healthpayerintelligence.com/news/private-payers-follow-cms-lead-adopt-value-based-care-payment
33. HITRUST. 2018 [cited 15 April 2018]. Available from: https://hitrustalliance.net/about-us/
34. Office of Inspector General. Oig.hhs.gov. 2018 [cited 19 April 2018]. Available from: https://oig.hhs.gov/oas/reports/region5/51600058.pdf
35. Work RVU Calculator [Internet]. Aapc.com. 2018 [cited 9 August 2018]. https://www.aapc.com/practice-management/rvu-calculator.aspx

Chapter 4
Legal and Regulatory Issues with Telemedicine Practice in the ICU

Kimberly L. Rockwell and Alexis S. Gilroy

Introduction

The regulatory and legal considerations pertinent to the provision of tele-ICU are robust and require careful consideration prior to implementing a tele-ICU program. Legal and regulatory topics governing telemedicine are primarily based in state-law authority (e.g., licensure, standard of care, prescribing authority, etc.), but several notable federal legal and regulatory considerations are often applicable (e.g., data privacy and security, remote monitoring device approvals, prescribing of certain medications, etc.). Importantly, many state and federal laws pertaining to the provision of health services via telemedicine are experiencing ongoing change, expansion, and specification, which require providers and institutions engaged in telemedicine to stay apprised of and monitor legal changes and correspondingly adapt ongoing programs to maintain compliance. Given this evolving legal and regulatory environment, this chapter provides a framework for highlighting the various state-specific legal and regulatory topics that are applicable to the tele-ICU framework, but providers and their advisors should review such topics relevant to

---

Authors are attorneys with the global law firm Jones Day; however, all information and opinions provided in this publication are personal to them and not necessarily that of the law firm. This should not be considered legal advice.

The authors would like to thank Luke Salisbury (a law student at the University of Michigan Law) for his significant contributions in the development of this publication.

K. L. Rockwell (✉)
Jones Day, Boston, MA, USA
e-mail: Klrockwell@jonesday.com

A. S. Gilroy
Jones Day, Washington, DC, USA
e-mail: agilroy@jonesday.com

M. A. Koenig (ed.), *Telemedicine in the ICU*,
https://doi.org/10.1007/978-3-030-11569-2_4

applicable jurisdiction(s) and consider the latest legal and regulatory actions and guidance available on the topics. For purposes of providing non-exhaustive examples, this chapter outlines several telemedicine-specific statutes, rules, and regulations applicable to tele-ICU outlays, including licensure and credentialing, data security and privacy, technology considerations, state restrictions on telemedicine care delivery, utilization of advance practice providers in the delivery of telemedicine services, business arrangement considerations, liability considerations, and specific issues to international telemedicine outlays.

State Licensure Issues

As a rule, healthcare providers practicing telemedicine across state lines must be licensed in every state in which patients receive their services. The Tenth Amendment relegates health and safety policy to the states. Accordingly, each state has vested medical boards with the power to require licenses for practicing medicine. Consequently, both medical and osteopathic boards across the USA require physicians engaging in telemedicine to be licensed in the state in which the patient is located at the time of the service [1]. This is pertinent to physicians in both centralized and decentralized models of tele-ICU if those physicians are servicing patients across state lines. Unfortunately, the physician licensure requirements and related renewals for any given state can be quite idiosyncratic and onerous, including high fees, criminal background checks, differing applications and documentation, letters of recommendation, certified copies of medical school and residency diplomas, various continuing educational requirements, tests, interviews, and other items. Such requirements make it time-intensive and expensive for physicians to achieve and maintain licensure in multiple states. There are, however, at least two rays of hope to this interstate licensing barrier that specifically affect physicians practicing telemedicine: state-specific telemedicine certificate/licensure and interstate medical licensure compact participation.

First, nine states – Alabama, Louisiana, Maine, Minnesota, New Mexico, Oklahoma, Ohio, Oregon, and Texas – issue special telemedicine licenses or certificates [2–12]. Such certificates or special licenses generally permit an out-of-state provider to render telemedicine services if certain conditions are met including that the provider (i) holds an active and unrestricted license to practice in another state, (ii) cannot open a physical office in the state or meet with patients in the state, and (iii) submit to jurisdiction and maintain compliance with the laws of the state providing the registration. For example, the Minnesota requirements provide that, in addition to not opening an office in the state, the physician cannot meet with patients in the state or take phone calls from patients within the state [5]. The statute also requires that the physician registers with the state medical board once per year as a telemedicine provider [5]. Unfortunately, this type of special telemedicine registration appears to be waning in popularity and use among the states, as some, like Tennessee, Montana, and Nevada, have revoked such options [12].

Despite the waning popularity of telemedicine-specific state registrations, there is another potential avenue to expedite multistate licensure for physicians engaged in interstate telemedicine services. In 2014 an Interstate Medical Licensure Compact ("Compact") was advanced by the Federation of State Medical Boards as an expedited process for licensure among states participating in the Compact. The Compact provides participating physicians with a full license to practice in each Compact state they select. The Compact, now active and operationalized through an independent commission, is a binding agreement among participating states. The independent commission, comprised of representatives of certain member states, was seated in October 2015 and began issuing letters of qualification in April 2017 [13]. Table 4.1 lists the specific physician eligibility criteria for participating in the Compact. As of June 2018, 21 states – Alabama, Arizona, Colorado, Idaho, Illinois, Iowa, Kansas, Maine, Minnesota, Mississippi, Montana, Nebraska, Nevada, New Hampshire, Pennsylvania, South Dakota, Utah, West Virginia, Washington, Wisconsin, and Wyoming – had adopted the Compact by legislation and are actively participating [13]. Five additional states had passed legislation, and participation in the Compact was currently in process but not yet active – District of Columbia, Maryland, Pennsylvania, Tennessee, and Vermont [13]. Finally, proposed legislation to adopt the Compact was pending in five additional jurisdictions – Georgia, Kentucky, Michigan, New York, and South Carolina – some of which may have adopted the legislation at the time of this publication [13]. To take advantage of the Compact, a physician must submit an application, prove eligibility with applicable documentation, and submit a $700 fee [13]. Once the physician is approved, the physician may obtain licensure in any of the participating states but must still pay the state-specific licensure fees [13].

As a corollary to state licensure requirements, only providers who are engaged in the "practice of medicine" as defined by a particular state are required to obtain licensure, which most likely includes mere physician-to-physician consultation in most states. Every state has its own definition of what it means to practice medicine, typically

Table 4.1 Physician eligibility criteria for licensure via the Compact

The physician:
Is a graduate of an accredited medical school or a school listed in the International Medical Education Directory
Passed each component of the applicable medical licensing examination within three attempts
Successfully completed approved graduate medical education
Holds specialty certification or a time-unlimited specialty certificate
Possesses a full and unrestricted license to engage in the practice of medicine issued by one of the member states approved to serve as a state of principal licensure under the Compact
Has no criminal history
Has no history of disciplinary action against a medical license
Has never had a controlled substance license or permit suspended or revoked
Is not under active investigation by a licensing agency or law enforcement authority

Interstate Medical Licensure Compact: A faster pathway to medical licensure, available at http://www.imlcc.org/do-i-qualify/ (accessed June 15, 2018)

based in statute, and often incorporating the concepts of (i) diagnosis, (ii) treatment, and (iii) prescribing for any disease or physical condition [14]. These state definitions are often intentionally broad but not all health-related activity amounts to the practice of medicine. Within the tele-ICU context, however, even mere consultation by an out-of-state provider who does not otherwise issue orders or prescriptions would likely be considered the practice of medicine in most jurisdictions and, thus, require state licensure. And though some states provide exception to licensure for provider-to-provider consultations, these exceptions are, by and large, intended for use only in rare and extraordinary circumstances and not as a safe harbor for a business model focused on the provision of ongoing medical services. Michigan, for example, limits the exception to consultations involving "an exceptional circumstance" [15], while Wyoming requires consulting physicians to notify the state medical board prior to their collaboration and limits the duration of their licensure exemption to a specific number of days [16, 17]. Thus, all providers engaged in delivering patient care via tele-ICU outlays must achieve and maintain licensure in each state where a patient receives that care.

Credentialing and Privileging

Credentialing

Credentialing is the process of reviewing and verifying the educational, training, and professional history of healthcare providers interested in providing patient care services at a healthcare facility. As a condition of state facility licensure, states typically require healthcare facilities to credential all providers prior to granting the provider privileges on the medical staff at the facility. Private and government payers similarly require healthcare facilities to credential providers as a condition of participation. Finally, the Joint Commission ("TJC") also requires participating facilities to credential providers. To comply with state, payer, and TJC credentialing requirements, providers engaged in delivering remote tele-ICU services are often required to be credentialed at the facility where the patient is located as well as the facility where the provider is physically located. This duplicative credentialing generates significant cost and requires often unnecessary time delays, which can be a significant barrier to adoption of telemedicine programs.

To address the downsides of this duplicative credentialing process and to facilitate greater adoption of telemedicine programming, the Centers for Medicare and Medicaid Services ("CMS") adopted a rule in July 2011 allowing for "credentialing by proxy" of telemedicine providers [18]. Under this rule, CMS expanded its conditions of participation rules so the originating site (i.e., the site where the patient is located) might, at their option, rely upon prior credentialing of the distant site (i.e., the site where the tele-ICU provider is located). Any originating site that is a Medicare-participating hospital with a telemedicine program may take advantage of this credentialing by-proxy mechanism, and eligible distant sites may be either Medicare-participating hospitals or TJC-accredited telemedicine entities.

Table 4.2 By-proxy agreement requirements

Agreement is written
Clearly identifies the scope of services provided and assures they are being provided in a "safe and effective manner" (*applies only if distant site is a non-hospital entity*)
Requirement that distant site utilizes credentialing and privileging procedures that meet the standards for Medicare-participating hospitals (*applies only if distant site is a non-hospital entity*)
Includes a current list of privileged practitioners subject to the by-proxy arrangement with scope of privileges
Requirement that each practitioner is licensed in the state of the originating site.
Requirement that distant site provide evidence of internal performance review of each practitioner subject to the by-proxy agreement
Requirement that originating site sends performance information, including adverse event information, and all complaints received about each practitioner are subject to the by-proxy arrangement

Department of Health & Human Services, Centers for Medicare & Medicaid Services, "Telemedicine Services in Hospitals and Critical Access Hospitals (memorandum), July 15, 2011, available at https://www.cms.gov/Medicare/Provider-Enrollment-and-Certification/SurveyCertification GenInfo/downloads/SCLetter11_32.pdf (accessed June 18, 2018)

Though this by-proxy credentialing process is optional, CMS requires the originating site and distant site to utilize a specific type of agreement to employ the model – the "by-proxy agreement." The by-proxy agreement must contain certain and specific features including, for example, ongoing reporting requirements by the originating site on clinical outcomes data (see Table 4.2 for a summary of requirements). And, while not required by the CMS rule, facilities engaging in by-proxy credentialing often find it helpful to incorporate agreement terms to address indemnification, confidentiality, records ownership, and physician withdrawal or resignation procedures. Notably, the by-proxy agreement is subject to review during audits and surveys – including TJC surveys – to confirm compliance with Medicare's conditions of participation.

The credentialing by-proxy mechanism can reduce go-live time from several months to several days for originating sites, allowing telemedicine providers to start delivering services more quickly and significantly reducing originating site start-up costs. Notwithstanding, few originating sites currently take advantage of this streamlined process. Because originating sites retain the ultimate responsibility for the privileging decisions of telemedicine practitioners delivering services at its facility, originating sites may be hesitant to rely upon the credentialing decisions of another institution. Furthermore, an originating site cannot take advantage of the credentialing by-proxy mechanism unless its bylaws so provide. And finally, while CMS credentialing by-proxy rules are mostly in harmony with TJC by-proxy credentialing requirements, TJC adopted a requirement in 2011 requiring both the originating and distant sites to be accredited by TJC to take advantage of the by-proxy credentialing process [19]. This additional requirement may limit the ability of originating sites to take advantage of by-proxy credentialing as telemedicine companies seek accreditation through alternative means. Ultimately, however, to the extent that originating sites can take advantage of the streamlined by-proxy credentialing procedures, it can reduce administrative burden and overhead in its start-up of tele-ICU services.

Scope of Telemedicine Provider Privileges

When engaging tele-ICU providers, the originating site must consider the scope of privileges that will be granted to tele-ICU providers who achieve credentialing. Studies of various tele-ICU models indicate that some tele-ICU originating sites require tele-ICU providers to issue orders and prescriptions directly into patient records, while other programs require the tele-ICU providers to make recommendations to on-site clinicians who then submit the orders [20]. Granting telemedicine providers a full scope of privileges to issue orders and prescriptions for patients directly into the originating site patient health record presents both risks and benefits versus using the tele-ICU providers in a more consultative role. The benefits of permitting tele-ICU providers to engage in a full scope of ordering privileges at the originating site include greater efficiency in initiating and implementing the orders and offloading the required work from on-site clinical staff. But, there are a host of legal risks and concerns with this practice model that entities wishing to engage in tele-ICU programming should consider at the outset.

First, the originating site hospital will absorb liability exposures for the care provided at its facility by tele-ICU providers. Limiting tele-ICU providers to issuing recommendations in consultation rather than permitting these providers to issue direct patient care orders creates some degree of separation between the recommending tele-ICU physician and the direct clinical decision-making process, thereby potentially reducing liability exposure. Furthermore, the ordering physician bears responsibility for ensuring that the order is properly applied and that the results of any diagnostic studies are evaluated and acted upon in a timely manner. These monitoring and follow-up responsibilities are much more easily executed by on-site personnel, which implicate patient safety and liability exposure.

Second, involving multiple physicians in active patient care, especially with multiple handoffs, is known to increase the risk of clinical errors and other patient safety events. This risk is theoretically greater when remote physicians are involved in the ordering process because (i) remote physicians may be unaware of formulary, procedure, and diagnostic study limitations and restrictions at the originating site; (ii) there may be role confusion as to which clinicians are responsible for follow-up on results of those orders or patient monitoring following medication administration; and (iii) it may be more difficult for remote physicians to ascertain all relevant and necessary clinical information prior to issuing such orders. Because patient adverse events may be the result of such issues, the originating site and tele-ICU providers may be inheriting greater liability for those clinical decisions. While telemedicine certainly does not, in and of itself, present a hindrance to the relevant standard of care (and could in certain circumstances advance the standard of care), these practical issues highlight the importance of written policies and protocols among originating sites and telemedicine organizations for anticipating and managing these issues.

Third, individual states may place certain limitations on telemedicine providers in the context of issuing orders. Such limitations are reviewed in more detail in section "State-Specific Requirements Pertaining to Telemedicine Services" of this chapter but may include technology-specific requirements for performing examinations, prohibitions on prescribing certain medications, and others, which may increase the administrative burden and complexity of engaging tele-ICU providers.

Fourth and finally, CMS and private payers have specific policies and regulations governing the medical necessity justifications for inpatient admission and other types of orders. These policies and regulations could potentially impact originating site and tele-ICU provider reimbursement if tele-ICU providers do not adhere to such policies and regulations. Furthermore, payers and CMS may prohibit client hospitals from seeking reimbursement for certain orders placed by remotely consulting tele-ICU physicians.

For each of these reasons, originating sites and tele-ICU providers should carefully consider the scope of privileges that the originating site should grant to remote tele-ICU providers who have been approved for credentialing.

State and Federal Privacy and Data Security Laws

The practice of telemedicine is especially vulnerable to exposing private patient health information due to its reliance on electronic data collection and storage along with the frequent distant data transfer necessary in telemedicine workflows. The addition of remote patient monitoring data exchange in the tele-ICU context further advances this exposure given the magnitude of digital data involved and flowing across multiple networks. Entities engaged in implementing tele-ICU programs must be mindful of several federal and state statutes and regulations that address these patient privacy and data security concerns.

The Health Insurance Portability and Accountability Act

Since its enactment in 1996, the Health Insurance Portability and Accountability Act ("HIPAA") dictates the privacy and security regulatory framework to protect identifiable patient health information when it is collected and shared by "covered entities" such as healthcare providers and health plans. HIPAA's privacy rule establishes limits on the use and disclosure of patient health information, while HIPAA's security rule imposes technical, physical, and administrative safeguards that must be implemented to protect the integrity and confidentiality of electronic patient health information. Table 4.3 is a non-exhaustive summary of some of the relevant and specific requirements under HIPAA's privacy rule and security rule. Every

Table 4.3 Various requirements of HIPAA privacy and security rules

HIPAA privacy rule	HIPAA security rule
• The Privacy Rule protects all "individually identifiable health information" held or transmitted by a covered entity or its business associate, in any form or media, whether electronic, paper, or oral • A covered entity must obtain the individual's written authorization for any use or disclosure of protected health information that is not for treatment, payment, or healthcare operations • A covered entity is permitted to use and disclose protected health information, without an individual's authorization only for a specific and narrow set of purposes • A covered entity must make reasonable efforts to use, disclose, and request only the minimum amount of protected health information needed to accomplish the intended purpose of the use, disclosure, or request • For internal uses, a covered entity must develop and implement policies and procedures that restrict access and uses of protected health information based on the specific roles of the members of their workforce	• The Security Rule requires covered entities to maintain reasonable and appropriate administrative, technical, and physical safeguards for protecting electronically protected health information (e-PHI) • Entities must ensure the confidentiality, integrity, and availability of all e-PHI they create, receive, maintain or transmit • Entities must identify and protect against reasonably anticipated threats to the security or integrity of the information • Entities must protect against reasonably anticipated, impermissible uses or disclosures and ensure compliance by their workforce • Entities must ensure the integrity and availability of e-PHI by ensuring that e-PHI is not altered or destroyed in an unauthorized manner and that it is accessible and usable on demand by an authorized person • Covered entities must review and modify their security measures to continue protecting e-PHI in a changing environment

U.S. Department of Health & Human Services, Summary of the HIPAA Privacy Rule, last revised May 2003, available at https://www.hhs.gov/sites/default/files/privacysummary.pdf (accessed June 18, 2018); U.S. Department of Health & Human Services, Summary of the HIPAA Security Rule, last revised July 2013, available at https://www.hhs.gov/hipaa/for-professionals/security/laws-regulations/index.html (accessed June 18, 2018)

healthcare provider and entity providing supportive tele-ICU services to such healthcare providers must ensure strict compliance with HIPAA as it relates to all tele-ICU devices, data transmission, and data storage sites under its control to avoid fines, penalties, and other sanctions.

The Health Information Technology for Economic Clinical Health Act

In 2009, the Health Information Technology for Economic Clinical Health Act ("HITECH") extended several HIPAA privacy and security requirements to certain "business associates" that "create, receive, maintain, or transmit" identifiable health information while performing a service or function on behalf of a covered entity. Though most patient-facing tele-ICU vendors likely qualify as HIPAA "business associates" subject to these regulations, it remains a nuanced and situation-based question, depending upon multiple variables. Table 4.4 provides a non-exhaustive

Table 4.4 Considerations for determining whether an entity is a business associate under HIPAA

"A business associate is a person or entity that performs certain functions or activities that involve the use or disclosure of protected health information on behalf of, or provides services to, a covered entity."
Business associate functions and activities may include:
Claims processing or administration
Data analysis
Processing or administration
Utilization review, quality assurance
Billing
Benefit management
practice management
Repricing
Business associate services may include:
Legal
Actuarial
Accounting
Consulting
Data aggregation
Management
Administrative
Accreditation
Financial
There are certain specific and technical exceptions to exempt certain entities from being considered a business associate notwithstanding its provision of services or functions requiring the use or disclosure of protected health information

The US Department of Health & Human Services, Business Associates, last updated July 2013, available at https://www.hhs.gov/hipaa/for-professionals/privacy/guidance/business-associates/index.html (accessed June 18, 2018)

summary of certain considerations for determining whether an entity is considered a "business associate" under HIPAA. Both originating and distant-site entities should consult with advisors knowledgeable in the application of the business associate rule to ensure that all required parties to a tele-ICU arrangement are aware of and compliant with HIPAA and HITECH regulations. As a practical matter, many originating site hospitals will require ICU vendors to enter into a business associate agreement, obligating the ICU vendor (at least contractually) to meet certain privacy and security requirements of HIPAA and notice obligations of a breach within specific time frames.

State Privacy and Security Requirements

In addition to federal HIPAA and HITECH privacy and security requirements, tele-ICU providers must consider state-specific privacy and security laws in both the originating site and distant-site state jurisdictions. According to the National Conference of State Legislatures, all 50 states and the District of Columbia have adopted privacy-specific legislation [21]. Some of these state rules necessitate greater security measures than those required by HIPAA [21]. California, for example, enacted a statute in 2009 requiring a provider to protect against unauthorized *access* to patient medical information – which goes beyond the HIPAA requirements that cover only unauthorized *uses* or *disclosures* [22]. Because federal law does not preempt more demanding state patient-related privacy and security standards, tele-ICU providers may need to implement additional security controls and procedures to assure compliance with requirements in multiple state jurisdictions.

Tele-ICU Device Technology, the FDA, and Safety

Tele-ICU service delivery requires extensive technology and hardware – including electronic medical records, audiovisual technologies, remote patient monitoring devices, and, in many cases, robots controlled by the remote provider that are designed to travel from bed to bed to evaluate sick patients. In 2013, there were 175 active robotic devices, 56 of which were known to be supporting ICU patients in 25 North American ICUs [23]. Such devices are often subject to the regulation of the Food and Drug Administration ("FDA") pursuant to the Food, Drug, and Cosmetic Act of 1938 and the Medical Device Amendments of 1976. The FDA's role is to ensure device efficacy and patient safety. To fulfill this role, FDA requires that device manufacturers implement robust quality and performance controls. Among other things, device manufacturers must register with the agency and may be required to seek pre-market approval from FDA for certain devices by demonstrating device safety and efficacy with clinical data. Regulated manufacturers must also adhere to the agency's "current good manufacturing practices" as well as other aspects of the agency's quality framework. And finally, manufacturers may be required to track and report adverse events and issue recalls when patient safety issues are uncovered. Healthcare providers who employ such medical device technology on behalf of patients must remain mindful of a device manufacturer's FDA obligations and ensure that all employed technology is warranted to comply with applicable FDA standards and regulations. Further, hospitals employing these technologies are encouraged to develop internal policies and procedures for monitoring and reporting adverse patient safety events involving the technology.

State-Specific Requirements Pertaining to Telemedicine Services

The majority of states have adopted statutes or regulations specifically addressing the delivery of healthcare services by telemedicine technologies. The specific requirements and restrictions vary significantly from state to state in both content and scope. But the categories of statutory and regulatory restrictions and requirements that entities engaging in tele-ICU services must consider include platform technology restrictions, requirements for physical examinations, telepresenter requirements, informed consent requirements, ordering and prescribing prohibitions, and standard of care thresholds adopted by the originating site jurisdiction. This section addresses each of these categories, in turn.

Technology Restrictions

Many states dictate the types of technology that providers may utilize in delivering telemedicine services within the state to accomplish the state's requirements for remotely establishing a provider-patient relationship. While some of the most permissive states expressly permit the use of asynchronous store-and-forward platforms in addition to more traditional real-time video and audio technologies, others only permit real-time audiovisual communication between the provider and the patient for at least the first encounter between the two. California, for example, is one of the more permissive states from this standpoint, while Arizona is one of the most restrictive. California expressly permits the use of "asynchronous store and forward" technologies in the delivery of telemedicine services [24], while Arizona expressly requires real-time audiovisual technologies to deliver telemedicine services [25]. Other states, such as Illinois and Michigan, are silent on the types of technologies either specifically permitted or prohibited. In such "silent" states, providers may engage in telemedicine services using a variety of technologies but are open to scrutiny by state medical boards without the certainty of explicit statutes or regulations on which to rely. Many tele-ICU programs utilize some form of real-time platform, whether it includes audio, visual, or just physiologic data such as cardiac monitoring or vital signs. As such, most tele-ICU programs are likely to meet the technology requirements of most states. Nevertheless, providers should be mindful of states that require real-time audio and visual components to engage in telemedicine services.

Potentially applicable to some tele-ICU programs, some state telemedicine practice standards exempt purely consulting providers from the application of the requirements. For example, Florida's medical board rule on delivering services using telemedicine specifically carves out consulting providers from the regulation [26]. However, activities such as direct ordering and prescribing by remote providers are likely to impair the utilization of these consultant exemptions, even where the orders are part of a consult activity, as the state regulators may view the order and prescription activities as beyond that of a typical consulting-only provider.

Physical Examination Requirements, Telepresenters, and Issuing Prescriptions

Many states have adopted vague requirements to conduct a "reasonable" or "adequate" physical examination prior to ordering or prescribing treatment for a patient via telemedicine. Though nearly every state at this point has amended its laws so that this physical examination requirement does not require an in-person physical examination, several states remain silent on the topic, while others retain Board of Medicine or Board of Pharmacy regulations that could be interpreted to require in-person examination or similar elements in order to write certain prescriptions. Some states, such as Ohio, exempt telemedicine providers from this requirement if the patient is receiving care at a hospital or when an on-site healthcare provider (i.e., a "telepresenter") is present with the patient at the initial telemedicine encounter [27].

By their very nature, tele-ICU programs involve the active engagement of on-site physicians or other practitioners actively providing direct patient care. Furthermore, for tele-ICU programs engaging tele-ICU providers in a purely consultative model of care, whereby telemedicine providers do not actively issue orders and prescriptions but rather provide guidance to on-site providers to issue such orders, this type of legal restriction would not necessarily be relevant or compliance should be easily achieved. That said, facilities looking to engage remote tele-ICU providers in issuing patient orders and prescriptions or to completely replace on-site intensive care physicians are advised to carefully consider the state-based physical examination requirements of the originating site jurisdiction. This is especially apparent for tele-ICU providers who are consulted to issue prescriptions for controlled substances and other drugs with increased abuse potential, which may be outright banned by states such as Minnesota which bans teleprescriptions for muscle relaxants, drugs containing butalbital, and controlled substances among others [28]. It is also important to remember that controlled substance prescribing is an issue of federal law under jurisdiction of the Drug Enforcement Administration ("DEA") pursuant to the Ryan Haight Act [29, 30]. But even while a telemedicine provider may be able to meet one of the exceptions within the federal requirements for prescribing controlled substances, providers must still maintain compliance with more restrictive state telemedicine laws and regulations on prescribing controlled substances.

Informed Consent

Given that telemedicine involves a mode of healthcare delivery with which many patients are unfamiliar, informed consent is both a best practice to mitigate general liability claims and a specific requirement by many state regulators. A number of states require some type of specific informed consent prior to the provision of telemedicine services. For example, Arizona, California, Kentucky, Louisiana, Mississippi, Nevada, Texas, and Vermont all require some form of written or verbal consent or affirmation in connection with a telemedicine engagement [31–38]. While model forms have been published by various organizations, providers must be mindful that specific informed consent requirements vary from state to state. Additionally, some government and private payers, especially Medicaid, also require telemedicine providers to adhere to specific processes and recording requirements with regard to obtaining patient-informed consent for telemedicine services.

As such, entities engaged in providing tele-ICU care should develop specific informed consent processes tailored to the ICU setting originating site state regulations, and payer requirements.

Standard of Care

Under historical standard of care constructs, the notion of physician discretion is central and judged against whether the data gathered would reasonably avail a physician of the necessary information given the attendant facts and circumstances to make an appropriate diagnosis and treatment decision. Not surprisingly, state regulators recognize that a physician's medical decision-making may be inhibited to some degree by the remote nature of the patient-physician encounter. As such, some state-specific regulations specifically address the standard of care to which physicians are subject when engaged with a patient by means of telemedicine. With the notion that a physician engages in telemedicine at his own risk, many states expressly indicate that physicians engaged in providing telemedicine services will be subject to the same standard of care as applied to in-person encounters, such as Minnesota [39]. This type of standard imports another risk on tele-ICU providers who must subsume the risks associated with what can be in certain circumstances less robust clinical information and examinations. Many states also adopt specific standards of engaging in telemedicine encounters to mitigate the associated risks. Such standards include the prescribing restrictions, technology requirements, and other specific conditions described earlier in this section with which physicians must comply or be subjected to medical board sanctions. As such, providers and entities engaged in providing tele-ICU services must be mindful of the specific standard of care promulgated by the state where the originating site is located. Here again, it can be helpful to develop applicable policies and protocols to manage the risks of engaging in remote telemedicine practice. Such procedures and policies should be derived from evaluating the activities necessary to meet the standard of care for particular telemedicine workflows used in tele-ICU among a team of clinicians (preferably involving some from an independent organization).

Utilization of Non-Physician Providers as Tele-ICU Providers

Studies indicate that telemedicine models enable greater levels of delegation to non-physician providers [40]. Indeed, it is clear that current tele-ICU programs utilize non-physician providers, including critical care nurses, to provide tele-ICU services remotely [20]. Many states place specific restrictions on the utilization of non-physician providers in the delivery of medical services. These restrictions can include specific requirements for the use of non-physician providers in the delivery of telemedicine, specific supervision requirements, and specific types of agreements that must be executed in order to utilize non-physician providers. Such restrictions often render the utilization of non-physician providers challenging, at best, for tele-ICU vendors.

Restrictions on Non-Physician Providers Engaging in Telemedicine

Generally speaking, telemedicine-specific statutes and regulations in several states are under the jurisdiction of state medical boards and pertain only to the provision of telemedicine services by physician providers [41]. In states where the statutes and regulation neither expressly prohibit nor permit non-physician providers to engage in telemedicine, tele-ICU providers should take caution and consider the overall posture of the state regulatory bodies before engaging non-physician providers in delivering tele-ICU services. Many states expressly permit nurse practitioners, physician assistants, and other types of non-physician providers to engage in telemedicine practice in addition to physicians [42, 43]. Few states expressly prohibit non-physician providers from engaging in telemedicine services, but the supervision and other practical aspects of utilizing non-physician providers (discussed below) can indirectly restrict utilizing such non-physician providers. Tele-ICU programs should be sure, before engaging non-physician providers to deliver medical services via telemedicine, that the specific non-physician provider to be utilized is permitted to practice telemedicine within the state and the bounds of that permission.

Specific Supervision Requirements

Every state has published statutes and regulations specific to the supervision of and delegation to non-physician providers though the specifics of those statutes and regulations vary significantly from state to state. The statutory and regulatory provisions, typically in place for years prior to telemedicine capabilities, include several different aspects of non-physician provider supervision. For example, some states, such as Georgia, explicitly limit the number of specific types of non-physician providers that a physician may supervise at any one time [44]. Approximately 22 states and the District of Columbia provide independent practice authority to nurse practitioners, while the remaining states require some level of physician supervision of nurse practitioners [45]. Some states require on-site or continuous supervision of certain types of non-physician providers, while other states permit remote supervision so long as the physician is available by telephone or electronic communication at all times. Colorado, for example, requires on-site supervision of physician assistants [46], while Florida permits physicians to remotely supervise physician assistants as long as the physician is continuously available through telecommunication technologies [47]. As one of the stricter states with regard to supervision of physician assistants, Colorado does not even permit a physician to supervise Colorado-licensed physician assistants unless the physician has "a regular and reliable physical presence in Colorado" [46]. Many states also explicitly indicate the types of quality assurance activities, chart countersignature processes, and prescriptive authority review protocols that physicians must implement when supervising a non-physician provider. Various of these state requirements may make it challenging for tele-ICU providers to engage in decentralized tele-ICU models with non-physician providers or to engage non-physician providers entirely. Some states, however, explicitly exempt certain types of healthcare facilities (e.g., hospital facilities, public health facilities, or facilities providing services to low healthcare access areas) from certain supervision requirements. As such, these idiosyncratic statutory and regulatory structures must be carefully reviewed by tele-ICU providers prior to engaging non-physician providers to ensure compliance with the originating site jurisdictional requirements in that regard. Direct engagement with the relevant state agencies may be helpful to obtain formal or informal approval to advance supervision programs discussed with the regulators, especially in jurisdictions demonstrating a desire to advance telemedicine activities though operating under dated legislative and regulatory requirements.

Delegation Agreements and Authority

In the event that a tele-ICU provider has decided to utilize non-physician providers to engage in delivering tele-ICU services, the tele-ICU should (as a best practice) and may be required under state law to execute a delegation and supervision agreement with the non-physician provider. Such agreements should include, among other things, clinical protocols, bounds of the supervisory relationship, emergency procedures for consultation, and quality assurance and chart review protocols. Several states require such delegation and supervision agreements to be filed with the respective state board, while other states require providers to make the agreements available to state boards upon request. Tele-ICU providers should review state-specific regulations and statutes related to the scope, content, and review procedures for such agreements prior to engaging the non-physician provider.

Business Arrangement Considerations

Hospitals looking to engage with an existing tele-ICU provider or entities looking to engage as a tele-ICU vendor must be cognizant of various business arrangements that may run afoul of state or federal laws and regulations related to physician payment, business organizational structure, and other business practices.

State Corporate Practice of Medicine and Fee-Splitting Laws

The organizational structures used by tele-ICU vendors are varied. While many tele-ICU programs originate from an affiliation with an academic medical center, there are many privately owned, independent tele-ICU vendors as well. This is important because more than half of the states in the USA prohibit the corporate practice of medicine and/or fee-splitting arrangements among healthcare providers [48, 49].

State corporate practice of medicine laws prohibits non-licensed persons or entities from dictating the provision of professional medical services. In other words, these states require that only licensed healthcare professionals have control over the provision of professional medical services and must, therefore, not be employed or controlled by non-healthcare professional individuals or entities. Similarly, state fee-splitting prohibitions restrict healthcare professionals from sharing revenue with non-healthcare professionals or entities. These laws are intended to protect the profession of medicine from laypersons who would interfere with the provider's medical decision-making. And though some states have adopted exemptions to these laws for traditional healthcare entities such as hospitals and health maintenance organizations, the practical result of these laws is that many tele-ICU vendors must take specific steps in certain jurisdictions to organize and execute services utilizing business models that conform with such specific state restrictions.

A typical contractual structure used by many private, independent telemedicine vendors (and even hospitals in some jurisdictions) to comply with state corporate practice of medicine doctrines is that of a management or administrative services arrangement. Under this type of arrangement, a general corporation provides all administrative and management services and equipment, technology, and facilities, while the licensed professionals – operating through an affiliated but unowned, professional corporation – practice medicine and provide medical services. This model is often referred to as the "friendly-PC" or PC/MSO structure. While this type of arrangement can successfully mitigate corporate practice of medicine and fee-splitting risks, the arrangement must be carefully crafted, entrusting key clinical decisions to licensed physicians and may require multiple tailored professional corporations if the services are provided across multiple jurisdictions. Further, hospitals advancing telemedicine services across different jurisdictions increasingly desire to operate utilizing a friendly-PC structure as it mitigates concerns for hospital facility licensing in multiple jurisdictions (in addition to mitigating impacts to the existing state facility licenses) and allows for more streamlined operations through a central business entity for the telemedicine business line.

Federal and State Anti-kickback and Self-Referral Laws

The federal laws and regulations referred to as the "anti-kickback statute" [50] makes it a crime for anyone to offer cash or in-kind payment as an award or inducement to healthcare professionals (or for healthcare professionals to accept such award or inducement) for ordering or prescribing any healthcare services or products purchased through federal programs such as Medicare, Medicaid, or Tricare. The federal self-referral law (known as the "Stark Law") [51] prohibits healthcare professionals from referring patients to or prescribing healthcare products from an entity with which the provider has a financial interest. Additionally, nearly every state has adopted state analogs to these anti-kickback laws and Stark Law. In addition to protecting consumers and payers from potentially fraudulent activities by healthcare providers, these laws serve, like state corporate practice of medicine and fee-splitting laws, as a mechanism to shelter healthcare professional clinical decision-making from financial or commercial influence by nonprofessionals. The practical effect of these laws is that all remuneration flowing from any healthcare entity or individual to a healthcare provider – including salary, bonuses, and all in-kind remuneration such as leased office space, equipment, and the like – must be evaluated for compliance with these laws.

Given these restrictions and requirements, arrangements involving (often expensive) donation or provision of telemedicine equipment at originating sites should be carefully considered as part of tele-ICU arrangements. The Office of Inspector General has indicated, for example, that a telemedicine vendor who provides discounted or free equipment to an originating site for the provision of telemedicine services could potentially run afoul of the federal anti-kickback statute in certain circumstances [52]. Thus, tele-ICU vendors and originating sites must take a thoughtful approach and seek advice of counsel when structuring their arrangements to ensure compliance with state and federal anti-kickback and self-referral laws.

Liability Considerations

The breadth of state and federal laws and regulations applicable to the provision of tele-ICU services makes the liability associated with non-compliance real and significant. Liability for non-compliance may arise from state medical board investigations and sanctions or federal agency investigations related to business arrangements, organizational structure, or inappropriate billing for tele-ICU services. In addition to these state and federal legal and regulatory compliance-based risks, healthcare providers are faced with the professional liability risks of engaging with relatively new and emerging medical delivery outlays that involve remote clinical care. Each of these liability considerations are discussed in this section.

State Board Sanctions

State medical boards have the authority and prerogative to investigate providers and entities engaged in the provision of tele-ICU services in the state for compliance with state laws and regulations associated with business entity structure, telemedicine technology requirements, practice of medicine restrictions, supervision of non-physician providers, and more. Many states have been quite active in pursuing investigations of and sanctions against telemedicine providers for a variety of these issues in recent years, although most are in the context of more novel "direct-to-consumer" telemedicine operations in contrast to more long-standing and generally clinically accepted tele-ICU practices. As of June 2018, the authors are not aware of any state actions against providers of tele-ICU services specifically.

Fraud and Abuse Issues

Both state and federal agencies have been increasingly active in evaluating telemedicine outlays in recent years for issues such as false advertising and physician incentive arrangements. While not specific to tele-ICU, recent notable state and federal actions provide insight for tele-ICU service organizations. On the federal level, the Department of Justice ("DOJ") chose to include Riordan, Lewis & Harden, Inc., a private equity firm, in its prosecution of a False Claims Act case against Diabetic Care Rx, one of Riordan's portfolio companies [53]. The violations alleged by the DOJ include forwarding patient information to telemedicine providers who worked on a per-consult basis and who had no physical or perhaps even verbal contact with the patient, in order to drive up short-term revenue from referrals [53]. On the state level, New York recently settled a dispute with DirectLabs and LabCorps regarding the testing of direct-to-consumer laboratory services [54]. These services were considered to be in violation of New York laws requiring laboratory tests to be carried out at the request of licensed medical practitioners. Of particular note was the process by which DirectLabs provided services to consumers. DirectLabs would automatically generate request forms using the name of a licensed chiropractor who had never had contact with the patient, charging only a $24 "access fee" [54]. Ultimately, while the authors are not aware of tele-ICU specific actions as of June 2018, it is instructive for programs to review telemedicine-specific fraud and abuse actions to be sure that certain arrangements have not already triggered federal or state authority scrutiny.

Professional Liability Risks

Providers understandably express concern that practicing via telemedicine in the management of critically ill adults could increase the frequency of malpractice claims and costs [23]. This concern is based upon the remote nature of the care being delivered, the limitations of the technology in providing all of the clinically relevant information to make informed medical decisions, and the fear that providing services via telemedicine puts providers in a less-defensible position [23]. Certainly, those concerns are important liability and patient safety considerations when designing tele-ICU programming and privileging of tele-ICU providers as discussed above. As of June 2018, however, there have been no cases published in the legal literature pertinent to services delivered in the tele-ICU context. This does not preclude the possibility that there have been cases that are settled prior to making it to court. But, at least one large case study to date indicates that the tele-ICU program, which utilizes continuous monitoring, direct observation of patients by tele-ICU providers, direct order writing by tele-ICU providers, and rigorous timely documentation review and action plans, has experienced a *reduction* in the frequency of ICU-related malpractice claims [23]. The case study is based upon a large multistate, nonprofit healthcare system that implemented tele-ICU services covering 450 ICU beds located in five states [23]. Implementation of the tele-ICU program throughout this system was associated with a reduction in ICU-related claims volume to less than half of what it had been prior to implementation of the continuous monitoring tele-ICU program [23]. Although this case study and lack of published malpractice cases involving tele-ICU services is promising, it is too early at this stage to draw conclusions that any model of tele-ICU care is expected to either increase or reduce the frequency and costs of professional liability claims.

Professional Liability Insurance Coverage

The scope of professional liability insurance coverage is generally dictated by contract, not state statutes or regulations. And while some professional liability insurers provide special riders for telemedicine coverage, many would historically only cover claims for face-to-face encounters for which the insurer agreed to cover the provider. Professional liability insurers may not even be licensed in states where patients are receiving telemedicine services from the provider. That said, a few states have proposed or adopted legislation requiring professional liability insurers to insure telehealth services in the same manner as they would the underlying face-to-face services. Hawaii, for example, requires that "every insurer providing professional liability insurance for a health care provider shall ensure that every policy that is issued, amended, or renewed in this State on or after January 1, 2017, shall provide malpractice coverage for telehealth that shall be equivalent to coverage for the same services provided via face-to-face contact between and health care provider and a patient" [55]. At minimum, tele-ICU providers must ensure that the provider's professional liability coverage extends to telemedicine services and care delivered to patients in the originating site jurisdiction.

The American Telemedicine Association Guidelines for Tele-ICU Operations

While various industry organizations have published models and guidance over recent years pertaining to telemedicine practice generally, the American Telemedicine Association published its *Guidelines for TeleICU Operations* in 2014

Table 4.5 Categories included in the ATA's Tele-ICU Guidelines

ATA's Tele-ICU Guideline categories
Administrative guidelines: These touch upon key leadership positioning; messaging; human resource management; healthcare professional licensure; privacy considerations; maintaining legal and regulatory compliance; fiscal management; and quality assurance programs
Clinical application guidelines: These guidelines touch upon the different types of service models and when and how they should be implemented; the types of patients that can be cared for; staffing models; workflow considerations; defining staff roles and responsibilities and integrating on-site and remote staff; orienting staff and maintaining professional competency; documentation in the heath record; educating families and patients about tele-ICU services and obtaining informed consent
Technical guidelines: These guidelines touch upon minimum requirements for technology platforms; mobile device use by healthcare professionals; data security measures; and infection control procedures

Davis et al. [57]

and updated them in 2016 ("ATA's Tele-ICU Guidelines") [56, 57]. Among other things, the ATA's Tele-ICU Guidelines touch upon many of the legal requirements and restrictions discussed in this chapter and serve as a helpful guidance document and comprehensive checklist for entities looking to implement tele-ICU programming. But equally as important, because industry guidelines often serve as the basis for standard of care considerations, the ATA's Tele-ICU Guidelines could potentially serve as a document for state regulators and state courts to view as informing the standard for tele-ICU programming and the standard of professional conduct for practitioners engaged in the provision of tele-ICU services. Importantly, the American Telemedicine Association is the largest telemedicine-focused industry organization and represents a large number of industry leaders and healthcare professionals, which makes its guidance document a natural resource for state regulators and courts when evaluating complaints or allegations against tele-ICU programs. As such, entities looking to implement tele-ICU programming would be well advised to consider the ATA's Tele-ICU Guidelines in designing their programming. Table 4.5 lists some of the specific categories of tele-ICU programming included in the ATA Tele-ICU Guidelines and should be considered by programs looking to implement Tele-ICU programming.

International Telemedicine Outlays and Considerations

Telemedicine outlays have proven to be successful in providing a variety of healthcare services to developing countries in need of readily available specialty healthcare providers [58]. There has also been at least one case report of an international tele-ICU program implemented in 2012 in Syria, a conflict area that was "too risky for direct engagement of even the most dedicated humanitarian organizations" [59]. These international outlays carry trans-jurisdictional legal risks and requirements similar to interstate outlays. This includes licensure requirements, telemedicine-specific restrictions, prohibitions or exemptions, data privacy legal requirements, and the like. The laws of many countries are, perhaps unsurprisingly, silent on the issues of licensure for international healthcare professionals and telemedicine-specific considerations. But several countries have adopted laws to actually facilitate the import of international telemedicine outlays into their respective countries. Saipan, for example, provides an explicit exemption from licensure for consulting by foreign licensed professionals and permits the delivery of healthcare services via a variety of remote technologies [60]. Moreover, international laws related to telemedicine are rapidly evolving as new technologies emerge and countries seek to capitalize on the telemedicine promise of greater access to vulnerable and low-access individuals across the globe. Entities exploring the option of implementing an international tele-ICU program must review country-specific laws related to licensure, telemedicine technology platform restrictions, data privacy and security laws, and other applicable laws and regulations prior to implementing these programs.

Practical checklist for evaluating legal consideration for Tele-ICU services
Evaluate whether the activity involves the practice of medicine or another regulated profession
Understand the applicable providers involved; confirm state licensure requirements and any corporate practice limitations in the states where you anticipate patients may be at the time of the service
Develop appropriate disclosures, terms of service, consents, privacy notices, and other documentation supporting a consistent demonstration of your proposed activity
Given the locations where you plan to provide the telemedicine services (e.g., the location of the patients), understand state-specific requirements for establishing the provider relationship, telemedicine-specific practice standards, and remote prescribing
Consider establishing a clinical team to evaluate the appropriate standard of care given the anticipated telehealth use case (see ATA and other industry guides as references) and a plan for ongoing quality review and updates
Consider technology that assists with compliance (e.g., verifying patient location, video or biometrics requirements, patient consent requirements)
Consider policies and training for medical staff on appropriate activities consistent with the standard of care and proposed activity to maintain compliance with legal and regulatory requirements
Make appropriate provisions for emergency situations, follow-up, and continuity of care (especially in any "direct care" offerings)
Develop a method for continuing to track requirements for multistate services (requirements evolve frequently)
Develop ongoing education and training around compliance topics (state-specific requirements, privacy and security requirements, standard of care best practices)
Evaluate specific reimbursement coverage eligibility and billing requirements
Consider payer contracts and incorporate appropriate provisions and engage with managed care contracting and compliance team to effectuate appropriate updates and ongoing coverage

References

1. Fish EM, Hickman SA, Chaudhry HJ. State licensure regulations evolve to meet the demands of modern medical practice. The SciTech Lawyer Am Bar Ass'n. 2014;10(3):18–22.
2. Ala. Code § 34024-502.
3. Ala. Admin. Code R. 540-X-15-.16.
4. La. Rev. Stat. § 37:1276.1.
5. Minn. Stat. § 147.032.
6. Ohio Rev. Code § 4731.296.
7. Or. Rev. Stat. § 677.139.
8. Or. Admin. R. 847-025-0000.
9. 22 Tex. Admin. Code § 172.12.
10. Ala. Code § 34-24-502.
11. Ala. Admin. Code R. 540-X-16.03, 540-X-15-.16.
12. State telehealth laws and reimbursement policies: a comprehensive scan of the 50 States and District of Colombia. Center for Connected Health Policy. Center for Connected Health Policy. 2018 http://www.cchpca.org/sites/default/files/resources/50%20STATE%20FULL%20PDF%20SPRING%202018%20-%20PASSWORD.pdf. Accessed 5 July 2018.
13. Interstate medical licensure compact, a faster pathway to medical licensure. http://www.imlcc.org/faqs/. Accessed 15 June 2018.
14. Marietta C, McGuire AL. Direct-to-consumer genetic testing: is it the practice of medicine? J Law Med Ethics. 2009;37(2):369–74.
15. Mich. Comp. Laws § 333.16171.
16. Wyo. Stat. § 33-26-103.
17. Wyo. Admin. Code § AI BM Ch. 7.
18. Medicare and medicaid programs: changes affecting hospital and critical access hospital conditions of participation: telemedicine credentialing and privileging. 76 Fed. Reg. 25550. 2011. https://www.federalregister.gov/documents/2011/05/05/2011-10875/medicare-and-medicaid-programs-changes-affecting-hospital-and-critical-access-hospital-conditions-of. Accessed 10 July 2018.
19. Final Revisions to Telemedicine Standards, Joint Commission Perspectives. 2012. https://www.jointcommission.org/assets/1/6/Revisions_telemedicine_standards.pdf. Accessed 18 June 2018.
20. Wilkes MS, Marcin JP, Ritter LA, Pruitt S. Organizational and teamwork factors of tele-intensive care units. Am J Crit Care. 2016;25(5):431–9.
21. Security Breach Notification Laws, Nat'l Conference of State Legislatures. 2018. http://www.ncsl.org/research/telecommunications-and-information-technology/security-breach-notification-laws.aspx. Accessed 18 June 2018.
22. Cal. Health & Safety Code §§ 1280.15-1280.18.
23. Lilly CM, Zubrow MT, Kempner KM, et al. Critical care telemedicine: evoluation and state of the art. Crit Care Med. 2014;42(11):2429–36.
24. Cal. Bus. & Prof. Code § 2290.5(a)(6).
25. Ariz. Admin. Code Sec. R. 20-6-1902.
26. Fla. Admin. Code Ann. r. 64B8-9.0141.
27. Ohio Admin. Code 4731-11-09.
28. Minn. Stat. § 151.37.
29. Ryan Haight Act 21 U.S.C.A. § 831 (West).
30. Controlled Substances Act 21 USC § § 801-904
31. Ariz. Rev. Stat. § 36-3602;
32. Cal. Bus. & Prof. Code § 2290.5;
33. Board Opinion Regarding the Use of Telemedicine Technologies in the Practice of Medicine. Ky. Bd. of Md. Licensure. 19 June 2014.
34. La. Admin Code tit. 46, § 7511;

35. 50-013-2635 Miss. Code R. § 5.3;
36. Nev. Rev. Stat. § 633.165(3) (osteopathic medicine);
37. Tex. Occ. Code § 111.002;
38. Vt. Stat. tit. 18, § 9361.
39. Minn. Stat. § 147.033.
40. Weiner J, Yeh S, Blumenthal D. The impact of health information technology an e-health on the future demand for physician services. Health Aff (Milwood). 2013;32(11):1998–2004.
41. Fla. Admin. Code Ann. r. 64B8-9.0141(1).
42. Del. Code Ann. tit. 24, § 1933 (West).
43. Del. Code Ann. tit. 24, § 1773(f) (West).
44. Ga. Code Ann., § 43-34-25.
45. American Association of Nurse Practitioners. State Practice Environment. https://www.aanp.org/legislation-regulation/state-legislation/state-practice-environment Accessed 15 June 2018.
46. 3 Colorado Code of Regulations R. 713-7:400-2.
47. Florida Annotated Statutes § 458.347.
48. Eric EJ. Understanding Corporate Practice of Medicine Laws by State. 2017. https://www.physiciansfirst.com/blog/corporate-practice-of-medicine-laws-by-state. Accessed 19 June 2018.
49. Ustin, M, Brass C. An examination of fee-splitting statutes in the context of value-based health-care. Bloomberg BNA Medicare Report 2015. https://www.manatt.com/uploadedFiles/Content/4_News_and_Events/Article_By_Us/MCR.Ustin-Brass.0605.pdf?elqaid=2774&elqat=2&elqTrackId=ae263478a4e64l7698edbbc88d5af037. Accessed 19 June 2018.
50. 42 U.S.C.A. § 1320a-7b (West).
51. 42 U.S.C.A. § 1395nn (West).
52. Advisory Opinion No. 99–14. Department of Health & Human Services Office of Inspector General. 2000. https://oig.hhs.gov/fraud/docs/advisoryopinions/1999/ao99_14.htm. Accessed 18 June 2018.
53. Jones Day Client Alert: DOJ Pursues PE Firm Based on Portfolio Company's Alleged Payment of Kickbacks. 2018. http://www.jonesday.com/doj-pursues-pe-firm-based-on-portfolio-companys-alleged-payment-of-kickbacks-02-27-2018/. 7 July 2018.
54. Press Release: A.G. Schneiderman Announces Settlements To Stop Prohibited 'Direct Access Testing'. 2015.https://ag.ny.gov/press-release/ag-schneiderman-announces-settlements-stop-prohibited-%E2%80%98direct-access-testing%E2%80%99. 7 July 2018.
55. Haw. Rev. Stat. Ann. § 671-7.
56. Davis TM, Barden C, Dean S, et al. American telemedicine association guidelines for TeleICU operations. Telemed J E Health. 2016;22(12):971–80.
57. Davis TM, Barden C, Dean S, et al. American Telemedicine Association Guidelines for TeleICU Operations. 2014. http://www.learnicu.org/SiteCollectionDocuments/Guidelines-ATA-TeleICU.pdf. Accessed 15 June 2018.
58. Wootton R, Bonnardot L. Telemedicine in low-resource settings. Front Public Health. 2015;3:3.
59. Moughrabieh S, Weinert C. Rapid deployment of international tele-intensive care unit services in War-Torn Syria. Ann Am Thorac Soc. 2016;13(2):165–72.
60. Saipan Public Health Law No. 15–105, Section 2203(f).

Chapter 5
Nursing and Provider Roles in the Tele-ICU

Timothy N. Liesching and Yuxiu Lei

Introduction

In the current technology revolution, one can easily communicate via video to family and friends across the world as if they were next door. It would seem, therefore, that implementing a tele-ICU should be straight forward, but it is far from simple because developing a well-coordinated tele-ICU extends far beyond the technology. It requires considerable strategic and operational planning. Such planning begins with establishing the right multidisciplinary team that includes caregivers (providers, nursing, and other clinicians) in addition to hospital administrative, technology, and operational personnel. Much of the strategic vision and operational planning will be addressed elsewhere in this book, but here we will consider the details of provider and nursing roles that should be considered while planning a tele-ICU program. Understanding these roles upfront is essential to a successful tele-ICU program.

Before exploring provider and nursing roles in the tele-ICU, it is important to understand the different tele-ICU models as clinical roles differ between such models and how these different models are staffed. The two major types of tele-ICU practice models, centralized and decentralized [1], are described in detail in Chap. 1.

T. N. Liesching (✉)
Department of Pulmonary and Critical Care Medicine, Lahey Hospital and Medical Center, Burlington, MA, USA

Tufts University School of Medicine, Boston, MA, USA
e-mail: Timothy.N.Liesching@Lahey.org

Y. Lei
Department of Pulmonary and Critical Care Medicine, Lahey Hospital and Medical Center, Burlington, MA, USA
e-mail: Yuxiu.Lei@Lahey.org

M. A. Koenig (ed.), *Telemedicine in the ICU*,
https://doi.org/10.1007/978-3-030-11569-2_5

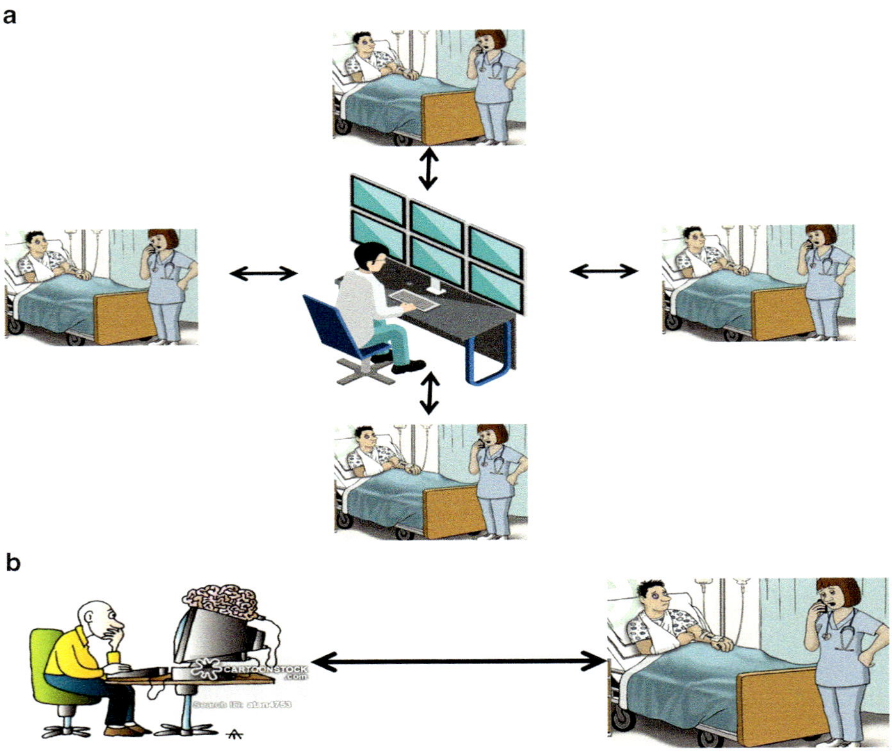

Fig. 5.1 Tele-ICU models (**a**) Centralized tele-ICU: A physician in tele-ICU center. (**b**) Decentralized tele-ICU: A physician in office or home

As shown in Fig. 5.1, the centralized tele-ICU model typically delivers continuous ICU care monitoring for a defined period of time such as 8, 12, or 24 hours per day to the originating site where the patients are located in the local physical ICUs. This model has also been referred to as the "Hub and Spoke" model with the "Hub" being the remote site and the "Spoke" being the originating site where the patient is located. The decentralized model is different as it typically involves scheduled care such as consultation, scheduled rounding, or response care in which patient evaluations are triggered by a specific alert or clinical event [1].

The caregivers in these two models include both providers and nurses. The tele-ICU team in the centralized model often includes one tele-intensivist and several tele-ICU nurses who proactively perform continuous monitoring according to a predetermined time period. In the decentralized care model, an intensivist, or a specialty physician, or an advanced practice provider (nurse practitioner or physician assistant) is located in a clinic unit, office, or home and accesses the remote ICU patients through a two-way audio-video system usually according to a predefined schedule.

Roles and Responsibilities During Strategic Planning and Implementation

Former US President Dwight Eisenhower was known for saying that "plans are worthless, but planning is indispensable." Likewise, the strategic and operational planning is the key to implementing a successful tele-ICU program. Members of such a planning team must include executive leadership, IT personal, human resources (including medical staff office), and other administrative representatives to address fiscal, documentation, and quality matters discussed elsewhere in this book. ICU clinicians and nurses should also be involved early in the design and implementation of the tele-ICU [2]. In fact, their participation in the Strategic Planning Team is essential for a successful program. Strategic Planning Team members should be chosen for their leadership in collaborative relationships that focus on transforming the delivery of quality care [3, 4].

Strategic planning takes time. It is not uncommon for the process to take 1–3 years to get a program from the conceptual phase to full implementation. The first steps of this process should include understanding the current care model and establishing specific program goals within a defined standard of care [1]. When exploring how to implement such goals, careful consideration must be given to the financial, quality, provider/nursing workforce implications, technological and institutional resources, and politics [5]. While provider and nursing members of the Strategic Planning Team have meaningful input on the financial aspects of a program, perhaps their biggest contribution lies with the quality of care, assessing the human resources needed for program implementation, ensuring the technology is "clinician friendly," and navigating institutional politics.

Provider and nursing members of the Strategic Planning Team carry the responsibility to ensure that the program's goals are not only best practice but that the delivery system is reliable and can be operationalized without execution risk. Knowledge of the patient population, current care delivery model and protocols, and best practice/standard of care will be important in this phase. It is necessary to evaluate the relevance of the current metrics measured and if any new metrics are necessary, as well as how the addition of tele-ICU is expected to improve the metrics [5].

With their clinical knowledge and experience, provider and nursing members of the Strategic Planning Team can provide guidance on workforce matters from the perspective of both the tele-ICU end and the local ICU sides. For example, does the remote tele-ICU location require to be staffed by MDs/DOs or critical care advanced practice providers and do current critical care providers have the capacity and willingness to participate; if not, what are the implications of recruiting new providers? [5] How recommendations from the tele-ICU team are carried out on the local end when it pertains to specific procedural recommendations, such as central line placement or intubations, also must be considered in the context of local resources. On the local ICU end, consideration needs to be given to whether the current MD/DO and nursing staff are capable of participating in tele-ICU care, how they maintain their bedside clinical expertise [5], and whether implementing a tele-ICU program will change the type of patient cared for in the local ICU such that the severity of illness extends beyond the clinical expertise of the local staff.

Most of the technological aspects may seem unimportant to the clinical leadership during the planning phase. However, the role of the provider/nursing leaders is imperative when the team is choosing a platform. Clinician knowledge is needed to evaluate each platform being considered for its clinical relevance and reliability. Only the clinical leadership can comment on whether a specific platform provides the necessary information to the tele-ICU provider and back to the local ICU to make an impact in patient care. Platforms also must be easy to use so that both the tele-ICU and the local providers can access each other without difficulty. In order to ensure program success, the provider and nursing members of the Strategic Planning Team should not shy away from insisting on making clinical relevance, reliability, and ease of use a priority when working with other members of the team in choosing a platform.

It will be important to gain the insight of the frontline ICU staff – not only for their practical input but to begin building support for a tele-ICU program [2, 6]. In order to select the most suitable service for a hospital, frontline physicians and nurses should be provided opportunity to understand the different models and provide input on their tele-ICU program. Surveying nurses on existing challenges in their current critical care practice and possible opportunities for improvements, for example, can yield valuable insight and result in engaged staff eager to participate at the time of implementation. Asking physicians to provide opinions about the different tele-ICU service models and their expectations on patient outcomes can provide the Strategic Planning Team helpful guidance to which model may be more likely to be successful. The Strategic Planning Team can collect input from frontline nurses and physicians to help identify the best fit for the specific ICU and the desired outcomes [7].

After the tele-ICU Strategic Planning Team makes decisions about the tele-ICU service model, nurses and physicians may be involved in more detailed aspects of workflow. A well-thought-out coordinated workflow is required in order to provide a meaningful ICU evaluation. In the case of an isolated critical care consult evaluation, the workflow starts with requesting the consult and notifying the consultant, who needs to have a workflow of how to remotely evaluate the patient and obtain the appropriate history and medical information. The consultant will then need a way to document his or her recommendations and communicate them to the bedside nursing staff and providers. There also needs to be a process for ordering tests and/or procedures. Orchestrating these steps requires developing workflows and educating all providers of the workflows well before implementation. There is not likely any single solution to organizing workflows that works as the best solution for all ICUs. One needs to consider local protocols and resources. Clinical representatives from both the originating and remote ends of the tele-ICU along with the tele-ICU medical director and operations director participating in clinical process design workshops may be helpful [8].

Finally, clinical leaders on the Strategic Planning Team should ensure that the detailed aspects of any workflow can be delivered by frontline clinicians reliably and without significant burden in excess of their current clinical responsibilities. Planning a complicated workflow may run the risk of low colleague engagement which will certainly hinder a program's success. In short, provider and nursing participation on the Strategic Planning Team is imperative as their input is needed to be sure that the tele-ICU is operationalized in a way that consistently provides added valuable patient care without unnecessary burden to staff.

Pre-initiation planning, when done well, is time consuming and labor intensive. Many programs have found it useful to assign a full-time point person to coordinate the multiple aspects of the planning phase and the implementation of the tele-ICU. Developing an education and training plan will need to be included in the implementation plan particularly for local critical care staff so that it is understood how tele-ICU services are provided. During this training and education phase, it is important for providers and nurses from the monitoring center to visit and meet the bedside teams on the local "side of the camera" during implementation so that they become familiar with each other as colleagues and build trust in person before meeting for the first time via a camera over patient care [8, 9]. A tele-ICU coordinator who can help organize the early planning stages, workflow development, education, and training, as well as facilitate introduction and familiarization among clinicians who will be on either end of the camera, will make a meaningful contribution to the program. Table 5.1 summarizes the roles during planning a tele-ICU program.

Operational Roles and Responsibilities

Nurses and physicians play essential roles in the tele-ICU operation. We will focus on their daily responsibilities in patient care from both remote and originating sites.

RN Roles in Centralized Model

In a centralized tele-ICU model, nurses in the remote site cover patient care 24 hours a day, 365 days a year [4]. Tele-ICU nurses practice "telenursing," defined as "the practice of nursing over distance using telecommunications technology" [4]. Tele-ICU nurses must possess high-level skills in communication, collaboration, decision-making, systems thinking, and computer literacy, in addition to qualifications as critical care nurses. Tele-ICU nurses' major role is making virtual rounds via the camera and assessing all patients [11]. They maintain standard monitoring such as electrocardiography and hemodynamic values and access to medical records, diagnostic images, and laboratory results. They use a color-coded acuity system to categorize patients on the basis of physiologic criteria and therapeutic

Table 5.1 Roles during planning a tele-ICU program

Topic	Nursing and provider role	Example
Goals	Understand the current ICU services and define specific goals desired that need to be achieved by a tele-ICU solution	Identify that current ICU has inadequate ICU provider available at night to answer medical management issues. Goal: Develop a remote tele-ICU program that provides access to a critical provider for management questions on all ICU patients at night
Tele-ICU model	Learn the pros and cons of various tele-ICU models, and analyze how their clinical outcome can contribute to addressing the program's goal	If overnight critical care management is needed, are the services so episodic that a decentralized model will suffice or does the frequency and acuity of the critical care management issues require more continuous monitoring with a centralized model
Quality	Determine	Whether the specialty and qualification of remote provider fits the acuity of patients in local ICUs
Workforce needs	Evaluate and determine	Remote nurse rounding twice during night or local nurse calling a remote tele-intensivist according to situation
Technology	Evaluate technology solutions with reliability and ease of use in mind	Choose the software (e.g., using historical ICU data of WBC, hematocrit, hemoglobin, platelets to develop a customized alert system [10]) and/or hardware (e.g., mobile bed, mobile robot, mobile cart)
Local drivers and politics	Commit to understanding and addressing institutional drivers and politics to improve buy-in and adoption	Invite tele-ICU providers or company officials to speak, discuss the possible collaboration to improve patient outcomes, and reduce costs
Workflows	Design workflows that are simple and reliable	A tele-ICU physician evaluates a patient with septic shock and, among other recommendations, determines that the patient would benefit from central venous access to deliver vasoactive drugs. A predetermined workflow at the local level is established so that it can be activated immediately; the patient can received the recommended action in a timely manner
Education/ training	Encourage adequate education and training. Set expectations. Encourage provider and nursing in person collaboration prior to implementation	Organize workshops, e-learning, surveys, team meetings

measures. They respond to alerts and alarms based on the lab results and vital signs. They interact with patients and family via the audio-video system. Tele-ICU nurses assist the bedside nurses as a second set of eyes and ears to observe patients [12]. They have instant access to the same information as bedside nurses via print and electronic resources. Tele-ICU nurses can also draft a detailed admission note or make notes in the electronic medical record, which is available promptly to all care providers from the remote site or originating site in the electronic medical record. Tele-ICU nurses promptly respond to questions and requests from bedside staff. For example, a bedside nurse may request a tele-ICU nurse to watch over another patient while the bedside nurse transports a patient off the unit to diagnostic tests.

In the new tele-ICU clinical care environment, tele-ICU nurses do not replace bedside nurses. The bedside nurse remains responsible for direct patient care [1]. The bedside nurse has a "second set of eyes" from tele-ICU nurses that provide clinical surveillance and support [12]. With mutual respect, bedside nurses may want to optimally use tele-ICU services including tele-nurses and tele-intensivists. Bedside nurses can push a button to activate tele-ICU service in many situations. For example, the bedside nurse may admit a patient from the emergency room at midnight when there is no on-site intensivist. A tele-ICU nurse can draft the admission note, while the bedside nurse is settling the patient's bed and taking vitals. The bedside nurse can request the tele-intensivist to check on the patient and order emergency medications or therapy. The bedside nurse also needs to educate the patient and family about the tele-ICU services and obtain consent from the patient and family to use tele-ICU services.

Bedside nurses at the originating site may participate in tele-ICU rounds. The night-shift tele-ICU nurse may give the bedside nurse (who just takes a new shift in the morning) an update of patient acuity status during the tele-ICU round. The bedside nurse also can learn about patients' recent interventions and ongoing treatment or plan from the tele-ICU intensivist who is leading rounds. Or the bedside nurse can get an update about patient status before the routine on-site rounds from the tele-ICU staff during the tele-ICU sign-out process as a pre-rounding activity. Most ICUs (80%) with a tele-ICU service reported <50% of providers and services have interactive (between tele-ICU staff and physical ICU staff) sign-out for all patients [13]. The tele-ICU intensivist can brief the interventions that he or she ordered for most unstable patients during off-hours. Such interactive pre-rounding processes help the bedside nurse better prepare to present the patient during on-site interdisciplinary rounds and decrease the duration of on-site rounding time. The tele-ICU nurse also can participate in the on-site rounds to assist the bedside nurse present the patient. For example, the tele-ICU nurse can tell the tele-ICU alerts and tele-ICU interventions that occurred when the bedside nurse was not present.

MD Roles in Centralized Model

Intensivists in tele-ICU are board-certified physicians with privileges and credentials in each participating hospitals. They provide oversight as well as interventions. A typical workflow includes (1) evaluating all new patients, (2) regular monitoring of the patients, (3) responding to "SmartAlerts," (4) supervising guideline and protocol management, (5) adjusting therapy to achieve objectives of care plans created by the bedside team, (6) responding to emerging or acute problems, and (7) being available to bedside physicians, house staff, and nurses [14]. The tele-intensivist prioritizes the issues and performs routine rounds in the physical ICUs via the real-time audio-video system [12]. The tele-intensivist evaluates patients' status using vital signs, progress notes, and lab results that are the same as on-site physician use. The frequency of tele-rounding depends on the acuity level of the patient. Most patients are reassessed every 1–4 hours according to acuity or as needs emerge [12]. As patient care conditions are identified, changes to the plan of care are discussed directly with the bedside team. The tele-intensivist may participate in the pre-rounding activity at his or her sign-out process before the on-site interdisciplinary round. During the pre-rounding activity, the tele-intensivist can brief the patients' acuity status, interventions, and further recommendations. The tele-intensivist may lead on-site interdisciplinary rounds with the beside team including nurses, residents, and pharmacists.

A tele-ICU service is not designed to replace local services, but to augment care through the leveraging of resources and the standardization of processes [1]. The ICU physician (intensivist, primary care physician, hospitalist, resident) is responsible for direct critical care with his or her regular schedule before implementation of tele-ICU. Optimal tele-ICU performance is strongly dependent on the partnership and integration between the tele-ICU and physical ICU team. A collaborative care delivery model should be established and maintained in order to achieve shared outcomes [1]. How physicians in the originating ICU collaborate with tele-ICU services should be already planned before implementation of tele-ICU [3]. Normally when an intensivist is available in the physical ICU, there is no need to schedule tele-ICU services. However, the on-site intensivist may have an effective and directed handover meeting with the tele-intensivist, who is taking over the night shift. Standardization of such handover processes may help improve the communication efficiency, accelerate patient care, and reduce medical errors [15]. An on-call attending intensivist overnight may have chances to interact with the tele-intensivist on emergency cases or critical clinical decisions. The primary care physician in the originating site may be contacted by a tele-intensivist regarding a patient's specific medical history during his/her off-hours. Specialty physicians including cardiologists, pulmonologists, neurologists, oncologists, anesthesiologists, and surgeons may co-manage ICU patients with the tele-intensivist according to the patients' specific comorbidities and acuity.

Approximately 83% of hospitalists have clinical responsibilities in the ICU [16]. Because of the shortage of intensivists in rural ICUs, hospitalists are increasingly involved in critical care delivery [17]. However, the hospitalist in the ICU may not be able to deliver sufficient critical care to patients with high complexity and acuity. They may have to practice medicine beyond their scope of training and experience and without enough support from a board-certified intensivist. In the ICU with no on-site intensivist, the hospitalist may collaborate with tele-ICU intensivist to perform interdisciplinary rounds. Hospitalists who follow their patients in the ICU can request the tele-intensivist's assistance in effective symptom management or consult with the tele-intensivist for urgent treatments. For example, the hospitalist can request the tele-intensivist to assist when performing central line insertion, arterial line insertion, intubation, or diagnostic ultrasound. Residents working in ICUs felt that tele-ICU not only improved patient care but benefited their training specifically with regard to ventilator management, initial management of an unstable patient, code supervision, and respiratory failure recognition [14]. Residents may also collaborate with the tele-ICU intensivist to perform interdisciplinary rounds.

RN Roles in Decentralized Model

In the decentralized tele-ICU model, there is no specific center to perform teleservices. This practice model is rather a process [1]. The on-site nurses participate in the scheduled virtual rounds, via traditional telephone or robotic tele-presence (RTP), which enables a direct face-to-face rapid response by the physician. The on-site nurses communicate better, are able to be involved in decision-making, and therefore improve work satisfaction when using RTP in scheduled remote rounds [18, 19]. The on-site nurses present the patients under their care and raise questions and concerns about patients' status or treatments. The on-site nurses also can activate tele-services by telephone, pager, or RTP in case of emergency. The calling/paging protocol should have been established before contracting a decentralized tele-ICU service [20]. Bedside nurses are familiar with calling/paging criteria such as unstable intracranial pressure, deterioration of Glasgow Coma Score, refractory hypotension, or hypoxemia. They report to the remote provider the patient's status, vital signs, and lab results and coordinate the treatment that is recommended by the remote provider. On-site nurses at the patient location provide hands-on assistance and may, if trained appropriately, serve as surrogate examiners. For example, the bedside nurse can shine a light into the pupils of an unresponsive patient or evaluate motor responses. The remote provider may or may not be able to view the patient's EMR directly. The on-site nurse may need to pull up images or lab results for the remote provider. If the remote provider is not able to document the tele-service directly in the patient's EMR, the on-site nurse will need to document the interventions in the patient's EMR.

MD Roles in Decentralized Model

The remote provider in a decentralized model (Fig. 5.1b) could be an intensivist, other specialty physician, or advanced practice provider. The remote provider utilizes telephone, computer, two-way audio-video system, or a mobile robot from various locations – clinic, office, or home – to provide clinical services. For example, physicians may use a mobile robot to perform off-shift rounding in the ICU from home [18–20]. The physician can activate the robot using software on his computer at home during nights or on weekends. The robot can patrol each room,

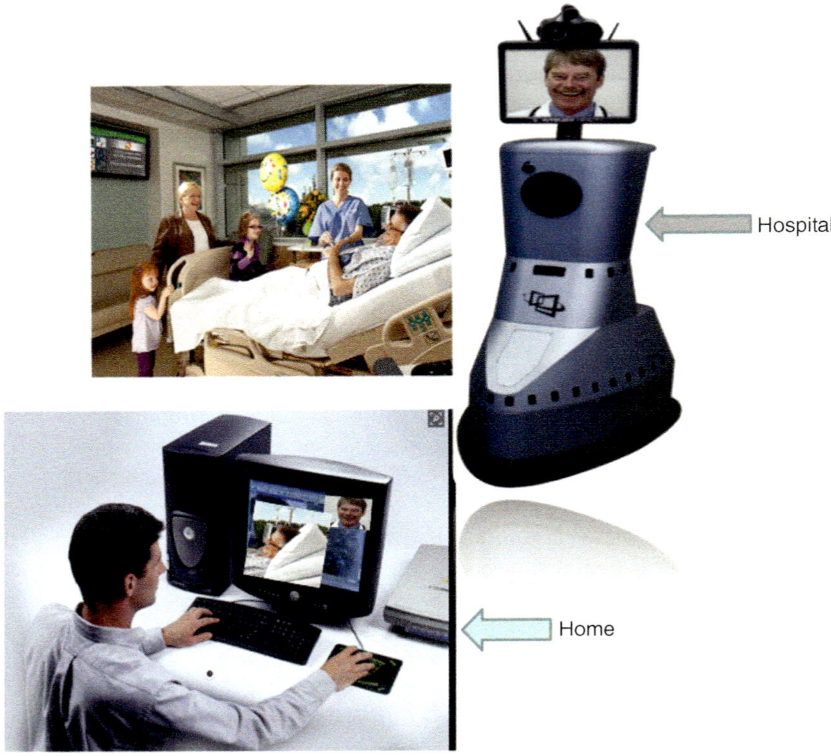

Fig. 5.2 A physician using a remote robot to examine the patient

and the physician can be displayed on the robot screen (Fig. 5.2) to enable face-to-face communication with patients and families, bedside nurses, and residents. The physician can review trends of physiologic variables such as cardiac output and treatment goals such as heart rate control and collaborate with bedside nurses and residents. In addition to routine patient rounds and ICU admissions, the remote physician can respond to the emergency calls or pages by activating the mobile robot using the computer from home. The mobile robot can also be used for ICU resident mentoring and education and family counseling.

Management Roles and Responsibilities

Operational Management

The tele-ICU medical director needs to overcome strong resistance to work with physicians and nurses in the physical ICU to empower the tele-ICU physicians to be actively engaged in patient management decisions [21]. The tele-ICU executive leadership should recruit leaders who can implement and sustain care models that support collaborative relationships between remote and originating sites to achieve the goal of enhancing patient care [1]. The tele-ICU medical director may work with the physical ICU director to achieve this goal through multiple strategies [12], such as (1) shared tele-ICU/physical ICU staff meetings, (2) providers from the remote site visiting the originating site and providers from the originating site visiting the remote site, (3) formal staff liaison positions, and (4) forming a partnership committee that allows providers from remote and originating sites to meet and identify potential problems and solutions [12]. The physicians and nurses in the originating site and remote site can learn about each other's qualifications and experiences through these mechanisms.

The organizations must also create guidelines about tele-ICU roles and responsibilities, appropriates staffing models, hours of operation, methods of communication, procedures around routine and emergency care delivery, and chain of command for escalation processes [1]. The providers from both remote and originating sites can work together as a team to develop protocols for the criteria for emergency tele-ICU activation, the methods for efficient communication, medication orders, therapy orders, resolving conflicts, etc. All protocols should be developed with the goals of achieving timely and appropriate management of patients with high acuity.

Communication

Communication between providers is extremely important in the high acuity and complex environment of caring for critically ill patients. Skilled and efficient communication is associated with better outcomes of patient safety [22]. The efficiency and accuracy of clinical information exchange between remote and originating site providers is the pivotal point of timely and successful versus delayed and failed intervention. Standardized communication tools provide a framework to organize messages. SAFE (Situation/Assessment/Findings and Figures/Express and Expect) was developed at Baylor University Medical Center [23]. The SAFE report was developed by interviewing experienced nurses and physicians about the effective communication style in their collaboration of patient care. If bedside nurses adopt the SAFE tool to communicate with tele-ICU physicians, they prepare for the dialogue and include information to be obtained and activities to be completed before calling. The bedside nurse then follows the structures in the table to report to the tele-ICU physician: **S** is the **S**ituation, a very brief and focused description of what is happening now and what prompted the call. **A** is **A**ssessment, the nurse's clinical impression of the patient's specific problem. **F** is Findings and **F**igures, explicit relevant data, or evidence that supports or leads to the clinical impression. **E** is **E**xpress and **E**xpect, which instructs the nurse to engage in dialogue about interventions to address the patient needs, such as orders for tests, medications, and treatments, or asking the physician to come see the patient.

SBAR is an acronym for Situation, Background, Assessment, Recommendation, a technique that can be used to facilitate prompt and appropriate communication [24]. SBAR may be a better communication tool for tele-ICU practice with complex situations requiring a clinician's immediate attention and action [25]. SBAR is a simple, straightforward tool:

- Step 1-**S**: Describe the **Situation** – What is the patient's current status? For example, HR 130, RR 22, sinus tachycardia on the monitor.
- Step 2-**B**: Include important **Background** information – What are the circumstances or medical history leading up to the situation? For example, the patient was admitted for COPD exacerbation.
- Step 3-**A**: Add your **Assessment** – What do I think the problem is? For example, acute respiratory distress.
- Step 4-**R**: Conclude with your **Recommendation** – What therapy or medication or procedure should we provide to the patient? For example, endotracheal intubation.

Once a standard communication tool has been adopted between the tele-ICU and physical ICU, the provider will expect the information in this format, and the speaker can communicate the message more efficiently. Many other communication tools for structuring written communication in the medical field have been developed such as SOAP (Subjective, Objective, Assessment, Plan) and APIE (Assessment, Plan, Intervention, Evaluation). SBAR may be the most appropriate communication tool for tele-ICU considering the urgency of clinical events in the ICU and widespread adoption of this tool. The standardized SBAR communication format can also be built into the communication software used for both originating and remote tele-ICU sites [26]. Clinical communication software, such as Vocera [27], can be used to communicate between remote and originating site providers either with voice or HIPAA-compliant secure text.

Medical Translation

For patients located in rural, underserved areas with high numbers of non-English speaking residents, a multi-lingual physician from a tele-ICU program will enhance the communication and therefore speed up diagnosis and treatment. There is immense inefficiency and potential danger in miscommunication between tele-ICU physicians and non-English-speaking patients. However, it is impossible to hire tele-clinicians who can speak all of the languages that patients are speaking. A remote medical translation service can solve this language barrier. Tele-health interpretation is a type of medical translation service that takes place during a telehealth appointment [28]. The interpreter is connected electronically with the tele-clinician and the patient. The interpreter will translate whenever the clinician or the patient says something so that everyone can understand each other throughout the appointment. Telephonic interpretation is the most practical way to connect the interpreter, clinician, and patient due to its low cost and convenience. Video interpretation is necessary for deaf or hearing-impaired patients [28]. American Sign

Language (ASL) services provide remote video interpreting. The interpreter for tele-ICU services should have specialized training in medical terminology. The initial set-up with a reputable language service provider can be incorporated in either tele-ICU center or originating site. To protect patients' confidentiality, the medical translation service provider should be HIPAA compliant.

Documentation and Billing

The procedures for clinical documentation of tele-ICU services must be established in compliance with organizational legal and risk management oversight [1]. The tele-ICU physicians, nurses, or pharmacists shall be able to write notes using direct interfaces between the tele-ICU and hospital EMR system, laboratory, pharmacy, and bedside monitor system. The goal of such documentation should be clarity of the tele-ICU clinical intervention and a complete clinical picture based on the available data in the tele-ICU. Documentation of tele-ICU services in the EMR should be prioritized to ensure the seamless flow of information between patient information systems to enhance clinical support and promote continuity of care.

The care team in the originating ICU site activates the tele-ICU service. The tele-ICU nurse reviews the patient information and documents a tele-ICU admission note in the patient's EMR. The tele-ICU intensivist can use a document template with structured data for the tele-consultation report. The document's header must contain at least the following: patient information; contact details of primary physician, private duty nurse, and other participants; document creation date; duration of service; and author identification [29]. The tele-ICU progress notes include patient's status change and acuity, the medication order, interaction with the patient and on-site care team, resolution, and care plan. The tele-ICU pharmacist documents the medication order, dosage, frequency, IV rate, etc.

Currently third-party payers do not pay for many tele-ICU services, especially those that employ centralized models. Hospitals need to budget for the cost of tele-ICU physicians and nurses who provide services from remote sites for patients in the originating ICUs [21]. As reviewed in Chap. 11 of this book, financial benefits may be achieved by increased case volume or reduced cost because of shortened length of ICU stay or reduced critical care complications [30]. The Current Procedural Terminology (CPT) codes for in-person critical care billing, as shown in Table 5.2 [31], are not applicable for tele-ICU services yet. The reimbursement rate

Table 5.2 Critical care billing CPT codes [31]

CPT Code	Definition
99291	Critical care, evaluation and management of the critically ill or critically injured patient; first 30–74 minutes
99292	Critical care, evaluation and management of the critically ill or critically injured patient; each additional 30 minutes (list separately in addition to code for primary service)

for critical care physicians at the originating site decreases as the length of ICU stay increases [32]. The physician time spent in activities outside of the unit such as telephone calls taken at home or office may not be reported as critical care. In 2008, in response to a request for new CPT codes to report tele-ICU services, the American College of Chest Physicians, American Thoracic Society, and the Society of Critical Care Medicine were asked to collect data to determine the pattern of usage for tele-ICU codes [33]. The survey data were collected from those centers monitoring patients in academic and community hospitals in urban, suburban, and rural settings. The survey showed that, per site per 12-hour shift, about 1.75 tele-ICU encounters could have been billed as critical care CPT code 99291 if the services had been provided in-person at the originating site. In this centralized model, the majority of tele-ICU services involved tele-ICU intensivists guiding patient care through nurses and other providers at the bedside and required far less than 30 minutes per episode.

Hospitals most commonly contract with a tele-ICU service center. The tele-ICU center pays the tele-ICU intensivist ($160–200/hour in 2007) [34] and nurses for providing remote coverage of ICU patients. In the centralized service model, the tele-ICU intensivist and nurses document the services. In decentralized service models, the on-site provider or nurse who requests the tele-ICU service typically documents in the patient's chart. The remote physician may then file a report or time card for documentation and reimbursement of the tele-consultation from the originating site. In this model, tele-ICU services are provided to the originating hospital, not directly billed to patients, and are considered part of the operational cost of the hospital [34].

Although physician reimbursement for telemedicine services is increasingly common [35, 36], few payers currently reimburse for critical care services provided via telemedicine, given the importance of bedside assessment in the ICU as well as concerns about overutilization and devaluation of critical care services [34].

Common Pitfalls

Acceptance and Common Issues

Young et al. reviewed staff acceptance of tele-ICU coverage and found that staff generally accepted the tele-ICU coverage with satisfaction score of 4.2–4.5 out of a five-point Likert scale (1 = poor acceptance, 5 = high acceptance) [37]. Nursing staff showed stronger resistance initially, but acceptance may improve over time [2, 38]. The bedside nurses might not take advice from tele-ICU nurses and might be reluctant to request tele-ICU services. Nurses could face conflict when advice offered remotely conflicts with treatment prescribed by ICU attending physicians [2]. There is need to focus on nursing education to adopt tele-ICU services [39, 40]. In a decentralized model, the majority of physicians believe that remote patient care is either "very valuable" or "valuable" in improving patient care and patient/family satisfaction [41].

The common problems for nurses were identified as follows [2, 8, 37]:

- Bedside nurses refused to take advice from tele-nurses or tele-clinicians.
- Advice offered by tele-ICU conflicted with treatment prescribed by ICU attending physicians.
- Bedside nurses avoided seeking help from tele-ICU proactively or only passively waited for tele-ICU services.
- Perception that tele-ICU "spied upon" them.
- Tele-ICU services interrupted their work and increased workload.
- More experienced nurses felt that tele-ICU is only helpful for new nurses.
- Low quality of audiovisual equipment and unfriendly technical system.
- Bedside nurses fear that tele-ICU nurses will replace them.

The common problems identified by physicians were as follows [37]:

- No need for tele-ICU services.
- Originating site physicians felt that tele-ICU failed to recognize when help was really needed.
- IT interface/security challenges.
- Physicians from originating site would not accept the tele-ICU interventions.
- Low quality of audiovisual system.
- Tele-ICU physicians had challenges of physical stress and boredom.
- Tele-ICU physicians became frustrated by the inability to directly intervene and by resistance encountered from originating site staff.
- Originating site physicians felt increased workload and responsibilities.
- Interruptions from tele-ICU services.

The success of collaboration between tele-ICU and physical ICU starts with initial visionary leadership and direction at the organizational level before the implementation of the tele-ICU program [3]. More specifically, the success depends on the organizational acceptance of tele-ICU, sufficient education and training, necessary clinical transformation of bedside practices, and clarification of responsibilities and authorities of each role involved in the collaborative care of ICU patients.

Differences of Opinion Between Remote and Bedside Providers

Sometimes advice offered remotely may conflict with treatment prescribed by ICU attending physicians [37]. The opinion about the diagnosis, treatment plan, medication or therapy, or end-of-life decision-making may differ because of considering different aspects of the patient's current status, past medical history, pathology or radiology interpretation, or patient code status. Conflicts between ICU intensivists may also be associated with burnout and depression for intensivists [42].

The conflict between tele-ICU and physical ICU intensivists may be more stressful. According to American Telemedicine Association (ATA) guidelines [1], the executive leadership must be appropriately positioned in the organization before or during the implementation of tele-ICU program. The leadership must participate in key decision-making forums with the authority to make necessary decisions. Either tele-ICU physician or bedside physician must resolve conflicts while focusing on patient safety and care quality. They may report to the tele-ICU program leadership with a mechanism that is nonpunitive and sensitive to assuring that the close collaborative relationship between the tele-ICU and ICU staff is not compromised.

Good communication involving primary care physicians, subspecialty consultants, pharmacists, pathologists, radiologists, nurses, and the patient and family is key to resolving conflicts. Physicians at both the remote and originating sites need to understand the source of conflicts first. If there are differing opinions about the diagnosis, for example, the providers can seek an opinion from the originating site pathologist or radiologist. Through discussion involving all the necessary personnel, a consensus regarding the diagnosis can be achieved. Conflict regarding medications or treatment strategy may be resolved by referring to specific guidelines or evidence-based protocols.

Where to Start

Read the Guidelines

In order to establish a common set of standards to ensure the safe delivery of tele-ICU care, all involved personnel should review the relevant guidelines for tele-ICU. The ATA updated the guidelines for tele-ICU operations in 2016 [1]. By definition, tele-ICU is not a separate medical specialty, but a tool or system to deliver critical care. Tele-ICU cannot replace local services, but augment care through the leveraging of resources and standardization of processes. The guideline emphasizes the collaborative relationships between originating and remote ICU sites to enhance patient care. The organization must create guidelines for such collaboration including the roles and responsibilities of staff at both sites, leadership, operation hours, communication pathway, workflow, and patient safety reporting. Tele-ICU staff must also follow the regulations to protect patients' privacy and confidentiality when managing the patients' medical records. The documentation of tele-ICU clinical interventions must be integrated in the EMR system and in compliance with organizational legal and risk management.

The ATA guideline advises incorporation of tele-ICU operations into ICU practice guidelines by other organizations such as Society of Critical Care Medicine, American Association of Critical-Care Nurses (AACN), the American College of Chest Physicians (ACCP), and the Critical Care Societies Collaborative. AACN provided guidelines for tele-ICU nursing practice [4]. Tele-ICU nurses must possess high-level skills in communication, collaboration, decision-making, systems thinking, and computer literacy, in addition to the knowledge, skills, and abilities required for bedside critical care nursing. The patient is the central component of all interactions between tele-ICU nurses and staff at the originating site. Tele-ICU nursing leaders, in collaboration with tele-ICU nursing staff, create policies to standardize tele-ICU procedures such as virtual rounding, patient and family communication and education, monitoring and response to alerts and alarms, management of bedside emergency situations, patient care hand-offs, documentation, debriefing about cases/events, downtime procedures, escalation processes to address real-time care concerns, etc.

Learn from Others

Lehigh Valley Hospital and Health Network (LVHHN) launched a tele-ICU program in 2004 [43, 44]. From 7 PM to 7 AM, a tele-intensivist and two critical care nurses work in the tele-ICU monitoring center located in Allentown, Pennsylvania. The tele-ICU monitoring center is equipped with multiple computer monitors (Fig. 5.3) [43]. The bedside nurses use the MetaVision charting system for automatic bedside data entry for vital signs, IV dosing, etc. The tele-intensivist and tele-nurses have bedside access to updated patient data. They can have a customized view of each patient, use note-writing tools to write progress notes into the EMR, read images through an interface with digital radiography, and order medications or treatments via an interface with computerized data entry (Fig. 5.4). In an example case, a patient (Joe) was transferred to an ICU bed after 7 PM. The ICU bed was equipped with high-resolution video, two-way audio, and an electronic bedside charting system. A bedside nurse (Sarah) came to measure Joe's vital signs and noted worsening tachypnea. Following the ICU protocol, Sarah pushed the button to activate tele-ICU services. The tele-nurse (Teresa) received the alarm and reported to the tele-intensivist (Dr. M) that Joe had a high respiratory rate. After reviewing the clinical findings with Sarah and looking at Joe's chest x-ray, Dr. M suspected decompensated congestive heart failure. Dr. M activated the audio-video system to

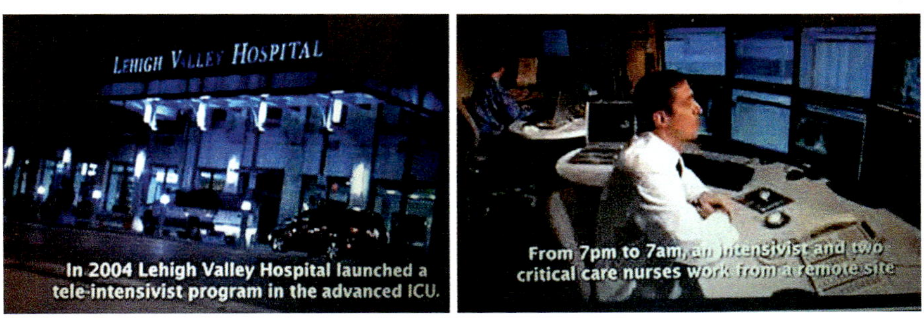

Fig. 5.3 A tele-ICU team is working in the tele-ICU monitor center in Lehigh Hospital

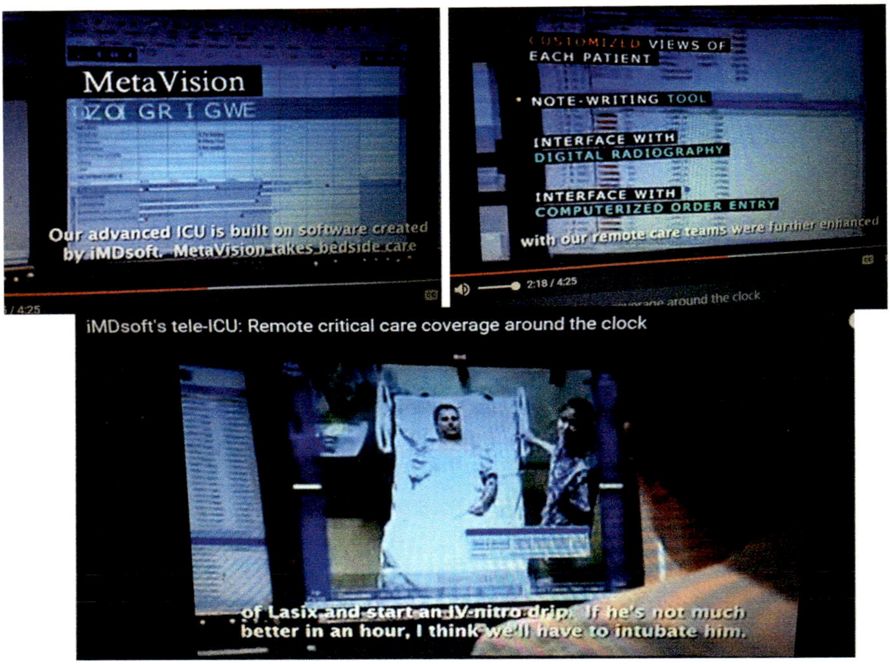

Fig. 5.4 Tele-ICU intensivist interaction with ICU patient

examine Joe with Sarah's assistance. Joe was able to interact with Dr. M on the screen at bedside (Fig. 5.4). After evaluating Joe and confirming the clinical findings, Dr. M told Sarah that he was ordering IV furosemide and a nitroglycerin drip. Dr. M also told Sarah that if Joe did not significantly improve after an hour, he would likely require endotracheal intubation. Dr. M entered the orders in the electronic software. The hospital pharmacy received the order, and Sarah started Joe on the medications according to the order.

References

1. Davis TM, Barden C, Dean S, et al. American telemedicine association guidelines for TeleICU operations. Telemed J E Health. 2016;22(12):971–80.
2. Kowitlawakul Y. The technology acceptance model: predicting nurses' intention to use telemedicine technology (eICU). Comput Inform Nurs. 2011;29(7):411–8.
3. Zapatochny Rufo RJ. The virtual ICU: pathway to improved performance. Nurs Manag. 2009;40(1):39–42.
4. American Association of Critical-Care Nurses. AACN Tele-ICU nursing practice guidelines. Aliso Viejo: American Association of Critical-Care Nurses; 2013.
5. Reynolds HN, Bander JJ. Options for tele-intensive care unit design: centralized versus decentralized and other considerations: it is not just a "another black sedan". Crit Care Clin. 2015;31(2):335–50.

6. Westbrook JI, Coiera EW, Brear M, et al. Impact of an ultrabroadband emergency department telemedicine system on the care of acutely ill patients and clinicians' work. Med J Aust. 2008;188(12):704–8.
7. Bartolini E, King N. Emerging best practices in tele-ICU Care Nationally. A NEHI ISSUE Brief/November 2013, https://www.nehi.net/writable/publication_files/file/nehi_issue_brief_final_emerging_best_practices_for_teleicu_1_.pdf.
8. Mullen-Fortino M, DiMartino J, Entrikin L, Mulliner S, Hanson CW, Kahn JM. Bedside nurses' perceptions of intensive care unit telemedicine. Am J Crit Care. 2012;21(1):24–31; quiz 32.
9. Stafford TB, Myers MA, Young A, Foster JG, Huber JT. Working in an eICU unit: life in the box. Crit Care Nurs Clin North Am. 2008;20(4):441–50.
10. Janz BA, Saeed M, Frassica J, Clifford GD, Mark RG. Development and optimization of a critical care alert and display (CCAD) system using retrospective ICU databases. AMIA Annu Symp Proc. 2005:994.
11. Williams LM, Hubbard KE, Daye O, Barden C. Telenursing in the intensive care unit: transforming nursing practice. Crit Care Nurse. 2012;32(6):62–9.
12. Goran SF. A second set of eyes: an introduction to tele-ICU. Crit Care Nurse. 2010;30(4):46–55; quiz 56.
13. Lilly CM, Fisher KA, Ries M, et al. A national ICU telemedicine survey: validation and results. Chest. 2012;142(1):40–7.
14. Ries M. Tele-ICU: a new paradigm in critical care. Int Anesthesiol Clin. 2009;47(1):153–70.
15. D'Empaire PP, Amaral ACK. What every intensivist should know about handovers in the intensive care unit. Rev Bras Ter Intensiva. 2017;29(2):121–3.
16. Lindenauer PK, Pantilat SZ, Katz PP, Wachter RM. Hospitalists and the practice of inpatient medicine: results of a survey of the National Association of Inpatient Physicians. Ann Intern Med. 1999;130(4 Pt 2):343–9.
17. Sweigart JR, Aymond D, Burger A, et al. Characterizing hospitalist practice and perceptions of critical care delivery. J Hosp Med. 2018;13(1):6–12.
18. Rincon F, Vibbert M, Childs V, et al. Implementation of a model of robotic tele-presence (RTP) in the neuro-ICU: effect on critical care nursing team satisfaction. Neurocrit Care. 2012;17(1):97–101.
19. Bettinelli M, Lei Y, Beane M, Mackey C, Liesching TN. Does robotic telerounding enhance nurse-physician collaboration satisfaction about Care decisions? Telemed J E Health. 2015;21(8):637–43.
20. Vespa PM, Miller C, Hu X, Nenov V, Buxey F, Martin NA. Intensive care unit robotic telepresence facilitates rapid physician response to unstable patients and decreased cost in neurointensive care. Surg Neurol. 2007;67(4):331–7.
21. Center NEHIMTCHT. Tele-ICUs: remote management in Intensive Care Units. https://www.nehi.net/writable/publication_files/file/tele_icu_final.pdf. 2007.
22. Goran SF, Mullen-Fortino M. Partnership for a healthy work environment: tele-ICU/ICU collaborative. AACN Adv Crit Care. 2012;23(3):289–301.
23. Dixon JF, Larison K, Zabari M. Skilled communication: making it real. AACN Adv Crit Care. 2006;17(4):376–82.
24. SBAR. https://en.wikipedia.org/wiki/SBAR. Accessed on March 2018.
25. Improving Clinical Communication Using SBAR. Available online. http://www.1000livesplus.wales.nhs.uk/sitesplus/documents/1011/T4I%20%283%29%20SBAR.pdf. Accessed March 2018.
26. Pimintel DM, Wei SH, Odor A. A software communication tool for the tele-ICU. AMIA Annu Symp Proc. 2013;2013:1139–48.
27. Clinical communication software. https://www.vocera.com/products/secure-texting-collaboration. Accessed on March 2018.
28. Lahiere B. Telehealth interpretation: help for rural non-english-speaking patients. Posted on Mar 24, 2017 at 10:41 pm. http://blog.spoken-here.com/telehealth-interpretation-providing-quality-healthcare-options-for-rural-areas. Accessed on 23 March 2018.

29. Finet P, Gibaud B, Dameron O, Le Bouquin Jeannes R. Relevance of health level 7 clinical document architecture and integrating the healthcare enterprise cross-enterprise document sharing profile for managing chronic wounds in a telemedicine context. Healthc Technol Lett. 2016;3(1):22–6.
30. Lilly CM, Motzkus C, Rincon T, et al. ICU telemedicine program financial outcomes. Chest. 2017;151(2):286–97.
31. Critical Care, Evaluation and Management Services (99291, 99292) Reimbursement Policy. https://www.modahealth.com/pdfs/reimburse/RPM041.pdf Accessed March 2018.
32. Ries M. Evaluating tele-ICU cost--an imperfect science. Crit Care Med. 2016;44(2):441–2.
33. McCambridge MM, Tracy JA, Sample GA. Point: should tele-ICU services be eligible for professional fee billing? Yes. Tele-ICUs and the triple aim. Chest. 2011;140(4):847–9.
34. Hoffmann S. Counterpoint: should tele-ICU services be eligible for professional fee billing? No. Chest. 2011;140(4):849–51.
35. Brown NA. State medicaid and private payer reimbursement for telemedicine: an overview. J Telemed Telecare. 2006;12(Suppl 2):S32–9.
36. Whitten P, Buis L. Private payer reimbursement for telemedicine services in the United States. Telemed J E Health. 2007;13(1):15–23.
37. Young LB, Chan PS, Cram P. Staff acceptance of tele-ICU coverage: a systematic review. Chest. 2011;139(2):279–88.
38. Grundy BL, Crawford P, Jones PK, et al. Telemedicine in critical care: an experiment in health care delivery. JACEP. 1977;6(10):439–44.
39. Pfrimmer DM, Roslien JJ. The tele-ICU: a new dimension in critical care nursing education and practice. J Contin Educ Nurs. 2011;42(8):342–3.
40. Barden C, Davis TM. The tele-ICU: a new frontier in critical care nursing practice. AACN Adv Crit Care. 2012;23(3):287–8.
41. Reynolds EM, Grujovski A, Wright T, Foster M, Reynolds HN. Utilization of robotic "remote presence" technology within North American intensive care units. Telemed J E Health. 2012;18(7):507–15.
42. Embriaco N, Hraiech S, Azoulay E, et al. Symptoms of depression in ICU physicians. Ann Intensive Care. 2012;2(1):34.
43. YouTube: iMDsoft's tele-ICU: remote critical care coverage around the clock. https://www.bing.com/videos/search?q=youtube+tele-icu+intensivist&view=detail&mid=CB6931B6C1077281B229CB6931B6C1077281B229&FORM=VIRE.
44. Lehigh Valley Hospital to Begin Using New State-of-the-Art Technology for Intensive Care Patient. Published for medical staff of Lehigh Valley Hospital. Medical Staff Progress Notes. https://scholarlyworks.lvhn.org/cgi/viewcontent.cgi?referer=https://www.bing.com/&httpsredir=1&article=1121&context=progress_notes. April, 2004;16(4).

Chapter 6
Structure and Design of the Tele-ICU

Spyridon Fortis and Matthew R. Goede

How to Build a Centralized Tele-ICU Program from the Ground Up

Building an ICU telemedicine program is not a uniform process, and its characteristics may vary depending on the needs of the ICUs supported by the tele-ICU. Large telemedicine vendors that provide service to several ICUs located in unrelated healthcare systems may need to adjust their operation and provide various levels of support to each ICU depending on the individual needs [1, 2]. On the other hand, telemedicine programs built to serve the needs of a small group of hospitals (e.g., hospitals affiliated with university medical centers or hospitals within a single health system) may provide similar service to all ICUs and may serve as a reference point to unify best practice across all locations [3].

In this section, we provide "practical" information on how to build a centralized tele-ICU program regarding (a) staffing requirements, (b) technology requirements, (c) designing tele-ICU hub, and (d) considerations for ICUs that will receive tele-ICU services.

S. Fortis (✉)
Pulmonary, Critical Care and Occupation Medicine, University of Iowa Hospitals and Clinics, Center for Comprehensive Access & Delivery Research & Evaluation (CADRE), Iowa City VA Health Care System, Iowa City, IA, USA
e-mail: spyridon-fortis@uiowa.edu

M. R. Goede
University of Nebraska Medical Center, Veterans Affairs VISN 23 Regional Tele-ICU Associate Medical Director, Omaha, NE, USA
e-mail: mgoede@unmc.edu

M. A. Koenig (ed.), *Telemedicine in the ICU*,
https://doi.org/10.1007/978-3-030-11569-2_6

Tele-ICU Staffing Requirements and Delineation of Roles

Some tele-ICUs are built to provide critical care expertise to ICUs with no intensivist [2, 4] while others to improve quality of care in high-resource ICUs of large tertiary facilities [5], or a combination or spectrum of the two. The staffing levels are therefore based on the services delivered at the individual sites. Telemedicine programs focusing on providing critical care expertise to sites without intensivists on-site will need to have a higher tele-physician-to-tele-nurse ratio. ICUs with available intensivists, at least during some portions of the day, may benefit from tele-ICU programs staffed predominantly by critical care nurses who are responsible for ensuring adherence to best-care practice. In some studies, large urban medical centers with in-house intensivists experience greater benefit from tele-ICU than rural small hospitals [5, 6]. Thus, adherence to best-care practices is a valuable deliverable of tele-ICU that impacts patient outcomes. Other innovative telemedicine programs have adopted a model that provides critical care in various settings [7] like the postanesthesia care unit [8] or the emergency department, identifying those patients that are suitable for ICU admission and monitoring those patients awaiting transfer to the ICU [9]. Other programs have expanded to patients in long-term acute care facilities to help with mechanical ventilator management [10]. It is hard to establish one standard staffing model for all tele-ICU environments. The role of tele-ICU nurses and physicians varies depending on the care model and the bipartite agreement between bedside ICUs and the telemedicine team. The ICU telemedicine care models according to the American Telemedicine Association (ATA) [11] are:

- *Continuous care model.* Continuous care model involves continuous monitoring of the patients without interruption 24/7 or for a specific period of the time (e.g., during off-hours).
- *Scheduled care model.* In scheduled care models, telemedicine consultations can be provided during scheduled time periods, e.g., during morning rounds.
- *Reactive care model.* In the reactive model, telemedicine staff may not be readily available but may be alerted by pager, phone call, etc.

These care models may be combined in various ways. For example, a tele-ICU may provide support based on the reactive care model during daytime hours when in-house intensivists are available at the bedside and based on the continuous care model during the night when the on-site critical care physicians are not available. The leadership of both the bedside ICU and the ICU telemedicine program should discuss prior to implementation what models of tele-ICU should be implemented. A written bipartite agreement that outlines the responsibilities of tele-ICU staff should be available. The authority of tele-ICU staff to intervene should be clearly defined and agreed upon by both parties. Direct intervention is associated with better ICU outcomes compared to monitoring and notifying the bedside staff, and therefore, this model is preferable [12]. Regular discussions between the two parties are essential. Ideally, visits of telemedicine leadership to the bedside ICUs and bedside ICU leadership to the tele-ICU clinical room before implementation help to clarify roles and abilities and identify the optimal care model [13]. Identifying the most appropriate care model is critical as it improves satisfaction in both bedside and remote staff. Having an easily available operation manual, e.g., on a frequently updated website, can facilitate the smooth operation of tele-ICU services as large tele-ICU programs that involve several unrelated ICUs may not provide the same service at the various ICUs. The manual should include information regarding the role of telemedicine staff for each ICU, along with contact and staffing information about the bedside ICUs and the remote hospitals' clinical capabilities, e.g., medical residents are in-house at night.

Role of Remote Nursing Staff

As in the physical ICU, the tele-ICU nurses are the "gatekeepers" of the unit. In general, one tele-ICU nurse is utilized for 20–70 monitored ICU beds [14, 15] and is responsible for initial assessments, ongoing evaluation, and advocacy for the safety and health of the patient. While there are no firm guidelines on the nurse-to-patient ratio, the needs of the site and the care model will set what will be a safe and efficient workload.

In continuous care models, remote nursing staff monitor physiological data, often using automated prediction tools that are built into the tele-ICU software. With the assistance of the computer algorithms, nurses are able to detect early signs of patients' deterioration and alert the bedside staff or the tele-intensivist (early warning model) [15, 16].

In several telemedicine programs, remote nursing staff ensure adherence to best-care practice and that may explain the improved outcomes in several tele-ICU programs after telemedicine implementation [3, 5, 17, 18]. Tele-ICU nursing staff support the local ICUs to ensure compliance in the following evidence-based practices: ventilator bundle, healthcare-associated infection, pressure ulcer prophylaxis, deep vein thrombosis prophylaxis, daily sedation interruption, glucose control, and cardiac prophylaxis. Table 6.1 shows the components of evidence-based practices in a typical ICU telemedicine program. When a compliance issue is detected, the tele-ICU nurse may inform the bedside staff or the tele-intensivist.

Tele-ICU nurses can also review new admissions and help with systematic acuity scoring, organ dysfunction scores, sepsis screening, and dietary assessment – often within the tele-ICU software. They may provide useful information to the tele-intensivist or bedside staff regarding the patient medical history, hospital admission, laboratory data, etc.

As many tele-ICUs recruit nurses with significant clinical and especially ICU experience, the tele-ICU nurses can serve the role of resource nurse to the bedside ICU nursing staff. Tele-ICU has the capability of extending many ICU nurses' careers by allowing them to continue in a clinical ICU role past a point when they can no longer physically perform a bedside nursing role.

Table 6.1 Evidence-based practices supported by ICU telemedicine

Adherence to lung-protective ventilation in acute respiratory distress syndrome
Catheter-associated urinary tract infection bundle
Cardiac prophylaxis
Central line-associated blood stream infection bundle
Daily sedation interruption
Deep vein thrombosis prophylaxis
Glucose control
Pressure ulcer prevention bundle
Sepsis bundle
Ventilator care bundle (bed elevation, stress ulcer prophylaxis, etc.)

Role of Remote Intensivists

For tele-ICU programs with less than 120 ICU beds, one intensivist is usually adequate. An additional intensivist can be added for programs with more than 120 beds [14, 15]. According to American Telemedicine Association guidelines, one intensivist could monitor 100–250 patients depending on the program operation [11].

In a continuous care model, the tele-ICU nurse or the telemedicine software alerts the tele-intensivist about derangements in physiological data. Physicians may communicate with bedside staff, discuss the case, and provide recommendations or may act directly depending on the bipartite agreement. The role of the remote intensivist may vary among various types of patients. Direct intervention staffing models may apply for medical patients, but monitoring and co-management staffing model may apply for patients that require specialized knowledge and skills like surgical or transplant patients. If direct intervention is selected, written protocols should be available to the tele-ICU, especially in patients with specialized care plans (cardiothoracic, bariatric, or neurosurgical).

In a continuous care model, remote intensivists may also review new ICU admissions depending on the bipartite agreement. In ICUs with no intensivist, the hospitalist may contact the remote intensivist, discuss the case, and formulate the appropriate plan. In ICUs with daytime intensivists, during the day, the tele-intensivist may review the chart, participate as a second opinion on rounds, ensure that best practices are implemented, participate in nutrition and antibiotic stewardship efforts, ensure that the care plan made on rounds had the intended effects, and receive sign-out from the bedside team at the end of the day shift. During the night, the remote intensivist may review new admissions with residents or hospitalists that are in-house.

In a scheduled care model, the remote intensivist acts as a consultant who reviews the cases with the bedside team, usually during rounds, and provides recommendations.

A surprisingly large amount of clinical care can be provided via telemedicine given the correct access to the electronic medical record (EMR) and high-definition bedside video teleconferencing (VTC) equipment. The main hindrance to delivery of critical care is the inability to lay hands on the patient and perform procedures.

Role of Advanced Practice Providers

The presence of nurse practitioners and physician assistants in ICUs is increasing [19]. Several tele-ICU hubs are staffing with advanced practice providers, in particular, at times where the remote sites have intensivists in-house. Utilizing advanced practice providers instead of physicians can reduce the operational cost of the tele-ICU substantially. Their focus is frequently on best-care practice adherence. Advanced practice providers may be responsible for ensuring adherence to, and the implementation of, best-care practice that is beyond what critical care nurses with effective care protocols can provide, e.g., mechanical ventilation and hemodynamic augmentation. There are some tele-ICU hubs that are staffed exclusively by advanced practice providers. A potential disadvantage of that model is that remote-site staff may often prefer to tele-consult with a physician instead of an advanced practice provider. Another potential disadvantage is the lack of a standard training pathway for advanced practice providers to obtain critical care expertise and skills.

Role of Administrative Staff (Relationships with Third-Party Provider Networks)

A significant amount of administrative time and workload is necessary to maintain the licensure, credentialing, and organizational compliance of the tele-ICU providers. Depending on the range of the program, sites that are covering multiple healthcare networks over multiple states will frequently need to employ individuals whose main responsibility is to maintain a working knowledge of the applicable laws, bylaws, regulations, and timelines to ensure smooth and continuous availability of providers. As billing options become available for tele-consultation and the delivery of acute inpatient telehealth, insurance contracts, and accountable care organization (ACO) memberships, will also have to be maintained. Maintaining various accounts that allow access to the EMR, picture archiving and communication systems (PACS), and clinical information systems (CIS) can also take a significant amount of time and a good working relationship with the various site information technology (IT) personnel.

Another administrative need is to maintain contracts and working relationships with software and hardware vendors. Technology invariably will fail or need to be upgraded. The smooth operation of the tele-ICU clinically requires a significant amount of advanced planning when it comes to implementing or replacing software and in-room equipment.

Technology Requirements

Smooth operation of ICU telemedicine requires uninterrupted function of VTC and access to the EMR, physiologic monitoring, and other systems that store radiographic images, electrocardiograms, etc. All interfaces should be user-friendly. Access to the patient end (bedside) should be uninterrupted and reliable [20]. Technical support and service lines should be available 24/7.

VTC and Broadband Requirements

VTC peripheral devices such as cameras, microphones, and speakers in both the bedside and tele-ICU hub are required for two-way communication. Ideally, the resolution of the cameras should be high definition to allow accurate visual exam of the patient, and to be able to read the patient identification band and intravenous pump, along with the ability to visualize and interact with the physiologic monitors and mechanical ventilator screens [21]. Cameras must include remote pan-tilt-zoom functionality. VTC devices have usually built-in echo and noise cancellation. Some VTC software may not have built-in echo cancellation and may require headsets or additional echo cancellation hardware. Video input needs to come through an installed digital video card or universal serial bus (USB) ports. Technological equipment for audiovisual communication may vary from proprietary hardware equipment to "bring-your-own device" to meet the needs for each individual program.

For high-quality video, data may be substantial, and when bandwidth is limited, data should be compressed to be transmitted using a codec device or software. Codec hardware are more efficient [22]. H.323 is the most commonly used VTC standard by commercial equipment manufacturers for a codec. The low performance of a codec software or device may be counteracted by high-quality cameras or monitors with high input and output ports. Bandwidth should be adequate to allow high-quality audiovisual communication. The minimum bandwidth required for tele-ICU audiovisual communications is unknown. It should be determined after consultation with clinical, IT, and biomedical staff. The bandwidth requirements depend on the peripheral devices and the codec.

Network security may be challenging because each site firewall may block the other site's network [22]. VTC hardware often have network security. When built-in security is not available, security can be provided by running virtual private network (VPN) software. If the tele-ICU hub location is not located in limited access rooms, timeout should not exceed 15 minutes.

EMR Access and Integration

The majority of ICU telemedicine programs have proprietary telemedicine software with clinical information systems (CIS) that integrate physiological data from real-time physiologic monitors and data from EMRs. The success of a tele-ICU program is frequently dependent on a full integration with the EMR and CIS [23, 24]. The most common ICU telemedicine software is eCARE (Philips). All tele-ICU software should have tools for early recognition of physiologic derangement, early sepsis recognition, handy interface and sign-out that improve efficiency of monitoring and in general tele-ICU operation.

Some tele-ICU programs do not have these types of software and work with the existing EMR within the systems they monitor. In that case, tele-ICU staff needs to have full access to the facility's existing CIS and EMR. Ideally, the telemedicine program should have full access to both. Data should be available from the time of admission to the hospital from any entry point.

Access to Peripheral Devices

Peripheral devices can be fixed – attached permanently to the wall – in the patients' ICU room or they can be part of a portable unit. Portable units are known as carts and may be used as the primary gate of communication or may serve as backup when the fixed peripheral devices fail. Carts operate within a wireless hospital environment and depend on personnel to push them and navigate them in the ICU. Semiautonomous portable units, known as robots, are also available and may have the advantage of being controlled remotely [25, 26]. Fixed peripheral devices can be connected to the hospital network with cable or through a wireless network. All peripheral devices must have their own Internet Protocol (IP) address and be connected to the network. Commercially available devices usually have software for Internet connection. Portable peripheral devices should be wireless and be connected to the network through a local area network (LAN) access point. That access point should be located in the center of the area that the portable device navigates.

Downtime Workflows

Workflow for planned and unplanned downtime should be built prior to telemedicine implementation [11]. Examples of planned downtime are construction in the ICU requiring temporary relocation of the ICU or planned software or hardware upgrades. In cases like those, a portable communication tower can serve as backup. Examples of unplanned downtime are Internet connectivity issues, failure of the tele-ICU software, facility disasters, and natural disasters. Workflow for those situations may vary depending on the care model and nature and duration of the downtime. Both sides of the tele-ICU system (bedside and telemedicine) should have established, published, and accessible downtime policies and procedures. Adequate two-way communication is essential during unplanned downtimes to help mitigate the situation. It may be possible for the tele-ICU to function in some diminished capacity given an effectively planned downtime policy.

Access to Imaging

Access to imaging is critical for the operation of ICU telemedicine programs [27]. Several vendors can offer image sharing through PACS. Preferable, all tele-ICU ends should be able to communicate with a common platform, usually with the use of Digital Imaging and Communications in Medicine (DICOM). Integrated PACS with the EMR can be more efficient but that requires the tele-ICU to have full access to the originating site EMR. Real-time access to image files is necessary in many crisis situations that arise in the ICU.

Remote Physiologic Monitoring Software

Almost every hospital has some type of remote physiologic monitoring, known also as telemetry, which enables the remote observation of cardiac rhythms. The difference between telemetry and remote physiologic monitoring needed for tele-ICU is that the latter receives input from several ICUs in various facilities and requires multiple physiologic parameters (continuous electrocardiogram, pulse oximetry, blood pressure, capnography) to be followed. That again creates challenges with data transmission and security. Because the data volume is smaller in comparison to VTC, it is easier to achieve real-time high-quality physiological data monitoring. Another challenge that may occur is whether the telemedicine software interfaces with various physiologic monitors. That is critical as the telemedicine software uses real-time physiological data from the monitors to alert the tele-ICU staff for physiologic derangement. Large or multiple screens in the tele-ICU hub workstations are preferable so the tele-ICU staff can review real-time physiological data for several patients simultaneously.

Designing the Workplace for Remote ICU Providers

Tele-ICU Hub (Command Center) Architecture

Although the architecture can vary substantially from a telemedicine command center to a physician office equipped with a personal computer, laptop, or smart device with headsets and the appropriate software, we will describe a typical tele-ICU hub that involves a clinical operations room with specialized hardware and software.

Telemedicine hub architecture is similar in both centralized and decentralized programs. The hub may include several tele-ICU workstations depending on the size of the program and the number of beds covered. Each hub should have at least two workstations even if they never operate simultaneously to allow for redundancy in case of hardware or software failure in one of the workstations. For each workstation, adequate space is required for optimal comfort and effective working space for the tele-ICU staff. Workstations should not be located behind or opposed to windows or opposed to other workstations as this would negatively affect VTC fidelity. The minimum distance between two workstations will be determined by the quality of microphones and headsets, along with necessary hardware space and space for the staff. This is important to avoid difficulties in communication between the hub and beside when more than one encounter is taking place simultaneously, as well as for patient privacy issues.

Ideally, a hub with several workstations should be hosted in a large room instead of multiple rooms to allow easy communication between the tele-ICU staff (tele-ICU nurse to tele-intensivist). This is also important for tele-ICU staff satisfaction. A survey in tele-ICU nurses showed that close communication between telemedicine staff is associated with higher satisfaction and creates an educational environment [28]. In decentralized telemedicine ICU programs, all hubs and sub-hubs should have audiovisual communication towers for continuous communication between locations. Printers and fax machines should be available at the hub or adjacent rooms. Figure 6.1 shows a proposed layout for a tele-ICU hub.

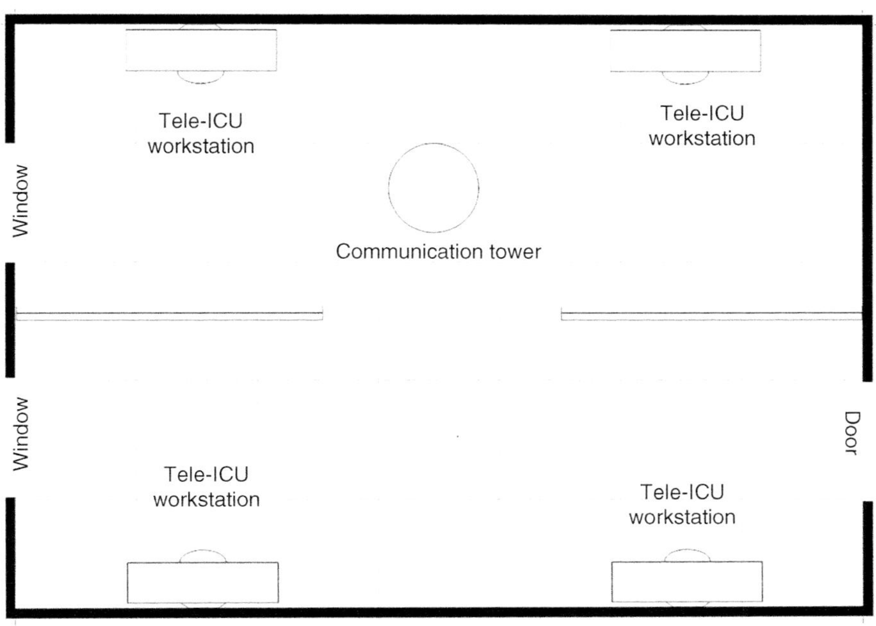

Fig. 6.1 Tele-ICU hub layout

Ergonomic and Employee Satisfaction Considerations

Telemedicine staff needs to be physically present in the hub at all times and for extended shifts. Confinement in a limited space is dissatisfying for the tele-ICU staff [28]. Therefore, large windows allowing for natural light are critical for staff satisfaction. Physical inactivity is also one of the main reasons for dissatisfaction among tele-ICU nurses. Ergonomic tele-ICU workstations can allow staff to shift between standing and sitting position while monitoring or communicating with the bedside ICU. Ergonomic chairs may also help alleviate complaints of back or neck discomfort after long shifts. It may be advantageous to obtain a formal ergonomic evaluation of the work area if there are multiple concerns about the working environment. Individual ergonomic assessments for employees may reveal that specialized padding or equipment is needed to prevent repetitive use injuries. Compact exercise equipment, such as treadmills that can be interfaced with the workstations, may be helpful as well.

Issues Related to Patient Privacy

In order to ensure patient privacy, workstations should not be located close to or opposed to each other. VTC devices that have noise cancellation headsets are preferred to help minimize the extraneous noise that occurs in the workroom. Access in the tele-ICU hub should be secure and limited only to the telemedicine staff. If that is not possible, timeout of the computers and their software should not exceed 15 minutes.

Patients and family should be informed about the operations of the tele-ICU. In most tele-ICU software, there is a feature to deactivate the audiovisual communication between the hub and ICU room when the patient or family declines tele-ICU involvement. This is an important feature in cases where the patient transitions to hospice or has a psychiatric or neurologic disorder, which is aggravated by the unique interaction that tele-ICU provides.

Building a Collaborative Work Environment

To build a collaborative environment among tele-ICU staff, critical care nurses, advanced practice providers, and physicians should be located in the same room either physically or virtually [28]. Staffing physicians and nurses together at a single location is ideal. However, as one of the advantages of tele-ICU is to stretch the valuable resource of intensivists and critical care nurses across a wider area, it may be necessary to use continuous VTC between hubs to allow for ongoing real-time virtual collaboration among the staff as if they are all in the same room. In large telemedicine centers, biographic information about the staff should be available and accessible to help facilitate interpersonal relationships between staff that may work with each other infrequently. Formal communication courses like crew resource management may be helpful as much of the communication may occur in a new and unique fashion over VTC.

Technology Requirements for Remote Providers

In decentralized telemedicine programs, equipment may vary from tablets and laptops to workstations [26]. In a typical centralized tele-ICU, the workstation consists of one to two real-time physiologic monitors, one to two screens for the tele-ICU software, one monitor for access the EMR, and one screen for imaging, electrocardiograms, and other studies. Figure 6.2 shows a workstation in an Iowa City tele-ICU sub-hub in the Veterans Health Administration VISN 23 Regional Tele-ICU Program. The workstation should be equipped with headsets and camera. Workstations should be connected to a power outlet with backup power in case of emergencies.

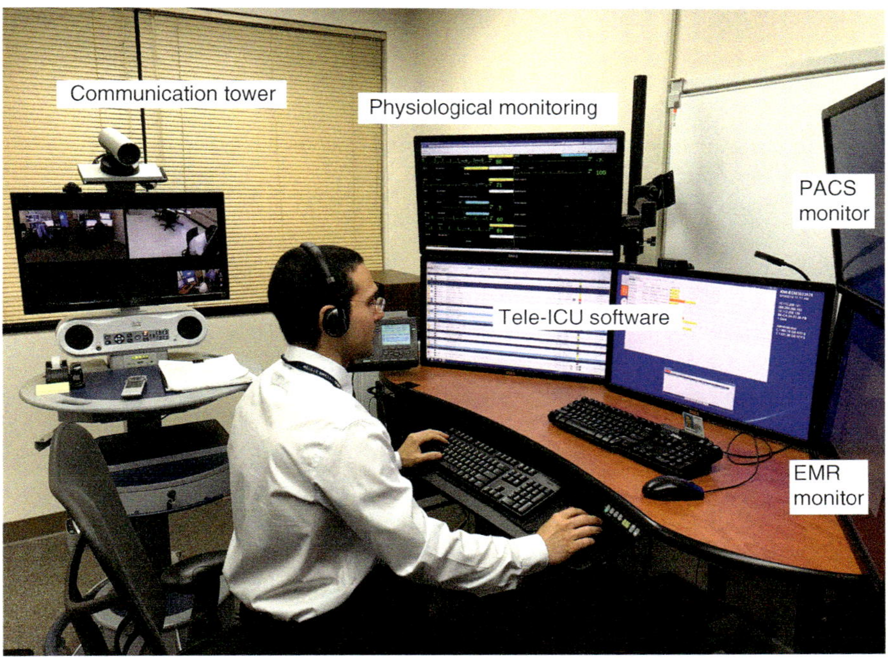

Fig. 6.2 Tele-ICU workstation in Iowa City Veterans Affairs Medical Center

Originating Site ICU Design Considerations for Hospitals Starting New Tele-ICU Practice

The optimal architecture of an ICU has been described previously [29]. In this section, we will focus on the optimal structure of an ICU that receives real-time telemedicine service. The ICU design must involve members from the hospital administration team, physicians, nurses, pharmacists, therapists, ancillary staff, architects, mechanical and electrical engineers, and members of the technology team.

The ICU consists of four major zones: (i) patient care zone, (ii) clinical support zone, (iii) unit support zone, and (iv) family support zone. Optimal design of the patient care and clinical support zones must be able to accommodate tele-ICU equipment, even when telemedicine implementation is not planned.

Patient Care Zone

Single-patient rooms are preferable for various reasons including patient safety and better sleep quality regardless of tele-ICU program presence. In addition, the room must be single-patient to avoid mixing up patients or audiovisual problems during the telemedicine encounter. The room should be large enough to allow a portable telemedicine tower/unit, in particular if it is the primary means of audiovisual communication. Ideally, the room should also be spacious enough to host the multidisciplinary ICU team with family presence. This is often not feasible due to space restrictions. In that case, multidisciplinary rounds can take place in the clinical support zone. The entrance to the room should also be constructed to limit visual communications interruption (e.g., an open door does not allow direct visual contact between the camera and patient). Continuous physiologic monitoring, like vitals and rhythm strip, and audiovisual communications are essential parts of the tele-ICU intervention. All contemporary ICUs have telemetry with a remote station where ICU staff can watch physiologic parameters without being physically in the patient room. That signal can be easily transmitted to another station in the tele-ICU hub, which can be located outside of the ICU.

The patient room should have a fixed or mobile video monitor and camera for VTC between the bedside and tele-ICU hub. The patient should have direct visual contact with the monitor from a supine position. The monitor should be large enough for efficient communication. The camera should be in a location that allows visual access to the patient, physiologic monitors, ventilator, and medication pumps at all times. Careful room design should limit the visual contract interruptions at a minimum.

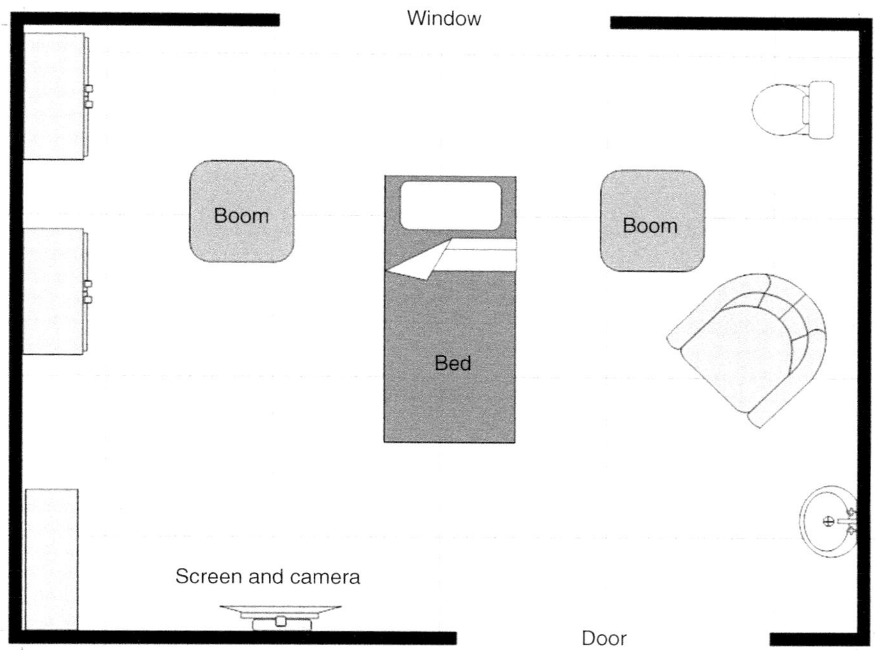

Fig. 6.3 ICU room layout

The microphone and speakers should be located in room areas that allow the patient and bedside staff to easily hear the tele-ICU staff without significant echo. The tele-ICU button for alerting the tele-ICU hub should be visible and easily accessible. Figure 6.3 shows a suggested layout of an ICU room with telemedicine.

Clinical Support Zone

The clinical support zone should be spacious enough to allow multidisciplinary rounds using a portable telemedicine unit if that is the preferable communication mechanism with the tele-ICU hub. A dedicated workroom where multidisciplinary ICU rounds with tele-ICU presence is preferable. The clinical support zone should also have a family room for communications with the tele-ICU (e.g., for end-of-life discussions). If there is no dedicated room for family communications or a workroom that can serve as such, a portable telecommunication device is required. The designated storage area for the portable telemedicine unit (if available) should be easily accessible.

Top Questions Physicians Should Ask Before Starting Tele-ICU Practice

Licensing and Credentials for Tele-Intensivists?

For physicians to practice in a particular state, they need to obtain a medical license for each state [30]. A tele-intensivist that works in a telemedicine programs that provides services in several states needs to apply for medical license in several states. Although there has been progress in the process of applying to several medical state boards through the Interstate Medical Licensure Compact, it is still a lengthy process with high cost. Similarly, credentialing in the various hospitals may require a lot of time. Large telemedicine programs and hospitals may often have dedicated staff for those matters, but rules and policies may vary and tele-intensivists may need to deal with this painful process. An advantage of telemedicine programs in the Department of Veterans Affairs (VA) is that a physician licensed to provide healthcare in the VA is authorized to provide care at any VA location in any state. More details regarding ICU telemedicine licensing and credentialing are provided in Chap. 4 of this book.

Combining Telemedicine with Bedside Practice?

A common problem for physicians that practice telemedicine is how they will combine that with bedside practice. Telemedicine assignments are usually for 8 or 12 hours, while ICU staffing may occur in 1- or 2-week blocks. Intensivists may need to schedule several telemedicine shifts back-to-back when they are not on a bedside ICU rotation. Future tele-intensivists need to plan how to reach the telemedicine command center. Tele-ICU hubs may be located in another state and lodging may need to be arranged together with tele-ICU shifts.

Top Questions Administrators Should Ask Before a Tele-ICU Practice Is Implemented

Do I Need Tele-ICU and Why?

Being tele-intensivists ourselves (the authors of this chapter) and great supporters of tele-ICU, we cannot say anything other than "yes." However, to answer this question, we need to briefly review the benefits of ICU telemedicine. Chapter 9 of this book discusses in details outcomes associated with tele-ICU, but in this section we would like to discuss the benefits of tele-ICU from a different angle. Tele-ICU is associated with a mortality benefit [1, 5, 31, 32], reduced length of stay [12, 32] and inter-hospital transfers [33], and likely reduced costs [34]. The ICU mortality reduction has a large range, but we would dare to say that the absolute mortality reduction in most tele-ICU programs ranges between 1% and 3% [5, 32]. Similarly, the length of stay is reduced approximately by 1 day [32].

Some studies report no benefit from tele-ICU programs [2, 35]. A very interesting counterintuitive observation is that the large urban academic hospitals benefit the most [6]. One would expect that the small rural hospitals with no dedicated on-site intensivist would experience the greatest benefit [36]. Although the explanation for this finding is not known and it can merely reflect the heterogeneity of telemedicine interventions and inherent difficulties in studying these interventions, we can make some assumptions. Large academic medical centers with large ICUs can group with a few other hospitals to create a financially sustainable program, while small hospitals need to create larger inter-hospital associations. The complexity in the operation of telemedicine programs that consist of several ICUs in unrelated hospitals is high, and the efficacy of tele-ICU may be low in this scenario. Why do large academic centers benefit from tele-ICU when they have in-house intensivists? This can be partially explained by an increase in best-care practice adherence like deep vein thrombosis prophylaxis, ventilator bundles, etc. [5]. Another reason is that ICUs preparing for telemedicine implementation may improve practices by adopting ICU protocols and policies, e.g., glucose control order sets and ventilator order sets [3, 5]. Apart from those benefits, early recognition and intervention of physiologic derangement may be another explanation for why large hospitals benefit from tele-ICU coverage. A study at the University of Massachusetts showed allowing tele-ICU staff to directly intervene rather than monitor and notify the bedside team is associated with reduced length of stay [12].

In addition, ICU telemedicine program can provide benefits beyond direct tele-ICU care. Using proprietary software administrators can obtain data regarding ICU outcomes and quality measurements for their ICUs or for the entire healthcare system [3]. This information can help strategic planning to improve care and operation at their facilities.

Taking all the above into consideration, we can assume that tele-ICU may improve outcomes via the following pathways:

- Improving the care provided by bedside ICUs by adopting protocols and policies
- Ensuring adherence to best-care practices
- Monitoring of ICU outcomes and quality measurements
- Intervening faster in patients with physiologic derangements
- Providing critical care expertise when the on-site intensivist is not available

Considering these potential mechanisms for tele-ICU to improve outcomes, administrators should decide whether they need a tele-ICU or not. Therefore, if you are the administrator of a single large hospital with relatively good ICU outcomes and you want to improve the outcomes of your ICUs, you may need to consider other alternatives like assigning a critical care nurse to ensure best-care practices. If you are the administrator of a large health system with several hospitals, a tele-ICU program may improve outcomes in the low-resource hospitals by adopting protocols and policies using telemedicine as a vehicle. Tele-ICU can be particularly helpful in large healthcare systems as it reduces cost not only by improving hospital outcomes but also by reducing the inter-hospital transfers to facilities outside the system.

Should We Build Our Own Tele-ICU?

Obviously this question refers to administrators of large healthcare systems [3]. Single hospital administrators have no other choice but to purchase telemedicine services from an outside vendor. Large healthcare system administrators have the option to purchase or build their own telemedicine program. Administrators should make that decision based on the characteristics of their health system. Building your own telemedicine program may be easier around a large academic hospital that can serve as the command center. Building your own tele-ICU may save money, but it will require effort, time, and skills [3].

What Care Model and Staffing Do We Need?

As we described above, a study at the University of Massachusetts showed that even in large academic centers, a continuous care model with full authority for the telemedicine providers to directly intervene improves outcomes [12]. Given the findings of that study, one can claim that every ICU should be overseen by a telemedicine program. However, that is not possible and it is counterintuitive that even the most-staffed ICUs need tele-ICU support. In many cases, on-site staff can provide the services that tele-ICU provides, e.g., a nurse to ensure adherence to best-care practices or an in-house ICU nurse or a nurse practitioner to monitor physiological data and intervene when there is a derangement.

Having those alternatives in mind, administrators should choose a model and staffing of tele-ICU depending on the particular ICU needs and characteristics. ICUs with an in-house intensivist 24/7 may benefit from a continuous care model telemedicine program staffed by a tele-ICU nurse, nurse practitioner, or physician assistant that encourages adherence to best-care practices. ICUs with available intensivists only during business hours may benefit from a continuous care morel with tele-intensivists during the night. A reactive care model may be sufficient for low-resource ICUs staffed by hospitalists with low acuity patients. The bedside team can request the support of the tele-ICU when challenging and high-complexity patients are admitted.

Is the ICU Telemedicine Program Financially Stable Long-Term?

The financial sustainability of the program depends on whether it returns the cost of its implementation and operation. Does the tele-ICU reduce length of stay and the cost of ICU patients? Does it prevent inter-hospital transfers from low-resource hospitals to hospitals outside of the healthcare system? Administrators should take these questions into consideration and plan ahead to ensure that telemedicine program can be maintained long-term. Chapter 11 of this book describes in detail the financial aspects of sustaining a tele-ICU program.

How Do I Recruit Tele-ICU Staff and What Are Their Characteristics?

Excellent collaboration and mutual respect between the bedside and offside teams is crucial. For that to happen, it will be ideal for all of the tele-ICU staff to also work in-person at the ICUs they service though telemedicine. Often, that is not possible due to long distances between the tele-ICU hub and bedside ICUs and other factors [3]. If that is not possible, full-time experienced ICU nurses can be recruited from the bedside ICU for tele-ICU positions.

Since recruiting tele-ICU staff can be challenging, several telemedicine programs have solved this problem by decentralizing the operation of the tele-ICU. This means creating more than one tele-ICU hub where they can recruit more staff.

Nurses should have extensive ICU experience as they need to recognize patients' acuity and alert the tele-intensivist or the bedside team appropriately [11]. Customer service skills are necessary as they often need to interact with healthcare providers that they have never met. Tele-intensivists should have similar skills [11]. Experienced intensivists are preferred because performing interventions with limited patient information and prior contact can be challenging.

Common Pitfalls in Design and Implementation of a New Tele-ICU Program

Integrating EMR and Telemedicine Software

The telemedicine software cannot integrate data from certain types of EMRs. Obviously, integration from ICUs with no EMR is impossible. A very common hurdle for the smooth operation of telemedicine programs, in particular large programs with several unrelated ICUs, is that they need to access several EMRs

[36]. As discussed above, that may increase the complexity of a telemedicine program and can decrease its efficiency. Administrators of telemedicine programs need to consider this challenge prior to implementation or expansion of a tele-ICU program.

Poor Collaboration Between On-Site and Off-Site Staff

Excellent collaboration between on-site and off-site staff is critical for the efficiency of telemedicine programs [37]. The American Association of Critical-Care Nurses (AACN) identified six standards adopted by the ATA guidelines that are critical for the optimal functioning of a tele-ICU program: skilled communication, true collaboration, effective decision-making, authentic leadership, appropriate staffing, and meaningful recognition [11]. The ATA guidelines also emphasize that skilled communication, true collaboration, and effective decision-making should be present in every tele-ICU program. This collaboration can be compromised by the fact that tele-ICU and bedside staff are not related. That can be prevented by recruiting tele-ICU staff that maintain bedside practice in the ICUs within the telemedicine program [3]. Clarification of the roles and responsibilities prior to implementation after discussion with the bedside ICU will help define expectations for the service [13, 37]. These concepts are discussed in more detail in Chap. 5 of this book.

In telemedicine programs with nurse practitioners or physician assistants, bedside staff may request to receive support only from tele-intensivists. This is something that needs to be taken into consideration prior to implementation. Dissatisfaction of the bedside ICU staff may lead to changes in the composition of the tele-ICU staffing model by increasing the physician-to-advanced practice provider ratio and operational cost. Unplanned increases in the operational cost may lead to a financially unsustainable telemedicine program.

Recruiting Telemedicine Staff

Since low-resource rural ICUs that suffer more often from inadequate intensivist coverage have a higher need for telemedicine, tele-ICU command centers may be located in areas that already have an intensivist shortage. For this reason, telemedicine programs may have difficulty recruiting staff. To overcome this challenge, some tele-ICU programs have decentralized their programs by creating hubs in areas located in large urban centers that can more easily recruit tele-ICU staff and/or leverage time zone differences.

Case Studies of Best Practices for Designing a New Tele-ICU Program

Several studies have shown that tele-ICU programs improve outcomes including mortality and length of stay [5, 6, 12, 33, 34]. However, as we already mentioned, it is difficult to define telemedicine interventions and measure their effects. In this section, we do not provide information about the most efficient ICU telemedicine program, but we present tele-ICU programs with unique characteristics: (i) a telemedicine program without a proprietary telemedicine software and very low cost, (ii) a build-your-own telemedicine program providing service to a different continent, and (iii) the University of Massachusetts ICU telemedicine program.

A Telemedicine Program Without a Proprietary Telemedicine Software and Very Low Cost

Fairview health system in Minnesota created its own ICU telemedicine program with a command center at the University of Minnesota Medical Center that provides support to 54 ICU beds in 5 hospitals [3]. The creators used the 24/7 intensivist in the University of Minnesota Medical Center to provide support to the off-site ICUs during the periods in which there was no intensivist available at the other hospitals. No tele-ICU proprietary software or outside vendor was used, but all hospitals shared the same EMR. "Off-the-shelf" technology was used. These factors brought the implementation and first-year operational cost of the program down to $45,000 per ICU bed [3] from $70,000 to 80,000 which is the average cost [38]. The annual operational cost was only $23,000 per ICU bed. A tele-ICU nurse was always present in the command center and performed quality improvement projects during the off-peak hours. Although the effect of the program on ICU outcomes has not been published, unadjusted mortality was lower the year after telemedicine implementation compared to mortality rates prior to telemedicine implementation. The telemedicine program also helped to unify practice among all the ICUs within the health system.

Build-Your-Own Telemedicine Program

A real pioneer telemedicine program is the one created by the Syrian American Medical Society to provide support to Syrian hospitals during the ongoing Syrian conflict [39]. The program was launched in 2012 with almost no cost. Initially, the creators who are physicians practicing in USA and Canada used everyday technology like laptops, free social media, and communication applications such as Skype and Viber to provide support to one Syrian hospital. Tele-intensivists were mainly pulmonary and critical care physicians that participated in the program without compensation. Later on, they purchased a commercial web-based EMR for $200 and expanded the program to more hospitals. In 2015, the Syrian American Medical Society received an $850,000 grant to expand ICU capacity in Syria including expansion of the tele-ICU program.

University of Massachusetts ICU Telemedicine Program

Of course, the University of Massachusetts ICU telemedicine program cannot be absent among the case studies for designing a tele-ICU program [5, 12]. It is probably the most studied and cited program in the USA. This model has been demonstrated to improve outcomes including mortality and ICU length of stay. The efficacy of the program is based not only on best-care practice adherence but also on timely tele-ICU interventions for physiologic derangements [12]. This program contains many important elements of tele-ICU operations and roles that are now considered the standard of care for every telemedicine program.

References

1. Lilly CM, McLaughlin JM, Zhao H, Baker SP, Cody S, Irwin RS. A multicenter study of ICU telemedicine reengineering of adult critical care. Chest. 2014;145:500–7.
2. Nassar BS, Vaughan-Sarrazin MS, Jiang L, Reisinger HS, Bonello R, Cram P. Impact of an intensive care unit telemedicine program on patient outcomes in an integrated health care system. JAMA Intern Med. 2014;174:1160–7.
3. Fortis S, Weinert C, Bushinski R, Koehler AG, Beilman G. A health system-based critical care program with a novel tele-ICU: implementation, cost, and structure details. J Am Coll Surg. 2014;219:676–83.
4. Sadaka F, Palagiri A, Trottier S, Deibert W, Gudmestad D, Sommer SE, Veremakis C. Telemedicine intervention improves ICU outcomes. Crit Care Res Pract. 2013;2013:456389.
5. Lilly CM, Cody S, Zhao H, Landry K, Baker SP, McIlwaine J, Chandler MW, Irwin RS, University of Massachusetts Memorial Critical Care Operations Group. Hospital mortality, length of stay, and preventable complications among critically ill patients before and after tele-ICU reengineering of critical care processes. JAMA. 2011;305:2175–83.
6. Kahn JM, Le TQ, Barnato AE, Hravnak M, Kuza CC, Pike F, Angus DC. ICU telemedicine and critical care mortality: a national effectiveness study. Med Care. 2016;54:319–25.
7. Barry ME, Hochman BR, Lane-Fall MB, Zappile D, Holena DN, Smith BP, Kaplan LJ, Huffenberger A, Reilly PM, Pascual JL. Leveraging telemedicine infrastructure to monitor quality of operating room to intensive care unit handoffs. Acad Med. 2017;92:1035–42.
8. Collins TA, Robertson MP, Sicoutris CP, Pisa MA, Holena DN, Reilly PM, Kohl BA. Telemedicine coverage for post-operative ICU patients. J Telemed Telecare. 2017;23:360–4.

9. Michael RM. Benefits of tele-ICU management of ICU boarders in the emergency department. HIMSS17 Annual Conference Education Sessions. 2017. https://www.himssconference.org/sites/himssconference/files/pdf/309_0.pdf
10. Mullen-Fortino M, Sites FD, Soisson M, Galen J. Innovative use of tele-ICU in long-term acute care hospitals. AACN Adv Crit Care. 2012;23:330–6.
11. American Telemedicine Association. Guidelines for tele-ICU operations. 2014. http://www.learnicu.org/SiteCollectionDocuments/Guidelines-ATATeleICU.pdf
12. Hawkins HA, Lilly CM, Kaster DA, Groves RH Jr, Khurana H. ICU telemedicine comanagement methods and length of stay. Chest. 2016;150:314–9.
13. Moeckli J, Cram P, Cunningham C, Reisinger HS. Staff acceptance of a telemedicine intensive care unit program: a qualitative study. J Crit Care. 2013;28:890–901.
14. Breslow MJ. Remote ICU care programs: current status. J Crit Care. 2007;22:66–76.
15. Huffenberger AM, Martin ND, Wiliiam Hanson C III. Telemedicine for the intensive care unit. In: Kaplan LJ, Martin ND, editors. Principles of adult surgical critical care. Cham: Springer; 2016.
16. Rincon TA, Manos EL, Pierce JD. Telehealth intensive care unit nurse surveillance of sepsis. Comput Inform Nurs. 2017;35:459–64.
17. Ruesch C, Mossakowski J, Forrest J, Hayes M, Jahrsdoerfer M, Comeau E, Singleton M. Using nursing expertise and telemedicine to increase nursing collaboration and improve patient outcomes. Telemed J E Health. 2012;18:591–5.
18. Olff C, Clark-Wadkins C. Tele-ICU partners enhance evidence-based practice: ventilator weaning initiative. AACN Adv Crit Care. 2012;23:312–22.
19. Garland A, Gershengorn HB. Staffing in ICUs: physicians and alternative staffing models. Chest. 2013;143:214–21.
20. Larinkari S, Liisanantti JH, Ala-Laakkola T, Merilainen M, Kyngas H, Ala-Kokko T. Identification of tele-ICU system requirements using a content validity assessment. Int J Med Inform. 2016;86:30–6.
21. Cruz M, Cruz RF, Krupinski EA, Lopez AM, McNeeley RM, Weinstein RS. Effect of camera resolution and bandwidth on facial affect recognition. Telemed J E Health. 2004;10:392–402.
22. Liu WL, Zhang K, Locatis C, Ackerman M. Internet-based videoconferencing coder/decoders and tools for telemedicine. Telemed J E Health. 2011;17:358–62.
23. Lilly CM, Fisher KA, Ries M, Pastores SM, Vender J, Pitts JA, Hanson CW 3rd. A national ICU telemedicine survey: validation and results. Chest. 2012;142:40–7.
24. Friedman LN, Halpern NA, Fackler JC. Implementing an electronic medical record. Crit Care Clin. 2007;23:347–81.
25. Adcock AK, Kosiorek H, Parich P, Chauncey A, Wu Q, Demaerschalk BM. Reliability of robotic telemedicine for assessing critically ill patients with the full outline of UnResponsiveness score and Glasgow coma scale. Telemed J E Health. 2017;23:555–60.
26. Reynolds HN, Rogove H, Bander J, McCambridge M, Cowboy E, Niemeier M. A working lexicon for the tele-intensive care unit: we need to define tele-intensive care unit to grow and understand it. Telemed J E Health. 2011;17:773–83.
27. Yoo SK, Kim DK, Kim JC, Park YJ, Chang BC. Implementation of a large-scale hospital information infrastructure for multi-unit health-care services. J Telemed Telecare. 2008;14:164–6.
28. Hoonakker PL, Carayon P, McGuire K, Khunlertkit A, Wiegmann DA, Alyousef B, Xie A, Wood KE. Motivation and job satisfaction of tele-ICU nurses. J Crit Care. 2013;28:315.e313–21.
29. Thompson DR, Hamilton DK, Cadenhead CD, Swoboda SM, Schwindel SM, Anderson DC, Schmitz EV, St Andre AC, Axon DC, Harrell JW, et al. Guidelines for intensive care unit design. Crit Care Med. 2012;40:1586–600.
30. Rogove H, Stetina K. Practice challenges of intensive care unit telemedicine. Crit Care Clin. 2015;31:319–34.
31. Lilly CM, Cody S, Zhao H, Landry K, Baker SP, McIlwaine J, Chandler MW, Irwin RS. Hospital mortality, length of stay, and preventable complications among critically ill patients before and after tele-ICU reengineering of critical care processes. JAMA. 2011;305:2175–83.

32. Wilcox ME, Adhikari NK. The effect of telemedicine in critically ill patients: systematic review and meta-analysis. Crit Care. 2012;16:R127.
33. Fortis S, Sarrazin MV, Beck BF, Panos RJ, Reisinger HS. ICU telemedicine reduces interhospital ICU transfers in the Veterans Health Administration. Chest. 2018;154:69.
34. Lilly CM, Motzkus C, Rincon T, Cody SE, Landry K, Irwin RS. ICU telemedicine program financial outcomes. Chest. 2017;151:286–97.
35. Thomas EJ, Lucke JF, Wueste L, Weavind L, Patel B. Association of telemedicine for remote monitoring of intensive care patients with mortality, complications, and length of stay. JAMA. 2009;302:2671–8.
36. Fortis S, Nassar BS, Resinger HS. Does size matter in ICU telemedicine? Chest. 2017;151:946.
37. Wilkes MS, Marcin JP, Ritter LA, Pruitt S. Organizational and teamwork factors of tele-intensive care units. Am J Crit Care. 2016;25:431–9.
38. Kumar G, Falk DM, Bonello RS, Kahn JM, Perencevich E, Cram P. The costs of critical care telemedicine programs: a systematic review and analysis. Chest. 2013;143:19–29.
39. Moughrabieh A, Weinert C. Rapid deployment of international tele-intensive care unit services in war-torn Syria. Ann Am Thorac Soc. 2016;13:165–72.

Chapter 7
Integrating Telemedicine Technologies in the ICU

Christian D. Becker, Mario Fusaro, and Corey S. Scurlock

Introduction

After deciding to implement tele-ICU services, one must begin planning the integration of telemedicine technologies in the ICU. This is a multifactorial process requiring significant preparation and a multidisciplinary approach. A common mistake is to leave this in the hands of information technology (IT) and administrative personnel alone. Clinical leaders of both the tele-ICU and bedside ICUs must be involved and become key stakeholders in all forms of the tele-ICU's operations, integration, and design to achieve overall success. In addition, executive sponsorship is vital, and agreement on its goal and "value" must be reached prior to onset of services. After go-live of the tele-ICU, the clinical leaders then must carefully examine and potentially redact protocols (workflows) based on output metrics to constantly look for areas of improvement and new opportunities for the tele-ICU to add benefit. At the end of this chapter, we present a case study in which design of a tele-ICU combined with proven business principles led to clinical and operational success.

C. D. Becker · M. Fusaro
Westchester Medical Center Health Network, Valhalla, NY, USA

New York Medical College, Department of Medicine, Division of Pulmonary, Critical Care and Sleep Medicine, Valhalla, NY, USA
e-mail: Christian.Becker@wmchealth.org; Mario.Fusaro@wmchealth.org

C. S. Scurlock (✉)
Westchester Medical Center Health Network, Valhalla, NY, USA

New York Medical College, Department of Anesthesiology, Department of Medicine, Valhalla, NY, USA
e-mail: Corey.Scurlock@wmchealth.org

M. A. Koenig (ed.), *Telemedicine in the ICU*,
https://doi.org/10.1007/978-3-030-11569-2_7

Models of Tele-ICU

Two prevailing models for tele-ICU delivery are the "Continuous Monitoring Model" (CMM) and the "Virtual Consultant Model" (VCM) [1]. CMM is considered an active monitoring modality whereby a coordinated team of nurses, doctors, and clerical staff are fed a continuous stream of fully integrated vital signs, labs, alarms, medications, as well as audiovisual communication with the bedside teams to augment patient care. This form is important for active monitoring, outcomes data collection, process improvement, and intellectual support. The episodic VCM is considered a reactive modality, whereby a remote presence is achieved via an audiovisual device aimed at tele-consultation without proactive monitoring of patient data. In this model, it is typically a clinician acting alone through technology without the added benefit of support staff. Without the intensive monitoring of the CMM, VCM is mostly useful for providing on demand cognitive support. However, it also can be instrumental in helping to facilitate discharge planning [2, 3]. The biggest difference between the two models is that CMM has a significantly higher implementation and ongoing capital cost. Often one sees VCM used in low-volume centers, such as critical access hospitals, while the CMM model is used in integrated delivery networks (IDNs).

The main CMM tele-ICU vendors are Philips®, Cerner®, and iMDSoft®. The prominent VCM vendors are InTouch Health®, Avizia®, Yorktel®, and Phillips® among many others. Telemedicine services via phone or tablet have also become much more prevalent with several companies offering mobile on demand virtual office visit platforms. Some organizations have implemented tele-ICU services using an amalgam of vendors [4]. Deciding between each platform is dependent on the organization's clinical needs, goals of the program, financial situation, and size of the institution.

Architectural Design of the Tele-ICU

Designing the physical layout of a tele-ICU should be a multidisciplinary process bringing together not only members of the architectural and technology teams but also clinical staff. Conforming the tele-ICU design to the communication pathways of the multidisciplinary tele-ICU team members is essential and should include clinician input from the beginning. Minimizing barriers to communication and flow of information upfront will pay off significantly after the program has been initiated. One may also wish to have visual dashboards with team goals, clinical data, etc. that will be clearly visible for the tele-ICU practitioners to review on a daily basis. Finally, details regarding ergonomics and prevention of repetitive use injuries along with eye and neck strain are also important.

Technical Integration

Tele-ICU has a myriad of functions including audiovisual communication, vital sign/note/lab/alert reporting, order entry, and clinical prediction tools, which are necessary for maximizing its effect. The most efficient way to achieve integration of tele-ICU technology depends on the existing hospital systems. Each native EMR has variable degrees to which it can fully integrate with a tele-ICU system. In some cases, full integration may not be necessary. In all cases, the uses of Health Level (HL) 7 standards are employed to allow the technical systems to communicate with each other. Before deciding on a platform, an important component of the planning process involves deciding which function(s) of the tele-ICU are most beneficial to the organization [5].

Interfaces

A near complete integration of the existing EMR is recommended to achieve maximum tele-ICU utility. As mentioned above, the building of HL7 interfaces include the following types:

- Lab interfaces
- Vital sign interfaces
- Medication interfaces
- Notes outbound interfaces
- Order entry interfaces

These interfaces typically serve to connect the telemedicine software with the EMR. Their accuracy and dependability is a key component to driving value and scaling efficiency for the telemedicine team. Vital sign alerts, medication dosing guidelines, and lab alerts are wholly dependent on access to these inputs. Crossover of vital signs from the hospital EMR to the tele-ICU platform is critical for CMMs, as the continuous flow of vital sign data is used to compile risk adjustment models, generate pathophysiologic alerts, and feed quality improvement databases. Complete integration is the ideal; however, it may not be feasible, and an alternative platform can be used concurrently. Because most tele-ICU platforms have a documentation manager and order entry, the organization must weigh the pros and cons of using this feature versus continuing use of the existing platform. Although double documentation should be minimized, certain aspects of the patient notes may benefit from redundancy across systems to facilitate sign out workflows.

Imaging

Integration of imaging clients usually consists of linking clinical decision support hotkeys to the native radiology software. As it takes a provider to interpret radiology images, tele-ICU software rarely uses the actual images in their algorithms, making full integration unnecessary.

Accessory Devices

All equipment, personal devices, peripheral devices, etc. should adhere to the IT policies of the organization as well as being HIPAA compliant. The clinicians providing the service must ensure that, if using personal devices, they have the latest security patches deemed necessary by the organization [6]. If using mobile devices, they *must* be enabled with a password or some other digital security feature and have a timeout of less than 15 minutes. They should also feature nationally recognized point-to-point encryption, be supported by ongoing maintenance plans and be in compliance with current infection control standards. Often, peripheral devices are used in patient care to supplement some of the data input regarding tele-ICU. If these devices are to be used, there will need to be integration achieved with a robust amount of IT support. Often these devices are not easily integrated with tele-ICU software, and the value achieved through potential perceived synergies is not present.

Downtime Procedures

As with nearly all technology, scheduled and unscheduled downtime procedures should be developed for the tele-ICU. The goal in drafting these procedures should be to ensure continual services in the event of a technology failure, planned system maintenance, or natural disasters. Commonly used downtime procedures involving the following:

- Redundant centers with geographical variation to avoid the effect of weather
- Reverting to the use of telephone in cases of system failure
- Activating bedside personnel in the case of technology failure

These workflows should be drafted in collaboration with the emergency planning departments of the organization as they will have similar goals.

Other IT Considerations

For optimal audiovisual clarity and to maintain patient safety, optimal bandwidths must be present within the hospital or care facility to support the telemedicine software. This requires the input of not only the clinical team but also biomedical and IT teams. Once the minimal bandwidth that will support optimal audiovisual performance has been determined, then each endpoint should be analyzed to ascertain that it conforms to these specifications. As care digitalization and convergence continues, healthcare IT executives, when designing their telemedicine programs, should not only be thinking of what their bandwidth requirements are today but what they will be 3 years from now. This is critical for program growth, scalability, and longevity.

Once the system is operational, customizations with the technology can be implemented to maximize tele-ICU benefits. Remote party multidisciplinary rounds have previously been conducted to improve ventilator usage including decreased ventilator duration, ventilator best practice adherence, and decreased ICU mortality [7]. Tele-ICU consultations have also been used internationally with a multidisciplinary initial evaluation of conjoined twins leading to transfer and successful separation procedures [8]. Tele-ICU service rounds have also been implemented in war-torn Syria employing American and European physicians to aid in ICU care [9].

Clinical Integration

After issues regarding technical integration of the tele-ICU are considered, then all eyes must be turned toward clinical integration. Often, this is more difficult than the technical integration and requires diplomacy and forward-thinking. Given the considerable extensive upfront investment required for a tele-ICU, care must be taken to ensure critical design elements are instituted so that it can maximize its value potential.

Implementation Pitfalls

In implementing a tele-ICU, several factors have been associated with success [10]. These include the following:

- Having the bedside ICU team be part of design and implementation
- Building support among staff prior to rollout

- Tele-clinicians visiting the ICU regularly
- Having agreement on best practices
- Having periodic meetings between the bedside tele-ICU staff
- Frequent and multidisciplinary review of performance data
- The presence of multidisciplinary rounds at the bedside

Additional authors have demonstrated the need for high-intensity staffing with the ability to intervene on patient care as potentially important factors for tele-ICU success [11, 12]. Others have found a lack of strong medical leadership in the tele-ICU to be associated with program failure [13]. When contemplating clinical integration of a tele-ICU, workflows need to be designed to minimize actual or perceived disruption to clinical services as well as to focus on areas in which the tele-ICU can best add value through care standardization, best practice implementation, second opinion services, and afterhours manpower support. We suggest a stepwise approach to this integration with building upon initial successes.

Workflow Redesign

Once the tele-ICU is operational, workflows must be continually examined to ascertain maximal value. Since tele-ICUs generate rich operational data, they lend themselves well to process improvement programs (Lean, Six Sigma, etc.) and a standardized approach. In a large multicenter study, Lilly demonstrated that tele-intensivist review of the patient chart within 1 hour of arrival to the ICU was associated with both decreased LOS and risk-adjusted mortality [13]. In our tele-ICU, after that study's publication, we specifically redesigned workflows to meet this 1-hour metric as reducing LOS and mortality are two core goals of our service. Periodic collaborative workflow re-evaluations incorporating eICU and bedside ICU personnel feedback may lead to incremental improvements or modifications to existing workflows.

Acceptance of Tele-ICU

Initially, some hesitation is reported among bedside staff; however, as trust forms, nursing satisfaction increases [14]. In a meta-analysis of tele-ICU coverage, overall staff acceptance was high with most tele-ICUs generating 4.2–4.5 on a standardized Likert scale [10]. Additionally when surveyed, residents said they wanted some form of tele-ICU in their post-training experience [2]. Data on family members acceptance suggests that a significant majority find the tele-ICU to be a positive feature of the overall care [2, 10]. The most common questions they generate regarding tele-ICU relate to how patient privacy is maintained, how care is augmented, and how the technology works [15]. The majority of family contact was noted to occur during the admission intake process. A study examining a remote telepresence robot reports that patient family members were pleased with increased access to a physician during "off" hours as well as timely discharge processes [2, 3].

Guidelines for Tele-ICU Implementation

The American Telemedicine Association (ATA) provides guidance for tele-ICU implementation in accordance with published best practices [6]. Several recommendations have been provided relative to formulation of a mission, best practices, and performance improvement. Recommendations guiding the initial planning phase of a tele-ICU begin with the creation of a shared vision. The parties most closely involved are nursing, physicians from both tele-ICU and bedside ICU, hospital administrators, vendor employees, and tele-ICU support staff. Tele-ICU is a collaborative process that can be tailored to meet institutional needs [5]. A multidisciplinary plan for tele-ICU structure and function must be devised and then that vision communicated to all relevant parties. Additionally, it is recommended that tele-ICU leadership be positioned to participate in key decisionmaking forums and have the authority necessary to affect change if needed.

The ATA also has recommendations for ongoing operations on fiscal responsibility, structured workflow procedures, and quality/outcomes assessment. These include establishment of an operational budget to include both upfront and recurring costs related to personnel, hardware/software licensing, supplies, and real estate. The budget should also reflect projected changes in costs. Additionally, revenue projections should be established based on contributions from payer reimbursement, grants, and the parent healthcare system. Other sources of revenue may be achieved through expansion of tele-ICU services outside of the hospital system.

Workflow protocols should be established with the goal of providing evidence-based, high-quality, consistent care. These include workflows that define step-by-step guidance which addresses normal and unexpected workday patterns. These may include active monitoring to pick up overlooked issues with patient's physiology, medications, or imminent patient danger. Additional workflows might address steps taken when system alerts detect patient concerns or routine technical issues.

While workflows help to ensure standardization of care, outcomes reporting and feedback are critical for assessing the effect of various quality improvement strategies. This helps to ensure the combined mission of providing high-quality patient-centered care while also controlling costs. ATA recommends establishment of metrics which are important for institutional benefit based on evidence-based practice. Those metrics should then be followed and reported to relevant parties such that a feedback mechanism can be implemented leading to enhanced practices and protocols, which lead to improved outcomes. These recommendations are in line with our experience and relevant literature.

Executive Sponsorship

As expressed in the ATA guidelines for Tele-ICU, the executive team and the clinical leadership should develop a shared vision of the tele-ICU and its role in enhancing care delivery [6]. Much of the executive's role involves:

- Communicating that vision throughout the healthcare system
- Placing the clinical leaders of the tele-ICU in key areas to affect change

Given the capital costs of creation and maintenance of the tele-ICU, a key component of the executive team's decisionmaking will be based on return on investment (ROI) and the sustainability of the program [16]. At this point, Medicare reimbursement in the ICU for telehealth services is limited to rural geographic areas [17], and private payer reimbursement varies based on state laws and payer policies. Therefore, other metrics of financial value must be defined in the creation of the program. These can include but are not limited to the following:

- Improved quality metrics that are a portion of value-based purchasing
- Reduced ICU nursing absenteeism
- Reduced ICU physician and nursing turnover
- Reduced transportation costs for system-wide ICU patients
- Costs savings associated with care standardization
- Costs savings associated with reduced length of stay (LOS)
- Costs savings associated with reduced litigation [13]
- Strategic positioning within the marketplace

A recent 10-year longitudinal study of 51,203 patients at an 834 bed academic medical center revealed that a tele-ICU combined with a capacity command center increased contribution margin by $52.7 million across their 7 adult ICUs [18]. Much of this benefit came from the adding of 1829 incremental cases. These incremental cases were able to flow through this existing ICU footprint of the hospital because of the impact that the capacity command center had on reducing LOS. If not for the program, the system would have had to build an additional 25 ICU beds at a projected cost of $30–60 million in capital expense.

While the benefits of a tele-ICU program can be myriad, it is important in program development to define the three to four most important benefits and to use those to shape a vision with the executive leadership team prior to starting the program. Using those benefits as a starting point to define goals and objectives for the program is key. Measuring and reporting on these metrics becomes a key role for the tele-ICU leadership team and is paramount to the overall program success.

Case Study in Tele-ICU Success

To illustrate and put into perspective the various concepts and building blocks for successful tele-ICU integration we have discussed above, we will highlight some of our successful tele-ICU clinical care standardization initiatives as well as a process

Fig. 7.1 Kotter's eight steps for "Leading Change"

1. Establish a sense of urgency
2. Form a powerful guiding coalition
3. Create a vision
4. Communicate the vision
5. Empower others to act on the vision
6. Plan for and create short term wins
7. Consolidate improvements and produce more change
8. Institutionalize new approaches

improvement initiative that actually targets the performance of the tele-ICU staff itself. At least initially, the tele-ICU is a potentially disruptive technology to existing organizational structures. For any tele-ICU-supported quality and process improvement initiative, we therefore closely follow Kotter's principles [19] for "leading change" (see Fig. 7.1).

A basic consensus exists in critical care on the need for consistent delivery of clinical best practices, which consist of five core practices with well-established clinical evidence:

(a) Lung protective mechanical ventilation
(b) Transfusion practices
(c) Venous thromboembolism prophylaxis
(d) Stress ulcer prophylaxis
(e) Glycemic control

Prior to implementation of tele-ICU services at our healthcare system (Westchester Medical Center Health Network, Valhalla, NY), we surveyed the existing approaches to delivery of best practices across a variety of subspecialty ICUs (trauma, surgical, medical, cardiac, cardiothoracic surgical, neuroscience, burn, and mixed medical/surgical). We found wide practice variations between the different subspecialty ICUs. We therefore established a sense of urgency to standardize the approach to best practices (Step 1). Next, we gathered the multidisciplinary clinical leadership of all ICUs (Step 2) to reach a consensus on criteria and goals for best practices (Step 3) and disseminated that consensus statement among all team members (Steps 4 and 5). After going live with tele-ICU services, we gathered performance data and instituted quarterly performance reviews with each individual ICU as well as the system as a whole. The performance reviews included key stakeholders of the multidisciplinary care teams as well as administrative leadership (Steps 4 through 7). As a result, we established collaborative workflows that informed the bedside teams about missing best practice items. In addition, the tele-ICU physician assumed responsibility to ensure compliance with best practices through an active collaborative approach with the individual bedside teams. Failure to provide established best practice therapies led to root cause analyses to determine where the workflow had broken down.

Quarterly performance reviews enabled the individual ICU stakeholders to compare the performance of "their" ICU over time and against all other anonymized ICUs in the system, creating a sense of urgency and competition, thereby fostering change and process improvement. Top performers were recognized, and the key elements of their collaborative tele-ICU to bedside ICU success were shared to benefit the underperformers (Steps 4 through 7). The collaboration between the tele-ICU and the different subspecialty bedside ICUs was individualized according to the relative ICU-specific care delivery features in order to maximize the value of the tele-ICU to bedside ICU collaboration (Steps 5 and 6). To enable the effective review of a plethora of relevant performance data and to show data trends over time effectively, we created visually intuitive, motion charts which allow comparisons between ICUs in different combinations of metrics over time (Step 8). For example, we created a motion chart depicting the compliance with venous thromboembolism prophylaxis (x axis) against compliance with stress ulcer prophylaxis (y axis) (see Fig. 7.2). Utilizing this innovative performance review system, we were able to incrementally increase the compliance rates with venous thromboembolism and stress ulcer prophylaxis to a consistent 100% (Steps 7 and 8).

On the tele-ICU operational side, as mentioned above, there is convincing evidence that tele-ICU conducted patient reviews including comprehensive audiovisual assessments within the first hour of new patients arriving in the ICU are associated with reduced mortality and LOS [13]. Similar to our best practice approach, we created visual tools to evaluate the timeliness of our tele-ICU nursing and physician staff in evaluating new ICU patients. Operational data of the tele-ICU system was processed to display the average duration from admission to first video evaluation (X axis) as well as the average duration of that first video interaction (Y axis) (see Fig. 7.3). Iterative performance reviews with the tele-ICU team as a whole as well as individual team members were again used to incrementally improve performance. Based on the initial video assessment times (Panel A for tele-ICU nurses, Panel D for tele-ICU physicians), we restructured the initial patient admission workflow to enable the tele-ICU to evaluate new ICU patients faster. Iterative performance reviews and further workflow optimizations led to a dramatic improvement in video assessment times for tele-ICU nurses and physicians to well within the window mandated by the evidence (Panels C and F).

Overall, it is important to stress that the essential underlying requirement for most of Kotter's steps to "leading change" is the timely use of performance data, as was found by Lilly [13]. The performance data has to be carefully vetted, its integrity ascertained and its presentation optimized for maximum effect.

Data integrity will allow the performance reviews and quality improvement discussions to focus on how to improve the performance and increase the quality of clinical care rather than on the data underlying the discussions themselves.

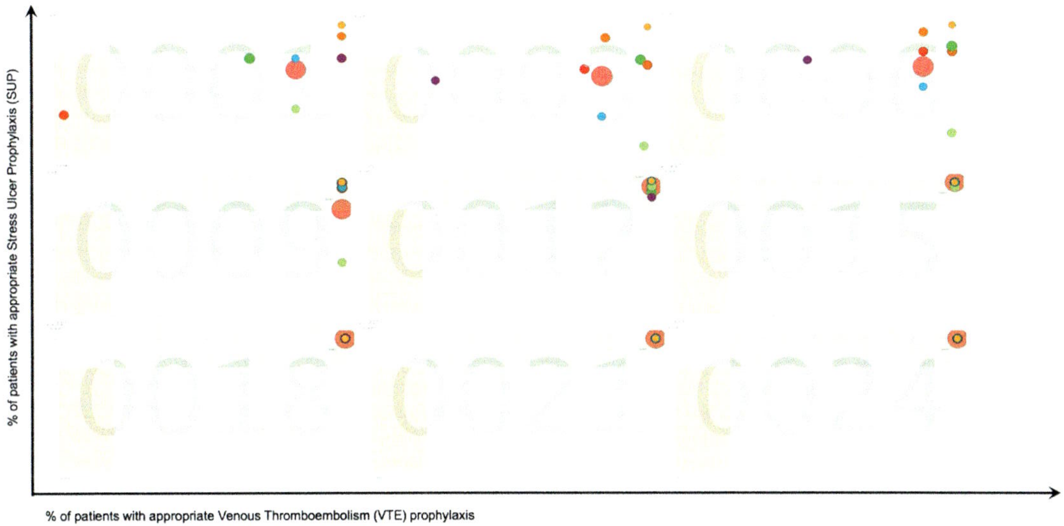

Fig. 7.2 Depicted are nine snapshots of the Best Practice Motion chart showing compliance with venous thromboembolism prophylaxis (x-axis) against compliance with stress ulcer prophylaxis (y-axis) (months 1, 3, and 6 on tele-ICU support (upper row), months 9, 12, and 15 of tele-ICU support (middle row), and months 18, 21, and 24 of tele-ICU support (lower row). The month is indicated by the large number displayed in the chart background. Each ICU is represented as an individually colored dot. The size of the dot corresponds to the number of patients admitted in the quarter. The x-axis depicts the % of patients with appropriate venous thromboembolism (VTE) prophylaxis. The y-axis depicts the % of patients with appropriate stress ulcer prophylaxis (SUP). ICUs which achieve >95% adherence to these best practices will be located in the green quadrant. ICUs which fall short in one of the two best practices will be located in the white areas of the plot, whereas ICUs which fall short in both SUP and VTE prophylaxis will be located in the red quadrants. The motion chart enables the user to intuitively visualize the performance over time of each individual ICU and the healthcare system ICUs as a whole (largest dot). It also enables the user to compare performances across different ICUs in an anonymized fashion. The month 1 and 3 graphs (upper left and upper middle) show the baseline distribution of system ICUs before any tele-ICU workflow interventions were instituted. Months 6 through 24 show the effect of the eICU-to-ICU collaborative intervention. Performance reviews were held with the stakeholders of each individual ICU at the beginning of each quarter (months 4, 7, and 10 for the first year and months 13, 16, 19, and 22 for the second year). Starting with month 6, the system ICUs start converging toward the green quadrant. Note that between months 18 and 24, no further improvement is possible, as all ICUs are superimposed at the 100%/100% mark. Performance reviews and additional vigilance in the eICU-to-ICU collaboration are ongoing to ensure that the effect is sustained. Note that the dynamic movement of motion charts cannot be adequately visualized in print format. The snapshot format is used to substitute for the dynamic motion

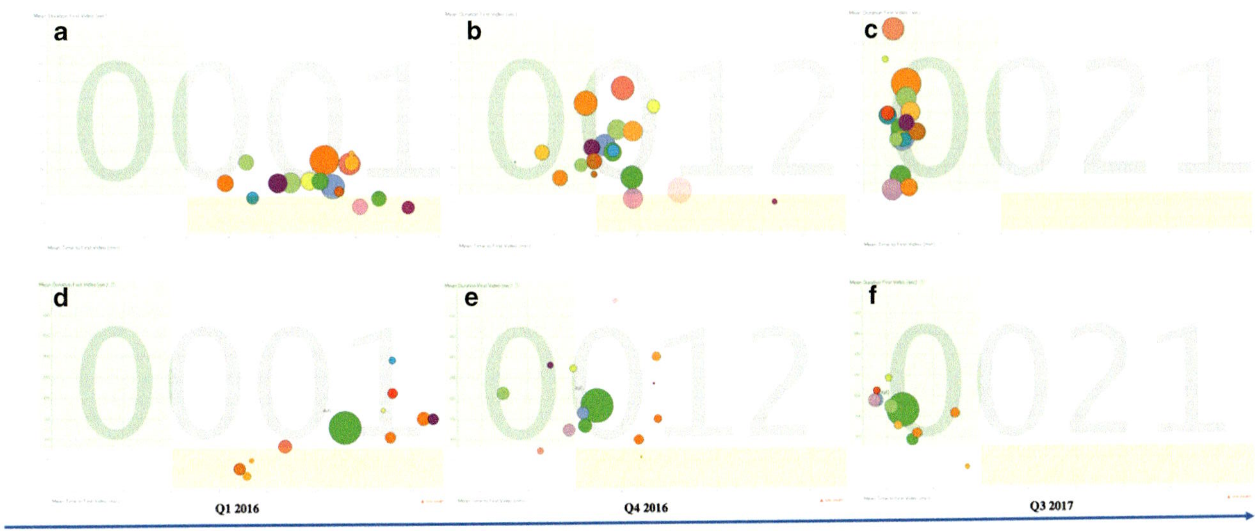

Fig. 7.3 Mean first video duration (FVD) (*y*-axis) plotted against mean time to first video (TTV) (x-axis) is shown for Q1 of 2016 (panels **a**, **d**, first month of study period indicated by 0001 in chart background), Q4 of 2016 (panels **b**, **e**, 12th month of study period indicated by 0012 in chart background), and Q3 of 2017 (panels **c**, **f**, 21st month of study period indicated by 0021 in chart background), for eICU nurses (**a**–**c**) and eICU physicians (**d**–**f**). The performance goal is indicated by the green quadrant representing timely (<60 minutes from admission to ICU) and comprehensive (>90 seconds) video review. Each eICU provider is represented by a dot (nurse upper row (**a**–**c**), physician lower row (**d**–**f**)). The size of the dot corresponds to the number of video interactions per quarter. Panels (**a**–**c**): *eICU nurse* distribution of Q1 of 2016 (**a**) shows variability in TTV more so than FVD. After repeated performance reviews TTV improved for all nurses (**b**). In response to further team and individual performance reviews, all nurses are moving towards evaluating newly admitted patients within 20 minutes of arrival to the ICU in Q3 of 2017 (panel **c**, green quadrant). Panels (**d**–**f**): *eICU physician* distribution of Q1 of 2016 (**d**) shows variability in both TTV and FVD and division into two groups: the first group with predominantly timely but short video encounters (lower left area of plot), and the other with predominantly delayed but comprehensive video interactions (upper right area of plot). After repeated performance reviews, panel (**e**) shows reductions in the meantime to first video (TTV) and an increase in mean first video duration (FVD), which is further accelerated in Q3 of 2017 following further QPRs, leading to reduction of provider-to-provider variability and consistent timely and comprehensive video reviews by physicians (panel **f**, green quadrant). Note that the dynamic movement of motion charts cannot be adequately visualized in print format. The snapshot format is used to substitute for the dynamic motion

References

1. Ramnath VR, Ho L, Maggio LA, Khazeni N. Centralized monitoring and virtual consultant models of tele-ICU care: a systematic review. Telemed J E Health. 2014;20:936–61.
2. Petelin JB, Nelson ME, Goodman J. Deployment and early experience with remote-presence patient care in a community hospital. Surg Endosc. 2007;21:53–6.
3. Vespa PM, Miller C, Hu X, Nenov V, Buxey F, Martin NA. Intensive care unit robotic telepresence facilitates rapid physician response to unstable patients and decreased cost in neurointensive care. Surg Neurol. 2007;67:331–7.
4. Fortis S, Weinert C, Bushinski R, Koehler AG, Beilman G. A health system-based critical care program with a novel tele-ICU: implementation, cost, and structure details. J Am Coll Surg. 2014;219:676–83.
5. Ries M. Evaluating tele-ICU cost – an imperfect science. Crit Care Med. 2016;44:441–2.
6. Davis TM, Barden C, Dean S, et al. American Telemedicine Association guidelines for teleICU operations. Telemed J E Health. 2016;22:971–80.
7. Kalb T, Raikhelkar J, Meyer S, et al. A multicenter population-based effectiveness study of teleintensive care unit-directed ventilator rounds demonstrating improved adherence to a protective lung strategy, decreased ventilator duration, and decreased intensive care unit mortality. J Crit Care. 2014;29:691.e7–14.
8. Fusaro MV, Becker C, Pandya S, et al. International teleconsultation on conjoined twins leading to a successful separation: a case report. J Telemed Telecare. 2018;24:482–4.
9. Moughrabieh A, Weinert C. Rapid deployment of international tele-Intensive Care Unit services in war-torn Syria. Ann Am Thorac Soc. 2016;13:165–72.
10. Young LB, Chan PS, Cram P. Staff acceptance of tele-ICU coverage: a systematic review. Chest. 2011;139:279–88.
11. Hawkins HA, Lilly CM, Kaster DA, Groves RH Jr, Khurana H. ICU telemedicine comanagement methods and length of stay. Chest. 2016;150:314–9.
12. Thomas EJ, Lucke JF, Wueste L, Weavind L, Patel B. Association of telemedicine for remote monitoring of intensive care patients with mortality, complications, and length of stay. JAMA. 2009;302:2671–8.
13. Lilly CM, McLaughlin JM, Zhao H, et al. A multicenter study of ICU telemedicine reengineering of adult critical care. Chest. 2014;145:500–7.
14. Goran SF. A second set of eyes: an introduction to tele-ICU. Crit Care Nurse. 2010;30:46–55; quiz 56.
15. Jahrsdoerfer M, Goran S. Voices of family members and significant others in the tele-intensive care unit. Crit Care Nurse. 2013;33:57–67.
16. Coustasse A, Deslich S, Bailey D, Hairston A, Paul D. A business case for tele-intensive care units. Perm J. 2014;18:76–84.
17. MedPac. Chapter 8: Telehealth services and the medicare program. *Report to the congress: medicare and the health care delivery system.* 2016:229. Available from: http://www.medpac.gov/docs/default-source/reports/chapter-8-telehealth-services-and-the-medicare-program-june-2016-report-.pdf?sfvrsn=0. Accessed 18 Aug 2018.
18. Lilly CM, Motzkus C, Rincon T, et al. ICU telemedicine program financial outcomes. Chest. 2017;151:286–97.
19. Kotter JP. Leading change. Harvard Business School Press. 1996. Available from: https://www.hbs.edu/faculty/Pages/item.aspx?num=137.

Part II
Quality and Outcomes of Tele-ICU

Chapter 8
Safety and Quality Metrics for ICU Telemedicine: Measuring Success

Ramesh Venkataraman and Nagarajan Ramakrishnan

Introduction

The word telemedicine implies the remote diagnosis and treatment of patients by means of telecommunications technology. Telemedicine has been deployed in the ICU setting for many decades and has been given several names in the literature (i.e., tele-ICU, virtual ICU, remote ICU, and electronic ICU (eICU)) and offers a means of optimizing intensivist coverage of ICU beds. These names all imply the provision of care by a remotely based team, comprised of intensivists, nurse practitioners, and ICU nurses through frequent two-way interactions with the bedside team and patients using audiovisual communication and computer systems. In this review, we will use the term tele-ICU to describe the use of telemedicine to provide ICU care.

Since the utility of tele-ICUs has been steadily increasing, one needs to be conscious of costs versus benefits while adding such monitoring to an existing system. In this chapter, we summarize the impact of tele-ICU on the safety and quality metrics.

Tele-ICU Models

Quality and safety of any tele-ICU service depends on the organizational and structural baseline of the ICU managed and the manner in which the tele-ICU coverage is provided. A high degree of variability exists in the manner in which tele-ICU coverage is provided, and this heterogeneity impacts analysis on patient

R. Venkataraman · N. Ramakrishnan (✉)
Department of Critical Care Medicine, Apollo Hospitals, Chennai, India
e-mail: ramesh@icuconsultants.com; ram@icuconsultans.com

M. A. Koenig (ed.), *Telemedicine in the ICU*,
https://doi.org/10.1007/978-3-030-11569-2_8

Table 8.1 Impact of tele-ICU on patient outcomes

Tele-ICU improves compliance with best practices and care bundles
The impact on ICU and hospital LOS and mortality is inconsistent
Teleconsultation enables improvements in care process of acute stroke
Teleconsultation enhances compliance with early sepsis bundles

outcomes and safety. These contextual variables include the type of hospital the tele-ICU service is provided to (academic vs non-academic), geographic location (urban vs rural), closed or open unit, etc. There are also several models of tele-ICU care delivery, and it is important to factor in the model of care provided when studies evaluating the quality and safety of tele-ICUs are interpreted. So, before we discuss the quality and safety metrics of tele-ICU, it is worthwhile understanding the various models of tele-ICU care delivery and the structure with which it is provided.

Broadly speaking, tele-ICU care can be provided as [1]:

1. "Continuous care model" in which monitoring of patients and titration of care happens continuously without any interruptions
2. Scheduled care model in which periodic consultations from a remote expert happens at prescheduled times (e.g., morning ventilator weaning rounds)
3. Responsive or reactive care model in which virtual visits are triggered by an alert

Some models incorporate various combinations of the above. The above models can be delivered through two major structures – centralized and decentralized tele-ICU. In the centralized tele-ICU, physicians, nurses, and clerical staff are connected to one or multiple facilities from a remote physical structure referred to as a "command center" or "monitoring center." In the decentralized tele-ICU, physicians and nurses can be located anywhere with internet access and monitor ICU patients digitally with the ability to provide audiovisual support when required [2]. It is likely that, when tele-ICU is provided in a decentralized manner on a scheduled or reactive care basis, improvements in quality and safety may be more difficult to establish.

It is clear that the data from one context cannot be generalized across all tele-ICUs. Apart from universal quality and safety metrics common to all ICUs, specific metrics needed for that particular context also need to me monitored and reported to comprehend the true impact of the tele-ICU service provided (Table 8.1).

Tele-ICU and Patient Outcomes

Tele-ICU care implementation should intuitively improve quality and safety of care provided to patients. First tele-ICU care can extend intensivist coverage to small rural ICUs without intensivist coverage. Second, even in ICUs with intensivists, tele-ICU provides for enhanced coverage time. Third, when used in a continuous care model, tele-ICU enables provision of proactive care by way of smart alert systems and allows for prompt interventions. Fourth, it provides for an additional layer of monitoring and supervision that could potentially capture errors, augment compliance to best practice bundles, and enhance safety and quality. Finally, it influences the existing care process by increasing nurse and physician staffing throughout the day [3].

The American Telemedicine Association (ATA) guidelines recommend tele-ICUs to "have in place a systematic quality improvement and performance management process that complies with all organizational, regulatory, or accrediting requirements" [1]. They recommend that quality metrics measured include administrative, technical, and clinical components needed for the effective provision of tele-ICU care. These metrics in turn should be utilized to implement technical, operational, and clinical changes that reflect advances in technology, practice patterns, and emerging clinical evidence.

Safety and Quality Metrics in Tele-ICU

The Critical Care Societies Collaborative categorized outcomes as provider-centered, patient-centered, and system-centered [3, 4] of which patient safety and quality belong in the patient-centered domain. Although mortality is the primary patient-centered outcome that matters the most and serves as the gold standard to ascertain the value of any intervention in the ICU, other equally important outcomes have been monitored and evaluated.

Identification of Problems and Timeliness of Intervention

The first logical step in enhancing quality and safety of ICU patients is in identifying physiologic derangements in patients promptly and intervening quickly to reverse them. Despite proactive care being the central theme of a continuous tele-ICU care model, no major studies have explored the relative proportion of proactive and reactive patient care interventions or the response time to intervention for physiologic derangements in an ICU with and without tele-ICU coverage. In one survey, only 6% of interventions were for preventing physiologic instability [5]. However, in another survey, investigators found that tele-ICU continuous monitoring identified gradually deteriorating trends and provided proactive care [6]. In a large multicenter observational study, review of new ICU admissions within 1 hour of admission and quicker alert response times have been associated with improved patient outcomes and have been used as quality metrics for tele-ICUs [7].

Compliance with Evidence-Based Care Bundles

Care bundles are designed to ensure the standard of care and optimize patient outcome by boosting the consistent implementation of a group of effective interventions. Care bundles work only when there is a high level of adherence to all components [8]. Often in clinical practice, compliance with implementation is suboptimal. Common barriers for implementation include staff shortages, staff perception of increased workload, time constraints amidst providing bedside care, and resistance to change. Tele-ICU care can potentially help overcome many of these barriers. Tele-ICU care intrinsically increases patient to physician and nurse staffing and provides for an extra pair of eyes to verify that all elements of a given care bundle have been ordered and implemented on a consistent basis. The tele-ICU model allows for sharing of workload and increases the efficiency of time utilization by enabling providers to perform two equally important parallel actions simultaneously. When a particular aspect of a care bundle is omitted, prompt identification by the tele-ICU team and notification to the bedside team and/or initiating that intervention when empowered can substantially increase the compliance. Most tele-ICUs also have the ability to capture data seamlessly, audit compliances with care bundle practices, and then provide frequent reports back to the bedside team. This feedback provides for an opportunity to constantly re-evaluate the quality benchmarks and helps fine-tune care processes persistently improving compliance with care bundles and standards of care.

Many studies have reliably documented that tele-ICU implementation enhances compliance with various best practices in the ICU [9–12]. In one study, the tele-ICU program enhanced compliance and recording of three ventilator bundle components (i.e., head-of-bed elevation, prophylaxis for deep venous thrombosis, and stress ulcer prophylaxis) [9]. Similarly, in another clinical trial, the addition of a night-shift tele-ICU pharmacist increased the percentage of patients receiving a daily sedative interruption trial [10]. Timely referrals to the organ procurement agency increased from 45% to 92% in one study when the tele-ICU team was authorized to make all referrals [11]. In a retrospective study, Kalb evaluated the effect of exposure to tele-ICU-directed ventilator rounds on adherence to lung protective ventilation, ventilation duration ratio (VDR), and ICU mortality ratio among several hospitals with variable baseline compliance. This study reported a steady increase in the compliance rates with statistically significant improvement in the third quarter after implementation [12]. More importantly, this improvement was sustained in the subsequent two quarters, and the tele-ICU-driven ventilator rounds decreased VDR and ICU mortality ratio. The tele-ICU can also function in the role of screening all mechanically ventilated patients twice per day for compliance with the ventilator-associated pneumonia (VAP) bundle. When a component of the bundle is missing, the tele-intensivist would either enter the necessary order or notify the bedside providers to address the oversight. When the tele-ICU team screened all ventilator patients for compliance with the VAP bundle in one study, compliance to the bundle increased to 99%, with a significant reduction in VAP [13].

Several studies have also evaluated the effect of tele-ICU on identification of sepsis and compliance with sepsis bundles [13]. Rincon evaluated the use of tele-ICU in defining the true incidence of severe sepsis using electronic screening for 161 ICU beds (36,353 admissions) in 10 hospitals [14] and documented a higher identification rate of patients with severe sepsis. Compliance with surviving sepsis guidelines increased significantly during the study period, with timely antibiotic administration increasing from 55% to 74% ($p = 0.001$), serum lactate measurement increasing from 50% to 66% ($p = 0.001$), initial fluid bolus of ≥20 mL/kg increasing from 23% to 70% ($p = 0.001$), and central line placement increasing from 33% to 50% ($p = 0.001$). Similarly, other studies have documented increased overall compliance with sepsis bundles [15, 16].

Mortality and Length of Stay

The studies that have evaluated the effect of tele-ICU services on important patient outcomes, such as length of ICU or hospital stay and mortality, have provided conflicting results. The variability in outcomes is largely due to variability in the type of client ICUs, baseline care process of the ICUs, acuity of patients, model of tele-ICU care provided, authority provided to the tele-ICU team, and the level of acceptance and implementation of the tele-ICU.

Initial research has been based on small, single-center studies with important limitations. In one of the early studies that evaluated outcomes related to tele-ICU, Grundy demonstrated that telemedicine was feasible, superior to consultations over the telephone, enhanced the educational value, and augmented the process and quality of care [17]. It is important to understand that, in this study, daily intensivist consultations via a two-way audiovisual link between a small private hospital and a large university medical center were utilized to provide tele-ICU care. Similarly, another study revealed decreased ICU complications, ICU length of stay (LOS), severity-adjusted ICU and hospital mortality, and ICU costs in a model of management by an intensivist during a 16-week period using video conferencing and computer-based data transmission [18]. All these studies had no or minimal baseline intensive care staffing, were based at single centers, and utilized a scheduled care model of tele-ICU.

Several large studies and systematic reviews seem to suggest important clinical benefits from tele-ICU coverage. In a large single-center study of over 6000 patients (7 different ICUs on 2 campuses), the tele-ICU intervention (compared with the pre-intervention period) was associated with improvement in implementation of stress ulcer prophylaxis (96% vs 83%, odds ratio [OR] 4.57, 95% confidence interval (CI) 3.91–5.77) and deep venous thrombosis prophylaxis (99% vs 85%, OR 15.4, 95% CI 11.3–21.1); lower rates of VAP (1.6% vs 13.0%, OR 0.15, 95% CI 0.09–0.23) and catheter-related bloodstream infection (0.6% vs 1.0%, OR 0.50, 95% CI 0.27–0.93); reduced mortality (OR 0.42, 95% CI 0.31–0.52); and decreased hospital LOS (9.8 vs 13.3 days, hazard ratio for discharge 1.44, 95% CI 1.33–1.56)

[19]. Tele-ICU was provided continuously in this study, and the tele-ICU intensivist reviewed all relevant medical information for new admissions, assessed patients using real-time video, and augmented the admission plan if needed. Continuous surveillance of patients with prompt response to alarms and prompt titration of plan of care was performed by the off-site intensivist along with regular communication with the bedside team. This study reported that faster response to alarms and review of the plan of care on the patients admitted overnight by the remote intensivist were associated with improved outcomes [19].

Significantly lower ICU and hospital LOS and mortality among patients who received tele-ICU care was noted in another multicenter study that included various types of ICUs across the USA (56 ICUs in 32 hospitals from 19 US healthcare systems) using a pre- and post-assessment methodology [7]. Review of patient care by the remote intensivist within 1 hour of ICU admission, adherence to ICU best practices, timely use of performance data, and faster reaction times to alerts were identified as the key elements of care that were associated with improved outcomes. A recent meta-analysis [20] combined studies that compared telemedicine-enhanced ICU care versus conventional ICU care and found a lower ICU mortality with a relative risk (RR) of 0.83 ($p = 0.01$); lower hospital mortality (RR 0.74, $p = 0.02$); and shorter mean ICU LOS of 0.63 days ($p < 0.0001$) in the tele-ICU group. This meta-analysis found no significant decrease in hospital LOS, however. Kahn performed a multicenter retrospective case-control study using Medicare claims data from 2001 to 2010 to determine the effectiveness of tele-ICU [21]. In this study, adjusted mortality at 132 tele-ICU adopting hospitals was compared to 389 non-adopting control hospitals, with one case being matched to three controls. There was a trend toward improved mortality, with urban hospitals showing the most benefit [21].

Although most studies seem to demonstrate positive outcomes with tele-ICU implementation, some studies provide contradictory results. A large systematic review and meta-analysis of more than 41,000 patients (13 studies at 35 ICUs in 27 hospitals) showed lower ICU mortality and LOS but not lower in-hospital mortality or hospital LOS [22]. However, this study had several important limitations. First, there was huge heterogeneity in the types and baseline staffing models of the covered ICUs. Second, tele-ICU provision was nonuniform across the centers with nearly half of the centers utilizing tele-ICU for evening and weekend coverage only. Third, the number of studies that provided data on in-hospital mortality was fewer which rendered the study underpowered for that outcome. Finally, there was a no consistent measurement, reporting, and adjustment for patient severity among the included studies.

Another multicenter before-and-after study found no significant differences in severity-adjusted ICU or hospital mortality or ICU or hospital LOS associated with the tele-ICU intervention [23]. However, in the subgroup of sicker patients, tele-ICU care improved survival. The tele-ICU coverage in this study, however, was partial (only between noon and 7 AM), and full authorization for tele-ICU providers to manage patients occurred only in 31% of patients, thus limiting its effectiveness. In another study, tele-ICU coverage did not improve ICU, non-ICU, or total mortality; hospital or ICU LOS; or hospital cost in a study of 4000 patients in two community hospitals [24]. More importantly, neither the continued presence nor the higher utilization of tele-ICU improved the mortality rate. It is likely that the low baseline mortality of patients and the variable intensity of tele-ICU coverage negated any potential positive outcomes in this study. Finally, Nassar evaluated the impact of tele-ICU on hospital LOS and ICU, hospital, and 30-day mortality within the US Department of Veterans Affairs healthcare system and found no outcome benefit with tele-ICU monitoring and care [25]. There were remarkable differences between the participating ICUs in their preparedness to adopt and implement tele-ICU which could have confounded the results.

Tele-ICU and Specific Patient Population

There are consistent data that telemedicine interventions in the ICU provide for important clinical benefits in specific patient populations. In a single-center retrospective review, when patients were managed collaboratively by tele-ICU intensivists along with bedside intensivists, they were moved out of the ICU faster compared to patients managed by the intermittently available surgical critical care group [26]. In a recent study done in a military hospital setting, initiation of tele-ICU coverage of the surgical ICU led to increased surgical admissions with higher severity of illness [27]. The authors postulated that presence of tele-ICU coverage enabled the surgeons to safely expand the surgical services provided to patients requiring perioperative ICU care, who previously may have been transferred out to another facility.

Another area in which teleconsultation has enabled improvements in care processes is in the care of acute strokes. Several studies have established the value of tele-neurology consultation in providing urgent consultations for confirming clinical findings, reviewing neuroradiological studies, and guiding treatment decisions regarding the role of thrombolytics for acute ischemic stroke [28–30]. Timeliness of care also improved in studies of sepsis treatment. In one study, when the emergency room was exposed to tele-ICU via an eICU cart, time to first dose of antibiotic, compliance with checking lactate levels, and length of emergency room stay all improved in sepsis patients [31].

It is intuitive that tele-ICU is likely to enhance the care processes when specific goals are targeted in a narrow patient population since it provides for immediate access to expertise, early recognition of warning signs, faster reaction time, and an additional layer of care delivery to scrutinize and rectify any oversights in the care process.

Staff Acceptance and Performance

For any intervention to be effective, it has to be accepted widely and integrated into routine practice. Tele-ICU acceptance will impact its ability to improve outcomes. When not adopted effectively, it can potentially disrupt care flow and interfere in the care provided. Tele-ICU training, understanding and expectations of the bedside staff, perceived need, and organizational factors such as availability of resources for local coordination have been identified as factors influencing the acceptance of tele-ICU before its implementation [32]. Studies that have evaluated staff acceptance of tele-ICU have provided variable results. However, most of the data is from studies that used a survey to assess this crucial aspect of tele-ICU care provision. One systematic review evaluated the acceptance of tele-ICU coverage among ICU staff and found that, despite initial ambivalence among nurses before implementation, the overall staff acceptance rate of tele-ICU coverage was high with a mean satisfaction score of 4.22–4.53 on a Likert scale of 1–5 [33].

Conclusion

There is increasing demand for ICU beds to accommodate the sick with a simultaneous shortage of intensivists [34]. Tele-ICU supplementation of traditional ICU care allows for leveraging the existing work force for maximum coverage and augmentation of quality and safety of care provided. Although the addition of tele-ICU service to any ICU intuitively enhances the care process, it has been a challenge to consistently demonstrate this improvement. Studies evaluating the effect of tele-ICU on quality and safety metrics predominantly seem to denote a positive effect on outcomes. Most studies have demonstrated a faster response to alerts, improved compliance with practice care bundles, and shorter duration of ICU stay. However, mortality benefits have been inconsistent among the studies. The continuous tele-ICU care model with a high level of involvement and authority to make and modify care plans seems to have the best impact on outcomes (Table 8.2). Intensivist review of new admissions within 1 hour of admission, more rapid responses to alerts and alarms, frequent review of performance data with the bedside team, higher levels of compliance with ICU best practice bundles, and frequent multidisciplinary rounds seem to improve patient outcomes. It is important to understand that almost all studies evaluating the impact of tele-ICU on outcomes have important limitations in that they are either single center or use a before-and-after implementation design and have variable baseline staffing in the ICU or variable models of tele-ICU care delivery. Safety and quality outcomes of tele-ICU vary based on the context of care provided which must be taken into account while interpreting the results of these studies.

Table 8.2 Factors associated with improved outcomes in tele-ICU

Acceptance of tele-ICU model by ICU staff
Daytime intensivist staffing of ICU
Level of tele-ICU involvement in patient care
Implementation of tele-ICU recommendations by the bedside team
Acuity and complexity of patients

References

1. Davis TM, Barden C, Dean S, Gavish A, Goliash I, Goran S, et al. American Telemedicine Association guidelines for teleICU operations. Telemed e-Health. 2016;22(12):971–80.
2. Reynolds HN, Bander J, McCarthy M. Different systems and formats for tele-ICU coverage: designing a tele-ICU system to optimize functionality and investment. Crit Care Nurs Q. 2012;35(4):364–77.
3. Kahn JM, Hill NS, Lilly CM, Angus DC, Jacobi J, Rubenfeld GD, et al. The research agenda in ICU telemedicine: a statement from the Critical Care Societies Collaborative. Chest. 2011;140(1):230–8.
4. Venkataraman R, Ramakrishnan N. Outcomes related to telemedicine in the intensive care unit. Crit Care Clin. 2015;31(2):225–37.
5. Lilly CM, Thomas EJ. Tele-ICU: experience to date. J Intensive Care Med. 2010;25(1):16–22.
6. Khunlertkit A, Carayon P. Contributions of tele–intensive care unit (Tele-ICU) technology to quality of care and patient safety. J Crit Care. 2013;28(3):315.e1–315.e12.
7. Lilly CM, McLaughlin JM, Zhao H, Baker SP, Cody S, Irwin RS, et al. A multicenter study of ICU telemedicine reengineering of adult critical care. Chest. 2014;145(3):500–7.
8. Horner DL, Bellamy MC. Care bundles in intensive care. Contin Educ Anaesth Crit Care Pain. 2012;12(4):199–202.
9. Youn BA. ICU process improvement: using telemedicine to enhance compliance and documentation for the ventilator bundle. Chest. 2006;130:226s–C.
10. Forni A, Skehan N, Hartman CA, Yogaratnam D, Njoroge M, Schifferdecker C, et al. Evaluation of the impact of a tele-ICU pharmacist on the management of sedation in critically Ill mechanically ventilated patients. Ann Pharmacother. 2010;44(3):432–8.
11. Cowboy EN, Nygaard SD, Robin Simmons JS. Compliance with CMS timely referral and organ procurement impact via tele ICU. Chest. 2009;136(4):15S–b.
12. Kalb T, Raikhelkar J, Meyer S, Ntimba F, Thuli J, Gorman MJ, et al. A multicenter population-based effectiveness study of teleintensive care unit–directed ventilator rounds demonstrating improved adherence to a protective lung strategy, decreased ventilator duration, and decreased intensive care unit mortality. J Crit Care. 2014;29(4):691.e7–691.e14.
13. Ries M. Tele-ICU: a new paradigm in critical care. Int Anesthesiol Clin. 2009;47(1):153–70.
14. Rincon TA, Bourke G, Seiver A. Standardizing sepsis screening and management via a tele-ICU program improves patient care. Telemed e-Health. 2011;17(7):560–4.
15. Patel B, Kao L, Thomas E, Young E. Improving compliance with surviving sepsis campaign guidelines via remote electronic ICU monitoring. Crit Care Med. 2007;35:A275.
16. Ikeda D, Hayatdavoudi S, Winchell J, Rojas A, Rincon T, Yee A. Implementation of a standard protocol for the surviving sepsis 6 and 24 hr bundles in patients with an APACHE III admission diagnosis of sepsis decreases mortality in an open adult ICU: 8. Crit Care Med. 2006;34(12):A2.
17. Grundy BL, Crawford P, Jones PK, Kiley ML, Reisman A, Pao YH, et al. Telemedicine in critical care: an experiment in health care delivery. JACEP. 1977;6(10):439–44.
18. Rosenfeld BA, Dorman T, Breslow MJ, Pronovost P, Jenckes M, Zhang N, et al. Intensive care unit telemedicine: alternate paradigm for providing continuous intensivist care. Crit Care Med. 2000;28(12):3925–31.
19. Lilly CM, Cody S, Zhao H, Landry K, Baker SP, McIlwaine J, et al. Hospital mortality, length of stay, and preventable complications among critically ill patients before and after tele-ICU reengineering of critical care processes. JAMA. 2011;305(21):2175–83.
20. Chen J, Sun D, Yang W, Liu M, Zhang S, Peng J, et al. Clinical and economic outcomes of telemedicine programs in the intensive care unit: a systematic review and meta-analysis. J Intensive Care Med. 2018;33(7):383–93.
21. Kahn JM, Le TQ, Barnato AE, Hravnak M, Kuza CC, Pike F, et al. ICU telemedicine and critical care mortality. Med Care. 2016;54(3):319–25.

22. Young LB, Chan PS, Lu X, Nallamothu BK, Sasson C, Cram PM. Impact of telemedicine intensive care unit coverage on patient outcomes: a systematic review and meta-analysis. Arch Intern Med. 2011;171(6):498–506.
23. Thomas EJ, Lucke JF, Wueste L, Weavind L, Patel B. Association of telemedicine for remote monitoring of intensive care patients with mortality, complications, and length of stay. JAMA. 2009;302(24):2671–8.
24. Morrison JL, Cai Q, Davis N, Yan Y, Berbaum ML, Ries M, et al. Clinical and economic outcomes of the electronic intensive care unit: results from two community hospitals. Crit Care Med. 2010;38(1):2–8.
25. Nassar BS, Vaughan-Sarrazin MS, Jiang L, Reisinger HS, Bonello R, Cram P. Impact of an intensive care unit telemedicine program on patient outcomes in an integrated health care system. JAMA Intern Med. 2014;174(7):1160–7.
26. Collins TA, Robertson MP, Sicoutris CP, Pisa MA, Holena DN, Reilly PM, et al. Telemedicine coverage for post-operative ICU patients. J Telemed Telecare. 2017;23(2):360–4.
27. Van Gent J-M, Davis KL, Henry N, Zander AL, Kuettel MA, Edson T, et al. The initial impact of tele-critical care on the surgical services of a Community Military Hospital. Mil Med. 2018;183:e494–9.
28. Schwamm LH, Rosenthal ES, Hirshberg A, Schaefer PW, Little EA, Kvedar JC, et al. Virtual teleStroke support for the emergency department evaluation of acute stroke. Acad Emerg Med. 2004;11(11):1193–7.
29. Pervez MA, Silva G, Masrur S, Betensky RA, Furie KL, Hidalgo R, et al. Remote supervision of IV-tPA for acute ischemic stroke by telemedicine or telephone before transfer to a regional stroke center is feasible and safe. Stroke. 2010;41(1):e18–24.
30. Silva GS, Farrell S, Shandra E, Viswanathan A, Schwamm LH. The status of telestroke in the United States: a survey of currently active stroke telemedicine programs. Stroke. 2012;43(8):2078–85.
31. Machado SM, Wilson EH, Elliott JO, Jordan K. Impact of a telemedicine eICU cart on sepsis management in a community hospital emergency department. J Telemed Telecare. 2018;24(3):202–8.
32. Moeckli J, Cram P, Cunningham C, Reisinger HS. Staff acceptance of a telemedicine intensive care unit program: a qualitative study. J Crit Care. 2013;28(6):890–901.
33. Young LB, Chan PS, Cram P. Staff acceptance of tele-ICU coverage: a systematic review. Chest. 2011;139(2):279–88.
34. Angus DC, Kelley MA, Schmitz RJ, White A, Popovich J. Committee on Manpower for Pulmonary and Critical Care Societies (COMPACCS). Caring for the critically ill patient. Current and projected workforce requirements for care of the critically ill and patients with pulmonary disease: can we meet the requirements of an aging population? JAMA. 2000;284(21):2762–70.

Chapter 9
Does ICU Telemedicine Improve Outcomes? Current State of the Evidence

Ricardo Teijeiro and M. Elizabeth Wilcox

Introduction

To date, the most convincing evidence to guide quality improvements in the ICU setting pertains to physician specialty training and medical staffing. Onsite staffing by intensivists has been associated with lower morbidity and mortality [1–4]. However, only 10–20% of ICUs in the USA are staffed by dedicated intensivists [5]. Each year, four million patients are admitted to an ICU, accounting for 30% of the costs in acute care hospitals [6]. Demand for critical care services has steadily increased over time, and the gap in intensivist number to meet that demand has only widened [5, 7]. Efficient methods for care delivery are needed. It is estimated that the full implementation of telemedicine in community hospitals would prevent 5400 to 13,400 deaths per year, with an annual cost savings of US$5.4 billion [8, 9].

R. Teijeiro
Instituto Nacional de Ciencias Medicas y Nutrición Salvador Zubirán, Mexico City, Mexico

Department of Medicine (Respirology), University Health Network, Toronto, ON, Canada

M. E. Wilcox (✉)
Department of Medicine (Respirology), University Health Network, Toronto, ON, Canada

Interdepartmental Division of Critical Care Medicine, University of Toronto, Toronto, ON, Canada
e-mail: elizabeth.wilcox@mail.utoronto.ca

M. A. Koenig (ed.), *Telemedicine in the ICU*,
https://doi.org/10.1007/978-3-030-11569-2_9

Understanding the Medical Literature as It Relates to Telemedicine

Telemedicine has been defined in multiple ways in the medical literature; it is the exchange of medical information via electronic communication when distance separates the providers from their patients [10]. More specifically, tele-ICU enables the provision of care to critically ill patients by healthcare professionals (i.e., intensivists) located remotely. Importantly, these different definitions must be considered when assessing the performance of tele-ICU in the literature.

Types of ICU Staffing Models

- Closed ICU model (high-intensity physician staffing): Mandatory transfer of responsibility for the care of every critically ill patient to an intensivist-led team or mandatory consultation by an intensivist [1, 4].
- Open ICU model (low-intensity staffing): Any physician can admit and care for patients without the involvement of an intensivist [1, 4].
- Decentralized tele-ICU: One or multiple medical facilities that may be accessed from remote sites [10].
- Centralized tele-ICU: One central ICU provides care via telemedicine and remote monitoring of several satellite ICUs [10].

Types of Tele-ICU Interventions

- Active: Continuous patient data monitoring with computer-generated alerts [11]
- High-intensity passive: Continuous patient data monitoring without computer-generated alerts [11]
- Low-intensity passive: No continuous data monitoring [11]
- Minimal delegation: Tele-ICU could intervene only for life-threatening situations [12]
- Full delegation: Routine orders, changes to treatment plans, intervene in life-threatening situations [12]
- e-ICU categories [13]:

    1. Initiates only emergency interventions for life-threatening conditions
    2. Category (1) and initiates minor non-emergent therapies (e.g., electrolyte replacement)
    3. Categories (1) and (2) and maintains therapies in existing patient care plan (titrate vasopressors, wean ventilator)
    4. Categories (1) and (2) and (3) and initiates new therapies as needed

The Impact of Tele-ICU on Outcomes

The majority of tele-ICU studies have employed a before-and-after observational design [12–30]. One study to date used a prospective, stepped-wedge design (see Table 9.1) [22]. Studies to date were structured around the hypothesis that tele-ICU implementation would reduce ICU and hospital mortality, as it would deliver an intensivist assessment to the bedside in a timely fashion. ICU mortality has commonly been the primary outcome in studies evaluating the impact of tele-ICU. Secondary outcomes evaluated would include in-hospital mortality, ICU as well as hospital length of stay (LOS) [14, 15, 17, 18, 31], rates of mechanical ventilation [21], nursing-staff satisfaction, adherence to ICU best practices [17, 20, 32], and cost [13, 15, 32–34].

Primary Outcome

To date, three meta-analyses [11, 35, 36] have pooled data from a total of 19 before-and-after observational studies with mixed results. Most recently, Chen and colleagues reported that tele-ICU reduced both ICU mortality (RR 0.83, 95% CI 0.72–0.96, $p = 0.01$) and hospital mortality (RR 0.74, 95% CI 0.58–0.96, $p = 0.02$) [35], whereas Young reported an associated reduction in ICU mortality but not lower in-hospital mortality [36]. As effect sizes varied between studies, it is possible that differing technology configuration, baseline ICU organizational characteristics (i.e., open vs closed ICU), and case mix of the implementation site as well as dose of the intervention (i.e., delegated authority or full implementation) are responsible for discrepancies. In one of the original tele-ICU implementation studies, Vespa and colleagues report on the use of a robotic telepresence to facilitate physician response time in assessing unstable patients in a neurocritical care unit [18]. The use of robotic telepresence was associated with reduced latency of intensivist face-to-face response for urgent pages (9.2 ± 9.3 minutes) as compared to conventional care (218 ± 186 minutes). Response time to specific emergencies included brain ischemia (7.8 ± 2.8 vs 152 ± 85 minutes) and elevated ICP (11 ± 14 vs 108 ± 55 minutes) [18]. This intervention allowed for the covering intensivist to respond more quickly to pages which resulted in decreased ICU LOS and cost [18].

An alternate implementation would be the use of tele-ICU to provide inpatient consultation where an intensivist is not immediately available. An example of this model would be that from Marcin and colleagues evaluating the impact of a regional pediatric tele-ICU program providing live interactive consultation to a rural adult ICU without pediatric intensivist coverage [31]. Tele-ICU consultations were sought in sicker patients, and the overall satisfaction with care was high among parents and healthcare providers with the intervention [31]. Given that approximately 40% of

Table 9.1 Characteristics of the included tele-ICU studies and the telemedicine intervention

Source	Patients (total/intervention), *n*	Units, *n*	Age (years) Mean (SD)		Sex (% men)		Intervention	Mortality, RR (95% CI)	Equipment used
			Standard care	Intervention group	Standard care	Intervention group			
Rosenfeld et al. [14]	628/201	1	62 (62.3)* 60 (55.6)*	61 (56.3)*	55 63	57	One of four intensivists available 24/7; interacted with patients and healthcare personnel via dedicated, computer-based video conferencing and data transmission equipment; available clinical data and stored physiologic data were reviewed at regular intervals; usually each 2 hours	0.22 [0.07, 0.71]	Spacelabs Medical, Seattle, Washington
Breslow et al. [15]	2140/744	2	61.3 (17.7)	60.1 (16.9)	56	49.7	Dedicated eICU facility off campus; all patients in MICU and SICU monitored from noon until 7 am (19 hrs/day) by eICU staff (board-certified intensivist); attending (admitting physician) determined level of intervention of eICU team, ranging from all decision-making authority to delegating some or all off-hrs decision-making authority to intensivist; regardless of category of intervention, the eICU reviewed all patient data at regular intervals (q4 hrs); remote intensivist assisted in the conduct of all codes	0.73 [0.53, 1.02]	VISICU Inc. (eICU CARE), Baltimore, Maryland

Marcin et al. [16]	429/47	1	65.8 (61.4) months	63.9 (62.1) months	NR	NR	Telemedicine consultation within 15 minutes of receiving page (portable telemedicine unit to University of California Davis Children's Hospital ICU and 5 consultants homes); available 24 hours a day, 7 days per week; live interactive consultation with physician, nurse, respiratory therapist, and parents; review of history, vital signs, lab work, radiology, monitoring devices, and telemedicine examination; telemedicine consultation with pediatric intensivist at the discretion of admitting physician	1.06 [0.13, 8.87]	Tandberg 800 video conference units
Howell et al [28]	5347/4647	NR	NR	NR	NR	NR	No details provided	0.9 [0.79, 1.10]	No details provided
Kohl et al. [17]	2811/2622	1	NR	NR	NR	NR	eICU, staffed by board-certified intensivists to an academic SICU	0.42[0.28, 0.61]	No details provided

(continued)

Table 9.1 (continued)

Source	Patients (total/ intervention), *n*	Units, *n*	Age (years) Mean (SD)		Sex (% men)		Intervention	Mortality, RR (95% CI)	Equipment used
			Standard care	Intervention group	Standard care	Intervention group			
Vespa et al. [18]	1218/640	1	NR	NR	NR	NR	Two physicians participated in the robotic telepresence program (RTP); live interactive consultation with physician; RTP rounds occurring 8 pm to midnight on weekdays and at 6 pm on weekends; review of trends in physiologic variables intracranial pressure, glycemic control, etc. were reviewed including prospective nighttime rounds was carried out by RTP; each patient was reviewed for a minimum of 5 minutes; a systematic paging protocol was established with general criteria defined that would require physician contact and the response goal to paging was answering the page within 15 minutes	1.09 [0.78,1.52]	Telepresence robot: InTouch Health, Santa Barbara, California; Integrated informatics: Global Care Quest, Aliso Viejo, California
Norman et al. [19]	1275/919	1	NR	NR	NR	NR	eICU team reviewed each patient and an electronic discharge tool daily; mixed MICU/SICU	NR	VISICU Inc. (eICU CARE), Baltimore, Maryland
Rincon et al. [29]	1818/499	4	NR	NR	NR	NR	No details provided	NR	VISICU Inc. (eICU CARE), Baltimore, Maryland

Thomas et al. [12]	4142/2108	6	60.2 (18.3)	59.3 (18.7)	51.0	52.9	Tele-ICU system consisted of remote office in administrative offices of healthcare system; equipped with eICU technology and staffed by two physicians from noon until 7 am Monday to Friday and 24 hrs per day on weekends as well as four registered nurses and two administrative technicians; rounds conducted based on subjective assessment of illness severity (severely ill, hourly assessments; moderately ill every 2 hrs; relatively stable every 4 hrs)	0.85 [0.69, 1.03]	VISICU Inc. (eICU CARE), Baltimore, Maryland
Zawada et al. [20]	7075/6379	5	NR	NR	NR	NR	Remote care center was staffed 24 hrs per day, 7 days per week, by 1 critical care nurse and a clerical support person; intensivists were present from 11 am to 7 am (20 hrs per day) to perform virtual rounds and evaluate proprietary alerts for vital signs, laboratory abnormalities, and gaps in best practices (Smart Alert prompts) and responding for requests from bedside nursing and physician staff	0.96 [0.57, 1.63]	VISICU Inc. (eICU CARE), Baltimore, Maryland

(continued)

Table 9.1 (continued)

Source	Patients (total/intervention), *n*	Units, *n*	Age (years) Mean (SD)		Sex (% men)		Intervention	Mortality, RR (95% CI)	Equipment used
			Standard care	Intervention group	Standard care	Intervention group			
McCambridge et al. [21]	1913/959	1	65.0	64.4	50.1	50.2	From 7 pm to 7 am, the telemedicine team admitted new patients, responded to telephone calls from ICU nurses about their patients, and responded to computer-generated events (emergency medical record's algorithmic event system: critical changes in physiologic parameters); responded to radiographic abnormalities; performed rounds for all monitored patients every 2 hrs	0.72 [0.58, 0.91]	Vistacom Inc, Allentown, Pennsylvania
New England Healthcare Institute [30]	927/1368	2	67 (17)	66 (18)	48	48	No details provided	2.07 [1.44, 2.97]	No details provided

Morrison et al. [13]	4088/2717	2	64.4 (17.8)	65.1 (18.6) 64.3 (19.0)	56	50.9 53.3	Admitting physician was responsible for establishing care plan; chose the extent of involvement in patient care provision of eICU care team (four categories for care provision defined a priori); regardless of physician category, the eICU intensivist reviewed all patient data at least every 4 hrs, made virtual rounds up to hourly on the sickest patients; eICU conducted rounds based on illness severity; access to laboratory values, and imaging studies; nurses provided additional triage through bedside rounds At one site eICU intensivist was encouraged to interact with house staff providing supervision and "real-time" teaching	1.15 [0.91, 1.46]	VISICU Inc. (eICU CARE), Baltimore, Maryland

continued)

Table 9.1 (continued)

Source	Patients (total/ intervention), *n*	Units, *n*	Age (years) Mean (SD)		Sex (% men)		Intervention	Mortality, RR (95% CI)	Equipment used
			Standard care	Intervention group	Standard care	Intervention group			
Lilly et al. [22]	6290/4761	7	62 (17)	64 (16.8)	57	57	Tele-ICU intervention implemented into seven different units in stepped-wedge design; Unit was already "closed" (intensivist-led); tele-ICU intensivist was an existing member of hospital staff; off-site team used tele-ICU workstations to monitor 5-minute-timed median vital sign values that were pulled into electronic flow sheet; care was serially reviewed, real-time audits of best practice adherence performed, reviewed nighttime admissions, monitored system-generated electronic alerts, audited bedside clinician responses to in-room alarms, and intervened when the responses of bedside clinicians were delayed; tele-ICU team participated in key critical care delivery processes throughout the entire day (24 hours every day)	0.80 [0.68, 0.91]	VISICU Inc. (eICU CARE), Baltimore, Maryland and APACHE (Cerner Healthcare Solutions, Kansas City, Missouri)
Willmitch et al. [24]	24656/18152	10	NR	NR	NR	NR	Tele-ICU facility operates 24/7 and is staffed by one intensivist, three critical care nurses, and one unit secretary	1.09 [0.78,1.52]	VISICU Inc. (eICU CARE), Baltimore, Maryland and APACHE (Cerner Healthcare Solutions, Kansas City, Missouri)

Sadaka et al. [25]	2823/2193	1	66.1 (14.5)	67.1 (15.3)	53	53	Hospital physicians were asked at the time of implementation to indicate their requested level of intervention from the tele-ICU between level I and II (level I, tele-intensivist could initiate interventions for any urgent/emergent conditions, evidence-based therapies, and hospital-approved protocols; level II, full order writing privileges and fully managed the patients)	0.48 [0.34, 0.68]	VISICU Inc. (eICU CARE), Baltimore, Maryland and APACHE (Cerner Healthcare Solutions, Kansas City, Missouri)
Lilly et al. [23]	118990/107 432	56	62.7 (17.6)	62.7 (17.4)	54.2	54.2	Variable implementation; no details provided	0.85 [0.80, 0.91]	Audio and video connections, an ICU-focused medical record and software for detecting evolving physiologic instability (Koninklijke, Philips N.V.); no other details provided
Nassar et al. [26]	6939/3355	8	67.1	66.5	96.9	97.6	In six ICUs, telemedicine staff were authorized to monitor patients and make interventions as they deemed appropriate; in two ICUs, the monitoring center staff could only intervene if requested	0.82 [0.59, 1.12]	No details provided
Fortis et al. [27]	97256/35113	306	64.5 (0.1)	65.9 (0.1)	96.1	96.7	No details provided	0.79 [0.71, 0.87]	No details provided

Median reported instead of means. Range used to calculate SD shown in parenthesis
NR not reported
*Range used to calculate SD shown in parenthesis

US hospitals are located in rural areas (American Heart Association; Facts on US hospitals. http://www.aha.org/aha/resource-center/statistics-and-studies/fast-facts.html. Accessed 25 August 2018) speaks to the possible sweeping impact that tele-ICU could have with full implementation. In a study evaluating the impact of a 15-hospital, rural, multi-state tele-ICU implementation program, smaller facilities reported improvements in quality of care, and, as a result, a reduced number of patients transferred to other hospitals [20]. With higher acuity scores, as care could be more comfortably provided for sicker patients, the raw mortality risk stayed the same or lower [20]. Of note, in the participating tertiary hospital, ICU and in-hospital mortality decreased as did LOS [20].

More recently, the tele-ICU intervention has been broadened to include a technology bundle that included a data monitoring system that generates alerts based on abnormal vital signs or trends in vital signs, in addition to audiovisual monitoring [12–15, 23, 26]. In these studies, patients were monitored continuously for 12–24 hours per day, with tele-ICU physicians, nurses, and other personnel rounding on all monitored patients every 1–4 hours and reviewing vital signs and laboratory results. However, in these studies the on-site attending (open units) or intensivist (closed units) was able to determine the level of involvement of the tele-ICU intensivist resulting in variable intervention saturation. In a study by Breslow and colleagues, initially most admitting physicians chose eICU category 1 or 2 in the initial intervention run-in period; however, by the end of it, most had chosen category 3 or 4 [15]. In an attempt to further tease out the level of tele-ICU team involvement in decision-making, Thomas and colleagues studied a 60-day period for four mixed, open, and closed ICU models and found 1446 orders to change care [12]. Comparing closed ICU and open ICU models, 5.3 and 18.5 orders per day were initiated, respectively [12]. In the open units, 26% of orders made by the tele-ICU team were determined to be high-level interventions (i.e., patients were severely ill, hemodynamically unstable) [12]. Apprehensive adoption of tele-ICU was also seen in a study by Morrison where initially only 20% of physicians opted for eICU category 3 or 4, but then, after a successive implementation period, this adoption increased to 50% [13]. Interestingly, utilization differed between implementation hospitals within the same study, with fewer physicians consistently choosing high-level involvement at one site, whereas at the other study hospital, physicians went from 25% opting for high-level involvement to 57% by the second wave [13]. In this study of what might be considered late adopters of an intervention, no reduction in mortality was seen [13].

In a rigorous study of what might be considered early adopters, 21 healthcare systems known to be implementing a tele-ICU program were invited to collect patient-level data as well as very granular data on structural and organizational characteristics of each ICU [23]. Although there was variable implementation of ICU admission procedures, the provision of technical support, involvement of the tele-ICU team on rounds, communication with caregivers, and other factors was again seen in this large sample of 118,990 adult patients from 56 ICUs. Adjusted ICU mortality was lower in the tele-ICU group (hazard ratio 0.74, 95% CI 0.68–0.79, $p < 0.001$) [23]. Although it was previously challenging to draw conclusions because studies provided varying levels of detail on the dose of interventions, those studies with continuous patient-data monitoring (active or high-intensity passive interventions) reported a significant decrease in ICU mortality (RR 0.78, 95% CI 0.64–0.95, $p = 0.01$) as compared to remote intensivist consultation only (passive intervention) with RR 0.64, 95% CI 0.20–2.07, $p = 0.45$ [11]. When only active interventions were considered, no effect on ICU mortality was found (RR 0.86, 95% CI 0.72–1.03, $p = 0.10$) and no difference from the effect in the passive group was found ($p = 0.62$ for test of interaction) [11]. These dated subgroup analyses were likely underpowered to detect a true dose-response effect [11], whereas the study by Lilly and colleagues was able to determine that certain individual components of the tele-ICU, specifically (1) intensive case review within 1 hour of admission, (2) timely use of performance data, (3) adherence to ICU best practices, and (4) quicker alert response times, were responsible for the mortality reduction seen [23].

Secondary Outcomes

A recent meta-analysis of 19 studies reported a significant reduction in ICU LOS (mean difference (MD) -0.63 days, 95% CI -0.72 to -0.17 days, $p = 0.007$) but not hospital LOS [35]. In a number of studies [22, 23, 25, 34], adjusted ICU LOS and hospital LOS were reduced after the introduction of tele-ICU. In a large study ($n = 6290$) by Lilly, ICU LOS was reduced from a mean of 6.4 days (SD 11) to 4.5 days (SD 6.7) from pre- to post-intervention [22]. Hospital LOS was reduced from 13.3 days (SD 17.1) to 9.8 days (SD 10), respectively [22]. The magnitude of the association of tele-ICU with shorter ICU and hospital LOS was greater for cases admitted after 8 PM [22]. Similar results with regard to time of admission, daytime as compared to evening, were found by Sadaka and colleagues [25]. Decreased LOS, combined with lower mortality, suggests that the bedside team when supported by the intervention may stabilize patients more quickly, facilitating recovery to rehabilitation and possibly expediting hospital discharge [22]. Corollary to this, however, several studies report no difference in ICU or hospital LOS with tele-ICU implementation [12, 13, 15, 26]. In fact, Thomas observed mean hospital LOS for the 3789 patients (91.5%) who survived to transfer was 4.3 days (95% CI 4–4.5 days) for the pre-intervention period as compared to the post-intervention period where the mean hospital LOS was 4.6 days (95% CI 4.3–4.9 days, increase of 0.3 days, $p = 0.13$) [12]. Similar results were seen for ICU LOS although different results were seen with high as compared to low severity of illness [12]. In another study, Breslow and colleagues showed that overall hospital and ICU LOS was unchanged. ICU and hospital LOS decreased in surgical ICU patients, whereas for medical ICU patients, hospital LOS was unchanged, while ICU LOS decreased [15]. In a large geographically dispersed network of hospitals within the Veteran Affairs Healthcare System ($n = 6939$), Nassar found no evidence that tele-ICU implementation reduced LOS. Stratification in this study by severity of illness also showed no significant difference [26].

In a study by McCambridge, implementation of a health information technology bundle with tele-ICU led to a reduction in ventilator use [21]. In general, patients with respiratory and neurologic diagnoses were more likely to be ventilated than those patients with a primary cardiology diagnosis [21]. In controlling for severity of illness and diagnosis by system, patients with neurologic or respiratory diagnoses were less commonly intubated in the intervention group [21]. At the same time, there was no significant difference in vasopressor use between patients when controlling for severity of illness of diagnosis category [21]. This might suggest that, with enhanced monitoring capacity, physicians are more comfortable leaving patients on noninvasive forms of mechanical ventilation which may contribute to reduced ICU and hospital LOS as well as decreased ICU-related complications (e.g., ventilator-associated pneumonia, ventilator-induced lung injury).

In the past decade, tele-ICU has employed an increasingly collaborative model of care that includes nurses, physicians, information technology, and administrative support personnel. Most studies measuring acceptance of the intervention have shown high acceptance for the increased ICU coverage. Thomas conducted a pre- and post-intervention attitude survey for physicians and found that the safety attitudes significantly increased after implementation [12]. Tele-ICU has increased the bedside team's confidence that patients were adequately covered. Another study conducted by Kowitlawakul measured the nurse's attitude through a survey. This study revealed that tele-ICU would be beneficial in units without adequate physician coverage [37]. Further, in a survey of more than 1200 nurses conducted by the AACN, almost 80% of the nurses surveyed said tele-ICU gives them an opportunity to improve patient care, and almost two-thirds said it improved their job performance [38]. Chu-Weininger showed that implementation of tele-ICU improved teamwork and the safety climate in certain units, especially among nurses [39].

Tele-ICU has consistently been associated with significantly higher rates of adherence to critical care best practices such as increasing appropriate and timely antibiotic administration, more frequent lactate measurement, and appropriate initial fluid boluses for severe sepsis [19]. Quality improvement and patient care have been improved by the implementation of tele-ICU and the resultant increase in adherence to evidence-based protocols not only for sepsis but for ventilator-associated pneumonia and blood transfusion [40–43]. In a study by Lilly and colleagues, tele-ICU implementation was associated with high rates of deep vein thrombosis prophylaxis and cardiovascular prevention best practice adherence as well as lower rates of bloodstream catheter-related infection and ventilator-associated pneumonia [22, 23]. In fact, the authors estimated that 25% lower hospital mortality and 30% lower ICU mortality can be attributed to adherence to best practices and complication measures implemented by tele-ICU [22]. In addition, when a patient's condition in the ICU acutely changed, the tele-ICU team prompted the bedside team when the timeliness of response was deemed unsafe and recommended antimicrobials and resuscitation for sepsis [18, 22, 23]. Further, it may be possible that tele-ICU supports more consistent ventilator weaning or a greater willingness to transfer patients out of the ICU on weekends and evenings.

Interestingly, Fortis and colleagues looked at the effect of tele-ICU on inter-hospital transfers using approximately half a million admissions from the Veteran

Affairs ICU database [27]. Over a 6-year period, transfers decreased from 3.5% to 2% in the tele-ICU hospitals. Reduction in transfers was seen across all severity of illness quartiles except the lowest acuity quartile, typically patients with gastrointestinal or respiratory diagnoses [27]. Results were consistent regardless of admission day (i.e., weekday as compared to weekend day) [27]. Furthermore, similar results were seen in centers with high as compared to low ICU volumes as well as centers with high and low baseline inter-hospital transfer volumes [27].

Cost of Implementation

One of the main barriers to widespread adoption of tele-ICU has been its implementation costs. Estimated start-up costs would include US $2–5 million per "command center" with an additional US $250,000 per ICU supported by the system [30, 44]. The projected annual operating cost of a tele-ICU network is approximately US $2 million, to cover ongoing maintenance, staffing, and licensing [33, 45, 46]. Advocates have estimated that as many as 50,000 lives and US $4.3 billion might be saved annually in the USA through more consistent intensivist staffing [46–48]. The current literature on tele-ICU demonstrates improved hospital financial performance and ICU financial performance in studies where the tele-ICU interventions were more active and fully integrated to the electronic medical records system or in ICUs with higher severity of illness [33, 45, 46, 49]. Studies showed that ICU costs were reduced by 25–31% in the tele-ICU intervention group [22]. Tele-ICU intervention may contribute to lowering care costs by preventing complications, decreasing LOS, and lowering the need for long-term care facilities [22]. The analysis of the individual cost elements demonstrated lower routine radiology and therapy costs, fewer subspecialty consultations, and expedited patient management with changes in the discharge patterns. Sixty-four percent of the difference in cost between the baseline and intervention periods was associated with higher incidence of complications in the baseline periods [14]. Mechanisms for the increased cost of operations relied on additional testing and consultation after tele-ICU involvement, which ultimately led to delayed ICU transfers [13]. Taken together, the implementation start-up costs of tele-ICU would run a hospital around US $50–100,000 per bed [33, 46] with a cost per patient for the hospital varying from US $2600 to US $5600 after tele-ICU program implementation [35]. The long-term cost-effectiveness of tele-ICU remains to be explored.

Addressing the Mixed Results of Clinical Trials Published to Date

The limitations of current knowledge to guide the deployment and implementation of tele-ICU are numerous. Misclassification of interventions limits generalizability. Furthermore, studies have been conducted solely in the USA. The future impact of tele-ICU likely depends on characteristics of the environment in which it is deployed; however, the possible benefit of such an intervention may be overshadowed by the costs of installation and maintenance, incident malfunction, and downtime, as well as the likely impact of redeployment of intensivists away from the bedside when there are already pre-existing labor shortages.

Effects of tele-ICU have been predominantly evaluated by means of before-and-after observational studies, from which conclusions regarding causality may be confounded by secular trends in case mix and other interventions (including those implemented at the time of the tele-ICU intervention). Consistently, observational studies have overestimated the effect of an intervention, and therefore widespread adoption of tele-ICU will depend on future studies. These studies should be designed when there is a robust understanding of system design and organizational factors on the participating facilities [50]. At the present time, existing data is insufficient to identify with certainty the components essential to success and how to make the intervention more cost-effective.

Important areas of research that would inform the design of such trials include [51]:

1. Individual level patient meta-analyses of existing studies to permit adjustment for hospital and patient-level characteristics to identify characteristics of patients and centers most likely to benefit from the tele-ICU intervention
2. Assessment of clinical equipoise (physician and nursing attitudes toward tele-ICU) and means to promote full adoption by qualitative methods
3. Pilot observational studies to establish the optimal telemedicine technology configuration and dose in the context of consistent structural and organizational characteristics before and after implementation

Current Tele-ICU Guidelines: A Guide to Hospitals Considering Implementation of a Program

The American Telemedicine Association (ATA) recently published a policy statement for the use of tele-ICU [10]. The purpose of this guide is to assist organizations in tele-ICU implementation through the provision of administrative, clinical, and technical guidelines. Core guidelines for tele-ICU operations as they pertain to administration are illustrated in Fig. 9.1 [10]. With regard to clinical application for the practice of tele-ICU, executive leadership, with both tele-ICU and bedside ICU leadership representation, should set goals for the program such as improved patient outcomes, leveraging resources and costs [10]. Operational hours of the tele-ICU team should be clearly communicated including the availability of tele-ICU pharmacists, educators, or others who may provide hours based on program goals. Furthermore, the scope of tele-ICU patient service would be determined by the executive, ICU, and tele-ICU leadership [10]. Consensus should be reached on tele-ICU workflow and optimal integrated strategies specific to the site of implementation. Adequate orientation, competency, and training as to the roles and

Administrative guidelines

Leadership: A clear vision should be articulated by executive leadership; leaders for tele-ICU should be recruited and appropriately positioned in order to participate in the program implementation and integration

Human resource management: The organization shall create guidelines describing the role and responsibilities, appropriate staffing models, hours of operation, methods of communication and escalating procedures for tele-ICU

Health professionals: Tele-ICU professionals should be fully licensed, registered and credentialed with their respective regulatory organization including federal and state regulations regarding prescriptive authority

Privacy and confidentiality: Organizations will incorporate the requirements for privacy and confidentiality in accordance with the Health Insurance Portability and Accountability Act and Health Information for Economics and Critical Health Act

Fiscal Management: Organizations will establish a budget that will include the costs of implementation (i.e. hardware, software, data lines, licensing fees, credentialing fees, personnel, supplies) as well as ongoing expenses

Management of patient records and documentation: Clear processes and policies for documentation, storage and retrieval of health records consistent with existing standards; clinical documentation of tele-ICU team should be in compliance with organizational legal and risk management oversight

Patient rights and responsibility: Patients and families should be informed and educated about the role of the tele-ICU team; the tele-ICU team should be respectful with use of audiovisual equipment in providing patient/family privacy and sensitivity

Quality and outcomes: Systematic quality improvement and performance management processes should be in place that comply with all organizational, regulatory, or accrediting requirements; quality indicators should include administrative, technical, and clinical components for tele-ICU; cost information should also be collected

Research protocols: Research involving tele-ICU patients should be encouraged and supported by the organization; research should be in compliance with the organization's institution research ethics review board

Physical considerations: Physical layout (including space, equipment placement, and secure examination space) including both tele-ICU and ICU suites should be addressed early in the planning process; input should be had from clinicians, technology engineers, and physical plant engineers; design should consider communication essentials

Fig. 9.1 Administrative guidelines. (Adapted from: Davis et al. [10]. Used with permission.)

responsibilities of tele-ICU should be accomplished prior to implementation [10]. In terms of technical guidelines for tele-ICU implementation, organizations should refer to the ATA Core Guidelines for Telemedicine Operations document (https://southwesttrc.org/sites/southwesttrc.org/files/ATA%20Core%20Guidelines.pdf, Accessed 23 August 2018).

Future Studies and Unanswered Questions

We suggest that differences between those studies showing a difference in ICU and hospital mortality or LOS and those that do not can be attributed to a number of factors. The earliest studies of tele-ICU explicitly noted that interventions needed to be more than just technology implementation to be effective. Furthermore, with expansion of the technology bundle over time, the emphasis has been more on care processes and team communication. Lilly and colleagues have overtly stated that a major component of tele-ICU implementation was a concerted effort for systems reengineering (i.e., computerized order entry, standardized protocols) in tandem with tele-ICU introduction [52]. It is necessary to promote a strong culture of collaboration between the bedside and tele-ICU staff because technology on its own is insufficient to yield benefit.

ICUs most likely to benefit from tele-ICU are those with comparably less robust infrastructure (e.g., intensivist staffing, advanced monitoring capabilities, or quality audit and feedback processes). In addition, tele-ICU may also be useful in hospitals that have ICU capacity strain [53–55], where intensivists are not caring for all critically ill patients or are not caring optimally because they have too many patients. In a recent effectiveness study, Kahn reported that hospitals with a significant mortality reduction with tele-ICU implementation were more likely to be large urban hospitals with high annual admission volumes suggesting that academic ICUs are differentially influenced by strain [56]. Higher ICU daily census has been associated with decreased compliance with hand hygiene, increased incidence of ventilator-associated pneumonia, catheter-related bloodstream infections, and postoperative complications [57–59]. Furthermore, the largest gains in ICU throughput, effectively relieving ICU strain, come from quality improvement initiatives [60]. These initiatives would be aptly supported by tele-ICU systems.

Determining the specific technological innovations that optimize care, however, must be tailored to each ICU. Better care requires better matching of ICU organizational weaknesses to tele-ICU strengths. This requires greater exploration. As a start, future studies adopting controlled before-and-after or stepped-wedge designs to control for secular trends, considering target ICUs with high patient acuity, low-intensity staffing, and no audit-feedback infrastructure, would be most informative.

References

1. Pronovost PJ, Angus DC, Dorman T, Robinson KA, Dremsizov TT, Young TL. Physician staffing patterns and clinical outcomes in critically ill patients: a systematic review. JAMA. 2002;288(17):2151–62.
2. Gershengorn HB, Harrison DA, Garland A, Wilcox ME, Rowan KM, Wunsch H. Association of intensive care unit patient-to-intensivist ratios with hospital mortality. JAMA Intern Med. 2017;177(3):388–96.
3. Kerlin MP, Adhikari NK, Rose L, Wilcox ME, Bellamy CJ, Costa DK, Gershengorn HB, Halpern SD, Kahn JM, Lane-Fall MB, et al. An Official American Thoracic Society Systematic review: the effect of nighttime intensivist staffing on mortality and length of stay among intensive care unit patients. Am J Respir Crit Care Med. 2017;195(3):383–93.
4. Wilcox ME, Chong CA, Niven DJ, Rubenfeld GD, Rowan KM, Wunsch H, Fan E. Do intensivist staffing patterns influence hospital mortality following ICU admission? A systematic review and meta-analyses. Crit Care Med. 2013;41(10):2253–74.
5. Angus DC, Kelley MA, Schmitz RJ, White A, Popovich J Jr. Caring for the critically ill patient. Current and projected workforce requirements for care of the critically ill and patients with pulmonary disease: can we meet the requirements of an aging population? JAMA. 2000;284(21):2762–70.
6. Halpern NA, Pastores SM, Greenstein RJ. Critical care medicine in the United States 1985–2000: an analysis of bed numbers, use, and costs. Crit Care Med. 2004;32(6):1254–9.
7. Cooper RA. There's a shortage of specialists: is anyone listening? Acad Med. 2002;77(8):761–6.
8. Coustasse A, Deslich S, Bailey D, Hairston A, Paul D. A business case for tele-intensive care units. Perm J. 2014;18(4):76–84.
9. Venditti A, Ronk C, Kopenhaver T, Fetterman S. Tele-ICU "myth busters". AACN Adv Crit Care. 2012;23(3):302–11.
10. Davis TM, Barden C, Gavish A, Goran S, Jackson W, Goliash I, Graley A, Herr P, Marcin JP, Morris JM, et al. Policy: American Telemedicine Association guidelines for teleICU operations. Telemed e-Health. 2016;22(12):1–10.
11. Wilcox ME, Adhikari NK. The effect of telemedicine in critically ill patients: systematic review and meta-analysis. Crit Care. 2012;16(4):R127.
12. Thomas EJ, Lucke JF, Wueste L, Weavind L, Patel B. Association of telemedicine for remote monitoring of intensive care patients with mortality, complications, and length of stay. JAMA. 2009;302(24):2671–8.
13. Morrison JL, Cai Q, Davis N, Yan Y, Berbaum ML, Ries M, Solomon G. Clinical and economic outcomes of the electronic intensive care unit: results from two community hospitals. Crit Care Med. 2010;38(1):2–8.
14. Rosenfeld BA, Dorman T, Breslow MJ, Pronovost P, Jenckes M, Zhang N, Anderson G, Rubin H. Intensive care unit telemedicine: alternate paradigm for providing continuous intensivist care. Crit Care Med. 2000;28(12):3925–31.
15. Breslow MJ, Rosenfeld BA, Doerfler M, Burke G, Yates G, Stone DJ, Tomaszewicz P, Hochman R, Plocher DW. Effect of a multiple-site intensive care unit telemedicine program on clinical and economic outcomes: an alternative paradigm for intensivist staffing.[Erratum appears in Crit Care Med. 2004 Jul;32(7):1632]. Crit Care Med. 2004;32(1):31–8.
16. Marcin JP, Schepps DE, Page KA, Struve SN, Nagrampa E, Dimand RJ. The use of telemedicine to provide pediatric critical care consultations to pediatric trauma patients admitted to a remote trauma intensive care unit: a preliminary report. Pediatr Crit Care Med. 2004;5(3):251–6.
17. Kohl BA, Gutsche JT, Kim P, Sites FD, Ochroch EA. Effect of telemedicine on mortality and length of stay in a University hospital [abstract]. Crit Care Med. 2007;35:A111.

18. Vespa PM, Miller C, Hu X, Nenov V, Buxey F, Martin NA. Intensive care unit robotic telepresence facilitates rapid physician response to unstable patients and decreased cost in neurointensive care. Surg Neurol. 2007;67(4):331–7.
19. Norman V, French R, Hassan E, Kabani N, Stone D, Griebel J Jr, Tragico E. Effect of a telemedicine facilitated program on intensive care unit length of stay (LOS) and financial performance. Crit Care Med. 2009;37(12):A3.
20. Zawada ET Jr, Herr P, Larson D, Fromm R, Kapaska D, Erickson D. Impact of an intensive care unit telemedicine program on a rural health care system. Postgrad Med. 2009;121(3):160–70.
21. McCambridge M, Jones K, Paxton H, Baker K, Sussman EJ, Etchason J. Association of health information technology and teleintensivist coverage with decreased mortality and ventilator use in critically ill patients. Arch Intern Med. 2010;170(7):648–53.
22. Lilly CM, Cody S, Zhao H, Landry K, Baker SP, McIlwaine J, Chandler MW, Irwin RS, University of Massachusetts Memorial Critical Care Operations Group. Hospital mortality, length of stay, and preventable complications among critically ill patients before and after tele-ICU reengineering of critical care processes. JAMA. 2011;305(21):2175–83.
23. Lilly CM, McLaughlin JM, Zhao H, Baker SP, Cody S, Irwin RS. Group UMMCCO: a multicenter study of ICU telemedicine reengineering of adult critical care. Chest. 2014;145(3):500–7.
24. Willmitch B, Golembeski S, Kim SS, Nelson LD, Gidel L. Clinical outcomes after telemedicine intensive care unit implementation. Crit Care Med. 2012;40(2):450–4.
25. Sadaka F, Palagiri A, Trottier S, Deibert W, Gudmestad D, Sommer SE, Veremakis C. Telemedicine intervention improves ICU outcomes. Crit Care Res Prac. 2013;2013:456389.
26. Nassar BS, Vaughan-Sarrazin MS, Jiang L, Reisinger HS, Bonello R, Cram P. Impact of an intensive care unit telemedicine program on patient outcomes in an integrated health care system. JAMA Intern Med. 2014;174(7):1160–7.
27. Fortis S, Sarrazin MV, Beck BF, Panos RJ, Reisinger HS. ICU telemedicine reduces interhospital ICU transfers in the Veterans Health Administration. Chest. 2018;154(1):69–76.
28. Howell GH, Lem VM, Ball JM. Remote ICU care correlates with reduced health system mortatality and length of stay outcomes. Chest. 2007;132(4):443S.
29. Rincon T, Seiver A, Farrell W, Daly MA. Increased documentation of ICD-9-CM codes and template-oriented monitoring and screening with tele-ICU. Crit Care Med. 2009;37(12):A5.
30. Institute NEH: Critical care, critical choices: the case for tele-ICUs in intensive care. 2010. https://www.nehi.net/writable/publication_files/file/teleicu_critical_care_critical_choices.pdf.
31. Marcin JP, Nesbitt TS, Kallas HJ, Struve SN, Traugott CA, Dimand RJ. Use of telemedicine to provide pediatric critical care inpatient consultations to underserved rural Northern California. J Pediatr. 2004;144(3):375–80.
32. Davis K, Perry-Moseanko A, Tadlock MD, Henry N, Pamplin J. Successful implementation of low-cost tele-critical care solution by the U.S. Navy: initial experience and recommendations. Mil Med. 2017;182(5):e1702–7.
33. Franzini L, Sail KR, Thomas EJ, Wueste L. Costs and cost-effectiveness of a telemedicine intensive care unit program in 6 intensive care units in a large health care system. J Crit Care. 2011;26(3):329.e321–6.
34. Lilly CM, Motzkus C, Rincon T, Cody SE, Landry K, Irwin RS, UMass Memorial Critical Care Operations Group. ICU telemedicine program financial outcomes. Chest. 2017;151(2):286–97.
35. Chen J, Sun D, Yang W, Liu M, Zhang S, Peng J, Ren C. Clinical and economic outcomes of telemedicine programs in the intensive care unit: a systematic review and meta-analysis. J Intensive Care Med. 2018;33(7):383–93.
36. Young LB, Chan PS, Lu X, Nallamothu BK, Sasson C, Cram PM. Impact of telemedicine intensive care unit coverage on patient outcomes: a systematic review and meta-analysis. Arch Intern Med. 2011;171(6):498–506.
37. Kowitlawakul Y. The technology acceptance model: predicting nurses' intention to use telemedicine technology (eICU). Comput Inform Nurs. 2011;29(7):411–8.

38. Kleinpell R, Barden C, Rincon T, McCarthy M, Zapatochny Rufo RJ. Assessing the impact of telemedicine on nursing care in intensive care units. Am J Crit Care. 2016;25(1):e14–20.
39. Chu-Weininger MY, Wueste L, Lucke JF, Weavind L, Mazabob J, Thomas EJ. The impact of a tele-ICU on provider attitudes about teamwork and safety climate. Qual Saf Health Care. 2010;19(6):e39.
40. Ries M. Tele-ICU: a new paradigm in critical care. Int Anesthesiol Clin. 2009;47(1):153–70.
41. Groves RH Jr, Holcomb BW Jr, Smith ML. Intensive care telemedicine: evaluating a model for proactive remote monitoring and intervention in the critical care setting. Stud Health Technol Inform. 2008;131:131–46.
42. Ikeda DH. The impact of using a standard protocol for the surviving sepsis 6 and 24 hr bundles in septic patients on total icu risk adjusted mortality. Crit Care Med. 2006;34(12):A108.
43. Loyola S, Wilhelm J, Fornos J. An innovative approach to meeting early goal-directed therapy using telemedicine. Crit Care Nurs Q. 2011;34(3):187–99.
44. Breslow MJ. Remote ICU care programs: current status. J Crit Care. 2007;22(1):66–76.
45. Yoo BK, Kim M, Sasaki T, Melnikow J, Marcin JP. Economic evaluation of telemedicine for patients in ICUs. Crit Care Med. 2016;44(2):265–74.
46. Franzini L, Thomas E. Costs and effectiveness of tele-ICUs in reducing morbidity and mortality in intensive care units. J Med Econ. 2008;11(1):165–9.
47. Young MP, Birkmeyer JD. Potential reduction in mortality rates using an intensivist model to manage intensive care units. Eff Clin Pract. 2000;3(6):284–9.
48. Milstein A, Galvin RS, Delbanco SF, Salber P, Buck CR Jr. Improving the safety of health care: the leapfrog initiative. Eff Clin Pract. 2000;3(6):313–6.
49. Yoo BK, Kim M, Sasaki T, Hoch JS, Marcin JP. Selected use of telemedicine in intensive care units based on severity of illness improves cost-effectiveness. Telemed J E Health. 2018;24(1):21–36.
50. Lilly CM, Fisher KA, Ries M, Pastores SM, Vender J, Pitts JA, Hanson CW 3rd. A national ICU telemedicine survey: validation and results. Chest. 2012;142(1):40–7.
51. Kahn JM, Hill NS, Lilly CM, Angus DC, Jacobi J, Rubenfeld GD, Rothschild JM, Sales AE, Scales DC, Mathers JAL. The research agenda in ICU telemedicine: a statement from the Critical Care Societies Collaborative. Chest. 2011;140(1):230–8.
52. Lilly CM, Thomas EJ. Tele-ICU: experience to date. J Intensive Care Med. 2010;25(1):16–22.
53. Gabler NB, Ratcliffe SJ, Wagner J, Asch DA, Rubenfeld GD, Angus DC, Halpern SD. Mortality among patients admitted to strained intensive care units. Am J Respir Crit Care Med. 2013;188(7):800–6.
54. Anesi GL, Liu VX, Gabler NB, Delgado MK, Kohn R, Weissman GE, Bayes B, Escobar GJ, Halpern SD. Associations of ICU capacity strain with disposition and outcomes of patients with sepsis presenting to the emergency department. Ann Am Thorac Soc. 2018;15:1328.
55. Brown SE, Rey MM, Pardo D, Weinreb S, Ratcliffe SJ, Gabler NB, Halpern SD. The allocation of intensivists' rounding time under conditions of intensive care unit capacity strain. Am J Respir Crit Care Med. 2014;190(7):831–4.
56. Kahn JM, Le TQ, Barnato AE, Hravnak M, Kuza CC, Pike F, Angus DC. ICU telemedicine and critical care mortality: a national effectiveness study. Med Care. 2016;54(3):319–25.
57. Hua M, Halpern SD, Gabler NB, Wunsch H. Effect of ICU strain on timing of limitations in life-sustaining therapy and on death. Intensive Care Med. 2016;42(6):987–94.
58. Wagner J, Gabler NB, Ratcliffe SJ, Brown SE, Strom BL, Halpern SD. Outcomes among patients discharged from busy intensive care units. Ann Intern Med. 2013;159(7):447–55.
59. Weissman GE, Gabler NB, Brown SE, Halpern SD. Intensive care unit capacity strain and adherence to prophylaxis guidelines. J Crit Care. 2015;30(6):1303–9.
60. Howell MD. Managing ICU throughput and understanding ICU census. Curr Opin Crit Care. 2011;17(6):626–33.

Chapter 10
Tele-ICU Patient Experience: Focus on Family-Centered Care

Ann Marie Huffenberger, Rebecca Stamm, and Niels D. Martin

Introduction

In this chapter, we explore how telemedicine can enhance the patient and family experience in the critical care setting. We start with a historical context for patient-family-centered care. We then discuss why the patient experience has become a strategic imperative, not only as it relates to moral, ethical, and exceptional hospital organization practice but also as it relates to associated financial incentives. Thereafter, we examine guidelines for patient-family-centered care and propose how centralized telemedicine operations might support hospitals within policies and procedures that foster patient-family connected health in the intensive care setting. Additionally, we propose constructs of satisfaction that are applicable for telemedicine and therefore creditable in efforts to design an instrument to measure patient-family satisfaction within telemedicine intensive care operations. Next, we present a vignette of a successful telemedicine collaboration that resulted in a high degree of patient-family satisfaction. Finally, in closing, we promote centralized telemedicine centers to begin the work of coordinating connected health activities to enhance patient-family-centered care 24 hours a day, every day of the year.

A. M. Huffenberger (✉)
Penn Medicine Center for Connected Care, University of Pennsylvania Health System, Philadelphia, PA, USA
e-mail: Ann.Huffenberger@uphs.upenn.edu

R. Stamm
Clinical Nursing Systems, The Hospital of the University of Pennsylvania, University of Pennsylvania Health System, Philadelphia, PA, USA
e-mail: Rebecca.Stamm@uphs.upenn.edu

N. D. Martin
Division of Traumatology, Surgical Critical Care & Emergency Surgery, Perelman School of Medicine at the University of Pennsylvania, Philadelphia, PA, USA
e-mail: Niels.Martin@uphs.upenn.edu

M. A. Koenig (ed.), *Telemedicine in the ICU*,
https://doi.org/10.1007/978-3-030-11569-2_10

Framework for Family-Centered Care

The notion of patient-centered care was first introduced by the Institute of Medicine (IOM) in 2001 as a visionary goal for twenty-first century healthcare and wellness [1]. Almost a decade later, in 2010, when the Patient Protection and Affordable Care Act (ACA) was signed into law [2], organizations began committing resources to realizing opportunities to improve the patient experience of care. One of the major drivers of the commitment to improve the patient-family experience is the ACA's focus on quality, thereby linking pay-for-performance incentives to value-based purchasing (VBP) care models.

To transform our healthcare delivery system, to achieve better health outcomes with more thoughtfully spent dollars, the Centers for Medicare and Medicaid Services (CMS) established four domains of quality under hospital VBP: safety, efficiency and cost reduction, clinical care, and person and community engagement. Person and Community Engagement is CMS's fiscal year 2019 renaming of the Patient and Caregiver-Centered Experience of Care. The four domains of quality are measured by Hospital Consumer Assessment of Healthcare Providers and Systems (HCAHPS) scoring. The intent of the HCAHPS is to provide a standardized survey instrument and data collection methodology for measuring patients' perspectives on hospital care [3]. The HCAHPS is available for distribution through authorized vendors, such as Press Ganey Associates, who holds the primary portion of the market share [4]. The HCAHPS is broadly distributed following most adult, nonpsychiatric inpatient stays throughout the USA. The HCAHPS are openly reported for each participating hospital with benchmarks against state and national averages. CMS ranks hospital performance on the approved set of measures [5], grouped into the respective quality domains and weighted, as represented in Table 10.1.

Each of the eight dimensions listed in Table 10.1 under Person and Community Engagement has defined performance standards. These standards are dynamic measures with threshold and benchmark percentage values that have been associated with increasing incentives. Thus, under hospital VBP, CMS rewards hospitals with incentive payments for the quality of care provided to Medicare beneficiaries, including person and community engagement [5].

Financially and operationally, a crucial factor is how CMS funds the hospital VBP program. It should be known that CMS funds the hospital VBP program by reducing hospitals' base operating MS-DRG payments, which it has been doing since 2013 in an incremental fashion (Fig. 10.1). To illustrate the operational drive for hospitals to earn 100% VBP incentive funds, an example of net loss revenue is calculated with an 80% VBP funds earned (Fig. 10.2).

While the complexity of healthcare finances is a minor consideration in the day-to-day work of clinicians, it is imperative that clinicians have a foundational understanding of hospital VBP, the associated domains of quality, and the coupled measures and dimensions. In countless ways, the transition to value-based care has opened a window to boost the patient and family experience, and it is the catalyst for the role of telemedicine in this domain.

Table 10.1 Hospital value-based purchasing domains, measures, and weights

Safety – 25%	Efficiency and cost reduction – 25%	Clinical care – 25%	Person and community engagement – 25%
CDI: Clostridium difficile infection	MSPB: Medicare spending per beneficiary	MORT-30 AMI: Acute myocardial infection, 30 day mortality rate	Communication with nurses
CAUTI: Catheter-associated urinary tract infection		MORT-30 HF: Heart failure, 30-day mortality rate	Communication with doctors
CLABSI: Central line-associated bloodstream infection		MORT-30 PN: Pneumonia, 30 day mortality rate	Responsiveness of hospital staff
MRSA: Methicillin-resistant *Staphylococcus aureus* bacteremia		THA/TKA: Elective total hip and/or knee arthroplasty, complication rate	Communication about medications
SSI: Surgical site infection and abdominal hysterectomy			Hospital cleanliness and quietness
PC-01: Elective delivery prior to 39 weeks gestation			Discharge information
			Care transition
			Overall rating of hospital

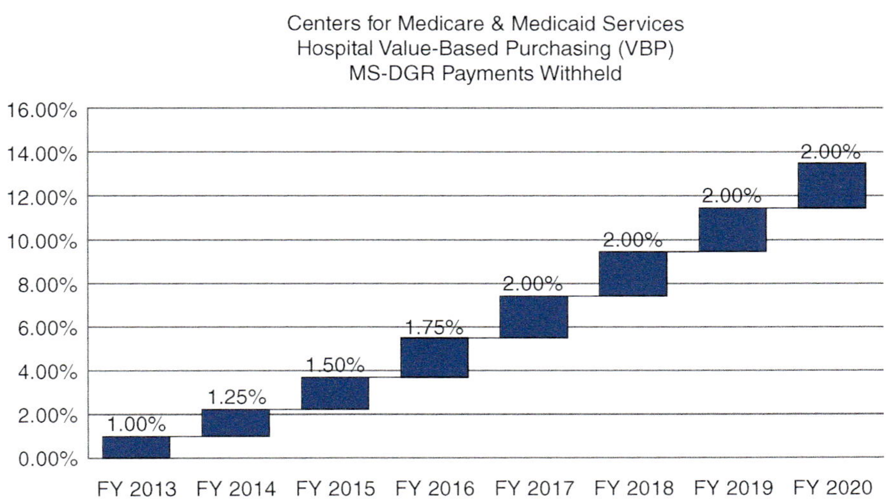

Fig. 10.1 Hospital value-based purchasing. Centers for Medicare and Medicaid Services payments withheld. Reductions in hospital base operating MS-DRG payments with an incrementally increasing proportion of lost revenue funds since 2013

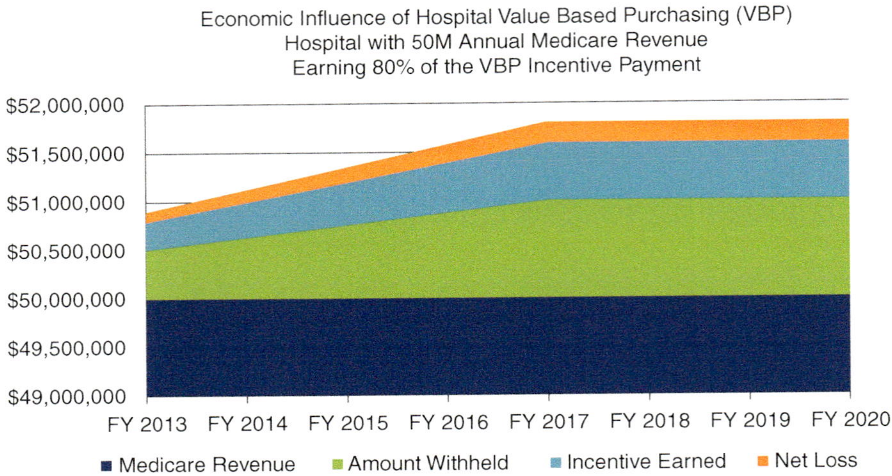

Fig. 10.2 The economic influence of hospital value-based purchasing on hospital revenue. As an example, for a hospital earning $50 million in annual Medicare revenue with the incremental MS-DRG annual payments withheld and 80% of the annual VBP incentive funds earned, there is still a net hospital loss

Business Case for Critical Care Medicine

Across the USA, the stakes are high for critical care medicine as some of the largest costs incurred in healthcare are associated with delivery of care in an ICU. Increased transparency in the ranking of hospital quality and outcome metrics has provided patients and families with metrics that were not readily available in past years. There is a strong economic drive to rank a notch better than competitors whether it be in cardiovascular, surgical, medical, trauma, neurological, transplant, or other clinical services.

Telemedicine obscures regional boundaries and introduces an opportunity for competitors to penetrate markets in which they were never considered a threat. For example, small community hospitals with geographically limited ICU resources can implement tele-ICU to provide real-time university intensivist expertise, thereby rendering 24/7 oversight of critical care through contemporary technology. From a patient-family perspective, tele-ICU can be a game changer as it promotes high-quality ICU services provided to the community in which they reside. In partnership, tele-ICU can rejuvenate market confidence in the community hospital [6] and, in that way, increase revenue [7] by supporting the right care, in the right place, at the right time [8], and – from a payer perspective – at the right cost. While there is much evidence pertaining to patient-family satisfaction with delivery of care in the ICU, there is a much less robust body of evidence showing how patient-family satisfaction relates to the delivery of the tele-ICU. An objective starting point for this chapter is to review the guidelines and evidence for family-centered care in the ICU and thereafter consider the opportunities and evidence of tele-ICU support for family-centered care goals.

Defining Family-Centered Care in the Intensive Care Unit

In 2017, the Society for Critical Care Medicine (SCCM) published guidelines for family-centered care in the ICU [9]. The SCCM guidelines were endorsed by prominent international organizations including the American College of Critical Care Medicine and the American Association of Critical Care Nurses [9]. SCCM defined family-centered care as "an approach to health care that is respectful of and responsive to individual families' needs and values" [9]. The SCCM established five areas of intervention for ICU teams to focus:

1. Family presence
2. Family support
3. Communication with family members
4. Consultations
5. Operational and environmental issues

SCCM asserted that there is likely some combination of interventions that improve family-centered care outcomes even further, although there is no evidence to report on the synergistic effects. While the 2017 family-centered care guidelines do not reference the role tele-ICU clinicians, in 2015, SCCM reviewed models of critical care associated with improved outcomes and recommended institutional support for quality improvement programs as well as institutional support for tele-ICU operations [10].

1.0 Family Presence

SCCM Guidelines for Family-Centered Care: Family Presence

SCCM guidelines for family-centered care	Opportunities for centralized tele-ICU operations
1.0 Family presence in the ICU	
1.1 Open or flexible family presence	Provide support to schedule on-demand family visits via secure telemedicine infrastructure that provides connectivity by one or more persons from one or more sites. Schedule family for teleconference into interdisciplinary team rounds. Schedule family for teleconference during or after resuscitation efforts
1.2 Participate in interdisciplinary team rounds	
1.3 Option to be present during resuscitation efforts	

There is wide acceptance that family presence is fundamentally key to family engagement and, when paired with educational programs in the ICU, open visitation has been shown to improve patient outcomes [11]. Ensuring an exceptional family-centered experience requires arming people with the skills, knowledge, and confidence they need to participate as informed partners [12]. Notably, there are stakeholder perspectives to consider in supporting an increased family presence in the ICU, and at the forefront of those stakeholders are the patient, family, ICU clinicians, and tele-ICU clinicians.

Patients who are critically ill are under stress receiving care that is largely focused on survival, and while patients have reported family visitation as a non-stressful experience that offers moderate levels of reassurance, comfort, and calming [13], they have also reported preference for some degree of visitation restrictions [14]. Patients have reported worrying about their visitor's travel time, disrupting their own rest, or intensifying their own pain during visitation [15]. Despite the evidence confirming that the nuances of visitation should be addressed in policies [16] and that ICUs should have procedures for patients to control visitation [16], there is also evidence emphasizing that flexible visiting policies lead to greater patient satisfaction with care [17].

For families, patient stays in the ICU can cause stress, anxiety, and depression [18]. Families have reported dissatisfaction with ICU care as it relates to poor communication, lack of comprehensible information, deficient emotional support upon entering an ICU room, and receipt of sensitive information in a location deemed not suitable [18]. Families have identified areas for ICU improvement that include better communication and provision for emotional support [19] to boost decision-making capacity and foster some degree of control over the care processes [20]. Notwithstanding, there is evidence to show flexible visitation increases family satisfaction and decreases family anxiety [21] and also promotes better communication that improves understanding of the patient care in ICU [22].

For ICU clinicians, open and flexible ICU visiting hours can be a challenge. It has been described that family presence negatively affects nursing workflows and that care in the ICU environment can be hindered [23]. Other nurses have conveyed that families can be obstacles in the provision of care, which validates their fears that open visitation policies increase workload demands [14]. Regardless of the challenges acknowledged, almost 80% of ICU nurses prefer unrestricted visitation policies [21], although it was reported in 2010 that 70% of hospitals had restricted family visitation policies [24]. Compounding the conflicts, evidence has shown that nurses enforced visitation policies inconsistently [16] and that discrepancies in the opinions and policies created contradictions and confusion between nurses and families [25].

While tele-ICU clinicians are physically located at a site distant from the ICU, seemingly absent and unaffected by the debate over flexible visitation, it is false to assume visitors do not affect the tele-ICU clinicians and their engagement with the ICU clinicians, patients, and families. While tele-ICU audio-video interactions use contemporary technology, there are human factors, such as situational awareness limitations, that can inhibit natural interaction between the virtual teams. For example, while tele-ICU clinicians can see and hear the activities occurring in and about the patient's bed, in practice, there are deficiencies in discerning activities that may be occurring outside the camera's view such as at the foot wall (directly under the camera mounting) and/or at the entrance to the ICU room (behind a curtain or door). Additionally, because there can be uncertainly in knowing whether the person in the room is a family, friend, neighbor, or foe, the richness and repetitiveness of tele-ICU to ICU interaction can be inhibited [26]. Without full situational context, tele-ICU clinicians are mindful of the risk in escalating anxieties or concerns at the bedside or, worse yet, breaching privacy or HIPPA considerations when communicating to clinicians with visitors in earshot.

For the aforementioned reasons, open and flexible visitation adds an element of adversity to the ICU and tele-ICU interactions. It has been described by some ICU nurses that tele-ICU can be intrusive and that it decreases patient privacy [27]. Tele-ICU nurses have expressed that ringing an audible doorbell when virtually entering an ICU room created frequent and repeated noise disturbance for patients and families. Communication between the patient, family, ICU clinicians, and tele-ICU clinicians can be challenging as evidenced by almost two-thirds of patients and families having reported that they were uninformed about existing tele-ICU operations [28]. For clinician colleagues, it is important to understand that without regular interaction, high levels of trust between team members cannot develop [29]. Trust is one of the predominant factors in successful collaboration, and consequently, one of the principal challenges in virtual team environments [29].

There are clear opportunities to optimize telemedicine utilization in supporting an open and flexible family presence. Tele-visitation is the virtual transportation of family to the bedside [30]. It is described as widely accepted by families and associated with reductions in patient stress [31]. Tele-visitation is promising for virtual participation during ICU rounds, and families have reported receptiveness [32]. Notably, tele-visitation can circumvent visitation challenges, which have been described as distance to hospitals [32], work or family obligations [32], timing of the hospital schedule [32], lack of personal time [33], and/or cost of travel [33].

2.0 Family Support

SCCM Guidelines for Family-Centered Care, Family Support

SCCM guidelines for family-centered care	Opportunities for centralized tele-ICU operations
2.0 Family support	
2.1 Option to assist in care of critically ill neonates	Provide support to schedule family access to ICU team members. For example, facilitate mutually agreeable timely family teleconference with the ICU attending physician, nurse, social worker, dietician, or pharmacist via secure telemedicine infrastructure that provides connectivity by one or more persons from one or more sites
2.2 Family education	
2.3 Peer-to-peer support in NICUs	
2.4 Family information about the ICU setting	
2.5 ICU diaries	
2.6 Reduce decisional conflict	
2.7 Improve communication	

Improving communication, providing education, and reducing decisional conflict are family-centered priorities to strengthen family support. While there is limited evidence that tele-ICU has played a direct role in supporting or educating ICU families, one might infer opportunity exists from the evidence of success outside of tele-ICU programs. Researchers [34] have illustrated 65 studies where telehealth had been used to support family caregivers. The types of patients varied but included patients with chronic disability [35], dementia [36], cancer [37], stroke [38], heart disease [39], spinal cord injury [40], brain injury [41], chronic disease [42], mental illness [43], and end-of-life care [44]. System tools included video conferencing, collaborative web-based platforms, interactive remote monitoring, and telephone technology such as phone calls or text messages, all of which were provided as a communication channel or social networking system to support families. Educational services have included family training by professional guides, videos, online chat sessions, emails, message boards, or resource rooms. Consultation services have included on-demand decision-making support for patients and families. Psychosocial and cognitive-behavioral therapy have provided problem-solving support and training to help families improve caregiving skills. Social services have provided long-term assistance with parenting skills to manage difficult children scenarios.

3.0 Communication with Family Members

SCCM Guidelines for Family-Centered Care, Communication with Family Members

SCCM guidelines for family-centered care	Opportunities for centralized tele-ICU operations
3.0 Communication with family members	
3.1 Interdisciplinary family conferences	Provide real-time collaboration with ICU care teams to support patient and family communication, provide tele-ICU guidance on clinical matters that reaffirm best practice, establish mutual trust, and reduce team conflict
3.2 Provide bereavement services	
3.3 Help clinicians to improve self-efficacy	

Tele-ICU teams have technology and clinical expertise that is aligned and positioned to facilitate virtual family conferences. While there is limited evidence that virtual family conferences occur in the ICU, there is evidence that virtual family conferences commonly occur outside of the ICU setting, with success. Family conferences have been shown to improve family satisfaction with communication, increase trust in clinicians, and reduce conflict between clinicians and family members [45]. Continual reassurance that a loved one is being cared for is associated with increased family satisfaction in the ICU [45].

Virtual interactive teleconferencing during patient rounds has been performed in a diversity of clinical settings with satisfied participants [46]. While patients and families appreciate and benefit from the personal interaction of in-person rounds, it is reported that tele-rounds have matched the performance of standard bedside rounds [47]. Additionally, almost two-thirds of queried patients preferred to be seen remotely by their own physician rather than by a covering colleague at the bedside [47]. Communication is centrally important to dying patients and their families. Virtual interactive teleconference has been used to support the family's decisions during the dying phases of life. If the family was not present at the patient's bedside when the death occurred, they have been, nonetheless, appreciative and relieved that the physician had a virtual presence during the patient's death [48].

Clinicians need family-centered training to facilitate clinician-family communication. For example, some organizations train clinicians to use the mnemonic "value" as an essential element to improve use of tele-ICU technologies for crucial discussions [49]. While the use of tele-ICU resources to enhance virtual family communication is progressive and not yet backed by strong evidence in practice, researchers have affirmed for decades that a key element of family-centered care is assurance that the design of processes for care delivery remains dynamic and that it is flexible, accessible, and responsive to family needs as they evolve over time [50].

4.0 Use of Consults

SCCM Guidelines for Family-Centered Care, Use of Consults

<table>
<tr><th colspan="2">4.0 Specific consultations</th></tr>
<tr><td>4.1 Palliative care consultation</td><td rowspan="6">Provide centralized support to schedule palliative care, ethical, spiritual, and other specialty team consultations on a secure telemedicine infrastructure that provides connectivity by one or more persons from one or more sites. Train tele-ICU to support patients and families by acting in the role of family navigator 24/7/365. Close the loop of communication with the ICU care teams by documenting interventions in the medical record</td></tr>
<tr><td>4.2 Ethics consultation</td></tr>
<tr><td>4.3 Learning materials for psychological support</td></tr>
<tr><td>4.4 Social workers within interdisciplinary teams</td></tr>
<tr><td>4.5 Family navigators to improve communication</td></tr>
<tr><td>4.6 Spiritual support</td></tr>
</table>

The use of specialty consults in the ICU is a recommendation for family-centered care; however, in practice, such consults are often impeded by resource limitations or logistical hurdles. Although technically feasible, there is no evidence to demonstrate tele-ICU operations have logically facilitated and/or coordinated palliative, ethics, social work, psychological, spiritual, or other care consults across the telemedicine infrastructures in which they operate on a day-to-day basis. However, palliative teleconsultation has been demonstrated in the home as support for traditional outpatient care in remotely monitoring and managing the symptoms of patients with advanced cancer [51]. As well, clinical ethics teleconsultation has been demonstrated on matters of transplant and donation ethics [52]. Furthermore, hospice teleconsultation has been established to improve access to high-quality support services at a lower cost [53]. Last, spiritual care teleconsultation has been endorsed in remote locations where few qualified professionals exist [54]. Researchers have affirmed that skepticism about whether these sensitive consultative services demand a more intimate level of care than can be provided by telemedicine have not been evidenced in practice [53].

There is evidence to show that a fully integrated nurse empowered to facilitate decision-making is a beneficial family-centered care intervention that it is well-received by ICU clinicians and families [55]. The role has been characterized as a family navigator [55]. When integrated with telemedicine, this role could have a broader scope of access than if assigned to a single ICU. This would separate the family navigator role from the bedside nurse, whose primary focus is on delivering care. It is reasonable to infer that tele-ICU nurses could function in the role of family navigator and could be more accessible as 24/7/365 virtual team members.

5.0 Operational and Environmental Issues

SCCM Guidelines for Family-Centered Care, Operational and Environmental Issues

<table>
<tr><th>SCCM guidelines for family-centered care</th><th>Opportunities for centralized tele-ICU operations</th></tr>
<tr><td colspan="2">5.0 Operational and environmental issues</td></tr>
<tr><td>5.1 Ensure standardized protocols</td><td rowspan="5">Uphold best practice protocols across ICU activities. Actively support ICU clinicians, guide, and mentor decision-making capacity to build confidence and trust. Highlight to families the benefits of tele-ICU as an added layer of clinical support available to loved ones. Encourage sleep-deprived families to go home and rest, offer options to coordinate on-demand telemedicine visits from home. Advocate for centralized monitoring of ICU environmental factors that negatively affect patient outcomes (noise, lighting, temp); remediate environmental issues in real time</td></tr>
<tr><td>5.2 Support nurses in their decision-making</td></tr>
<tr><td>5.3 Policies to promote family-centered care</td></tr>
<tr><td>5.4 Environmental hygiene practices</td></tr>
<tr><td>5.5 Consider family sleep deprivation</td></tr>
</table>

While there are fundamental differences in how tele-ICUs operate [56], the majority of tele-ICU operations aim to support the bedside clinicians in ICU decision-making and therefore do not have direct engagement with family members. However, standardized protocol adherence could assist in compliance with family-centered care goals. There is evidence to support that tele-ICU operations have had long-standing success in ensuring compliance with other ICU protocols, such as sepsis [57] or ventilator management [58].

Tele-ICUs can directly or indirectly play a role in monitoring ICUs for environmental hygiene practices to optimize the patient and family experience. This includes deployment of sensor devices to remotely monitor sound, light, noise, temperature, and other key environmental considerations in an ICU. Sound and light have been previously shown to be effectively monitored remotely in the ICU setting [59]. As hospitals implement policies to promote family-centered care in the ICU, administrators should consider how tele-ICU can support the healing environment by ensuring compliance with environmental policies.

Technological Considerations in Optimizing the Patient-Family Experience

Hospitals should consider the architectural framework of the infrastructure they deploy to provide tele-ICU services. From a family-centered care perspective, an open architecture is favorable. An adaptable infrastructure supports connectivity by one or more persons, from one or more sites, typically connected to cellular or Wi-Fi services [60]. With multiple people able to connect from the hospital, office, or mobile device, consultative services are easily enabled from inside or outside the constraints of a hospital network. This type of robust telemedicine functionality is superior in building the interactive, collaborative relationships that are necessary elements of patient and family communication success.

ICU Design Considerations in Optimizing the Patient-Family Experience

Besides the "behind the walls" architectural framework, there are a few other basic technology considerations that are key in optimizing the patient-family experience with tele-ICU services. Key elements include the location of the camera, quality of acoustics, and placement of the display monitor. The camera itself should have a comprehensive wide angle for initial viewing, which will mitigate situational awareness deficiencies for the tele-ICU team. Thereafter, the camera should effectively pan, tilt, and zoom (PTZ) to focus on specific areas, such as the patient or the ventilator.

Information technology technicians should work closely with the vendors and the clinicians to modify camera settings to optimize wide-angle view options. Camera settings may need to vary for ICU rooms that are smaller or larger and for ICU rooms that have ceiling height limitations. Deficiencies in the placement of the camera and/or the ability to provide wide-angle view options may negatively affect patient-family interaction. Camera placement and camera settings are an important element of patient-family experience with tele-ICU services.

Acoustics, including speaker placement, and configurations to diminish latency, minimize background noise, and provide echo suppression are all essential elements.

Speakers and microphones should be placed close to the ICU bed so that patients can hear and be heard. The same is necessary for families or bedside clinicians. Acoustics should provide high-quality performance that avoids any tendency for one person to speak over the other or introduces any hesitancy for another person to speak back. Acoustics should be practical enough to discern individual interactive communications in times when multiple individuals are speaking, such as during an emergency situation. Furthermore, acoustics should be effective in ICU rooms that have heightened levels of background noise related to equipment, television, radio, or other environmental considerations. Lastly, acoustics should be effective when joining multiple parties, from one or more sites, on a single telemedicine platform. Hospitals should not underestimate the finer intricacies of high-quality acoustic performance, in particular, in older ICUs that may have structural ceiling or physical plant limitations.

A third basic technology consideration is the display monitor placement. Ideally, clinicians can easily visualize each other without turning attention from the patient, and patients can easily visualize family members who tele-visit from home. It is common for the tele-ICU display monitor to be placed on the wall at the foot of the hospital bed. However, installation considerations should ensure room curtains, ceiling-mounted lift equipment, and other clinical equipment do not obstruct the display monitor. Alternate display methods include more than one display monitor, a mobile display monitor, and/or a display monitor that is integrated with the TV monitor in the ICU room.

Optimizing the Patient-Family Experience with Translation Services

There is evidence that non-English languages continue to grow as a core distribution of the national fabric in the USA [61]. For patients and families who do not speak the English language, there are commercially available certified medical interpreters, who provide integrated telemedicine language interpretation [62]. Hospitals that deploy these telemedicine services have access to on-demand interpretation, which reportedly provides high-level accuracy in more than 300 spoken languages. Additionally, some telemedicine services provide certified medical interpreters to communicate with deaf and hard-of-hearing patients, something that cannot be done with telephonic translation services.

Telemedicine Etiquette

The collaborative nature of virtual teams introduces an added layer of complexity to the ICU environment. To ensure the patient-family experience is top notch, hospitals must commit to addressing and resolving the challenges associated with virtual teams. In a recent publication, interviews conducted with ICU and tele-ICU teams, key operational and cultural barriers to success were identified as (a) unrealistic expectations of the operational capabilities, (b) lack of trust, (c) poorly defined leadership, and (d) lack of communication policies [63]. Tele-ICU nurses reported they spend 26% of their time communicating, although 15% received incorrect information from ICU nurses and 40% were not informed about a change in patient status [64]. Tele-ICU nurse attributes [65] that were rated extremely important included (a) proficiency with software tools, (b) effective listening skills, (c) ability to foster collaboration, and (d) ability to prioritize patient issues. While there is little evidence to define perfect tele-ICU etiquette, it is widely accepted that the yeoman's work in operationalizing a well-integrated tele-ICU is strengthening communication so that trust is established primarily. Researchers have advocated that tele-ICU operations consider unique strategies to ensure effective communication across multiple ICU cultures [66].

Strategies to Improve Tele-ICU Acceptance and Adoption

It is clear that successful integration of tele-ICU is a complex interprofessional responsibility. Researchers [67] have reported barriers to tele-ICU adoption such as significant variability in training, poor understanding of expectations and accountability, infrequent interaction, deficiencies in pivotal trust, and lack of resources dedicated to integration. Moreover, there is a perception that hospital executives are unaware of the scale of tele-ICU implementation which is a principal barrier to mobilizing resources to support the long-term integration of tele-ICU operations [67]. Actions to facilitate tele-ICU adaption include well-defined accountability, measures to enhance collegial teamwork, site visits to the tele-ICU, standardized clinical pathways, consensus on thresholds to engage the tele-ICU staff, distinct escalation protocols, collaboration on process improvement projects, and dedicated resources to support the integration of services long-term.

Despite the aforementioned challenges, signs of early adoption do occur fairly rapidly in many ICUs. With extensive access to patient data and remote ability to conduct real-time visualization, it is reasonable to infer that tele-ICU yields a unique and complementary form of clinical support. Notwithstanding, researchers have cautioned that resistance to an integrated tele-ICU solution degrades performance [68]. For that reason, it is advised that organizational stakeholders remain unambiguous with frontline clinicians about their support for the tele-ICU [69]. Hospitals should establish accountability for integrated operations and decide how deficiencies in collaboration will be tackled [70].

How to Measure Patient-Family Satisfaction with Tele-ICU Program?

As tele-ICU operations continue to grow, there is a necessity to ensure the means are available to evaluate the success of these programs. The challenge is that patient-family satisfaction remains loosely defined. Without agreed upon dimensions on

Table 10.2 Constructs proposed for defining patient-family satisfaction with telemedicine [71]

System quality	Healthcare		Net benefits	Information quality	Others
Ease of use	*Process*	*Outcomes*	Cost	Information completeness	Reuse
Reliability	Interaction with provider	Service quality	Ease of scheduling	Privacy	End user support
Environment	Treatment	Comparison of care quality	Duration		
	Relationship with provider	Medical outcomes	Provider benefits		
			Usefulness		

what constitutes satisfaction with telemedicine, there is difficultly interpreting and comparing results of studies that have been performed [71]. While Press Ganey Associates has developed a telemedicine survey for medical practices, with specialized questions to capture deeper insights around key components of virtual visits, their new survey offering is not specific nor applicable to tele-ICU operations. Researchers [71] have defined five constructs of patient-family satisfaction identified from existing measurement instruments that may be helpful in discerning telemedicine satisfaction, see Table 10.2. The next step in research will be validating which constructs of patient-family satisfaction are applicable in designing an instrument to measure patient-family satisfaction with tele-ICU operations.

Top Questions Hospital Administrators Should Ask

To ensure success with the implementation of tele-ICU operations, hospital administrators should consider the following questions, directly aimed at maximizing the utility of telemedicine for enhanced patient-family satisfaction:

1. A pervasive foundation of executive sponsorship is required and should include leadership from physicians, nursing, hospital operations, information technology, finance, regulatory affairs, change management, telemedicine, and critical care teams. Once the sponsor team is identified:
   (a) What are the tele-ICU patient-family satisfaction goals?
   (b) What metrics will be used to measure tele-ICU patient-family satisfaction?
   (c) What formulas will be used to capture the return on investment for tele-ICU patient-family satisfaction?
   (d) What resources are necessary to sustain the tele-ICU patient-family satisfaction goals?
2. Is there consensus to deploy an open telemedicine architecture that is adaptable to communication from inside or outside the constraints of a hospital network?

(a) In addition to 1a, 1b, 1c, and 1d, what resources are necessary to facilitate secure on-demand telemedicine encounters?

(i) What department is best prepared to manage the virtual care telemedicine facilitator team?

While the stated questions may seem apparent to sound business practice, it is worth mentioning that a number of tele-ICU programs across the USA have terminated operations because the goals, metrics, or formulas were deemed non-sustainable in an increasingly cost conscious market. Due diligence in planning and executing intelligently to broadly capture value is an operational imperative. Thereafter, value should be continuously reappraised in parallel with the reappraisal of workflows to ensure that operations remain agile enough to embrace new value propositions that present over time, such as Person and Community Engagement.

Vignette to Maximize Patient Satisfaction

Mr. Reilly was admitted to the ICU overnight. He and his wife enjoyed dinner and a movie earlier in the evening. After the meal, he developed hives but was not initially concerned as he had no known allergies. As the movie progressed, he became more concerned. As he felt his hives worsening and throat become irritated, he wondered if his airway was becoming compromised. He and his wife drove to the local emergency room where, unbeknownst to them, an urban academic medical center had long-standing tele-ICU operations. By the time Mr. Reilly was admitted to the ICU, he had become increasingly anxious over whether or not he was going to require intubation. Given the clinical presentation, the ICU nurse felt safest to preemptively intubate and protect his airway. However, the ICU physician recommended continuing medical management and holding off on intubation until clinically mandated. The patient's wife sensed disparity between the clinicians and became panic stricken with uncertainty over the best clinical approach. The bedside clinicians were unable to lessen tensions and summoned the tele-ICU intensivist for consultation. The tele-ICU intensivist led a virtual care team meeting. Perceived as an impartial expert, the tele-ICU intensivist reviewed the risks and benefits of immediate care options. After 20 minutes, Mr. Reilly and his wife felt calmer, better informed, and needed time to reflect on the situation. After another 10 minutes, Mr. Reilly and his wife requested another meeting with the tele-ICU intensivist. In the short time that had passed, they felt that the symptoms had worsened and early intubation should occur. The tele-ICU intensivist reassured Mr. Reilly and his wife that the ICU team would provide excellent care for them. All parties agreed to proceed with the procedure in a controlled setting. The tele-ICU team continued to monitor the situation overnight. In the day that followed, clinicians expressed gratitude for the collaboration. Upon transfer to the floor, Mr. Reilly and his wife expressed that the patient-family care experience was exceptional.

Conclusion

Tele-ICU operations have been an intricate part of hospital operations in the USA for over a decade. While these programs have been a mainstay of exceptional ICU care in past years, the future of connected health is logistically broader. Hospitals are adopting innovative solutions to achieve superior Person and Community Engagement outcomes. Tele-ICUs operating under a centralized hub, where ancillary resources are available, have full potential to support domains of community engagement. Maximizing the utility of telemedicine for enhanced family-centered care is imperative in supporting standardized, well-coordinated, high-quality, cost-efficient care that has become increasingly essential to hospitals operating in value-based care environments. FaceTime, Skype, WhatsApp, and other video solutions are increasingly popular for conferencing outside hospitals. Our patients, families, and clinicians need policies, procedures, and technologies to support in-hospital, on-demand connectivity. The connected health options for ICU care are endless: visitation, consultation, collaboration, harmonization, education, and care coordination – all virtually available to the patient, family, and clinical team at any time of the day or night, operationally coordinated by the centralized telemedicine resource team.

References

1. Institute of Medicine. Crossing the quality chasm: a new health system for the 21st century. Washington, DC: National Academy Press; 2001.
2. Affordable Care Act. Public Law 111–148—March 23, 2010. Retrieved from https://www.gpo.gov.
3. Centers for Medicare and Medicaid Services. What is the purpose of the HCAHPS Survey? 2017. Retrieved from https://www.cms.gov.
4. Zusman EE. HCAHPS replaces Press Ganey survey as quality measure for patient hospital experience. Neurosurgery. 2012;71(2):N21–4.
5. Centers for Medicare and Medicaid Services. Hospital value based purchasing. 2017. Retrieved from https://www.cms.gov.
6. Potter AJ, Natafgi N, Ullrich F, A Clinton MacKinney MS. Perceptions of the benefits of telemedicine in rural communities. Perspect Health Inf Manag. 2016;1:1–13.
7. Goedken CC, Moeckli J, Cram PM, Reisinger HS. Introduction of Tele-ICU in rural hospitals: changing organisational culture to harness benefits. Intensive Crit Care Nurs. 2017;40:51–6.
8. Institute of Health Care Improvement. The right care, right setting, and right time of hospital flow. 2017. Retrieved from http://www.ihi.org.
9. Davidson JE, Aslakson RA, Long AC, Puntillo KA, Kross EK, Hart J, et al. Guidelines for family-centered care in the neonatal, pediatric, and adult ICU. Crit Care Med. 2017;45(1):103–28.
10. Weled BJ, Adzhigirey LA, Hodgman TM, Brilli RJ, Spevetz A, Kline AM, et al. Critical care delivery: the importance of process of care and ICU structure to improved outcomes: an update from the American College of Critical Care Medicine Task Force on Models of Critical Care. Crit Care Med. 2015;43(7):1520–5.
11. Melnyk BM, Alpert-Gillis L, Feinstein NF, Crean HF, Johnson J, Fairbanks E, et al. Creating opportunities for parent empowerment: program effects on the mental health/coping outcomes of critically ill young children and their mothers. Pediatrics. 2004;113(6):e597–607.
12. Wynn JD. The value of exceptional patient experience. N C Med J. 2016;77(4):290–2.

13. Gonzalez CE, Carroll DL, Elliott JS, Fitzgerald PA, Vallent HJ. Visiting preferences of patients in the intensive care unit and in a complex care medical unit. Am J Crit Care. 2004;13(3):194–8.
14. Bélanger L, Bussières S, Rainville F, Coulombe M, Desmartis M. Hospital visiting policies–impacts on patients, families and staff: a review of the literature to inform decision making. J Hosp Admin. 2017;6(6):51.
15. Carroll DL, Gonzalez CE. Visiting preferences of cardiovascular patients. Prog Cardiovasc Nurs. 2009;24(4):149–54.
16. Smith L, Medves J, Harrison MB, Tranmer J, Waytuck B. The impact of hospital visiting hour policies on pediatric and adult patients and their visitors. JBI Database System Rev Implement Rep. 2009;7(2):38–79.
17. Azzil R, Bambi S. Open intensive care units: a feasible option? The opinions of patients, relatives and health care workers. Assist Inferm Ric. 2009;28(2):89–95.
18. Azoulay E, Pochard F, Kentish-Barnes N, Chevret S, Aboab J, Adrie C, et al. Risk of post-traumatic stress symptoms in family members of intensive care unit patients. Am J Respir Crit Care Med. 2005;171(9):987–94.
19. Schwarzkopf D, Behrend S, Skupin H, Westermann I, Riedemann NC, Pfeifer R, et al. Family satisfaction in the intensive care unit: a quantitative and qualitative analysis. Intensive Care Med. 2013;39(6):1071–9.
20. Osborn TR, Curtis JR, Nielsen EL, Back AL, Shannon SE, Engelberg RA. Identifying elements of ICU care that families report as important but unsatisfactory: decision-making, control, and ICU atmosphere. Chest. 2012;142(5):1185–92.
21. Simon SK, Phillips K, Badalamenti S, Ohlert J, Krumberger J. Current practices regarding visitation policies in critical care units. Am J Crit Care. 1997;6(3):210–7.
22. Roland P, Russell J, Richards KC, Sullivan SC. Visitation in critical care: processes and outcomes of a performance improvement initiative. J Nurs Care Qual. 2001;15(2):18–26.
23. Monroe M, Wofford L. Open visitation and nurse job satisfaction: an integrative review. J Clin Nurs. 2017;26:4868.
24. Institute for Patient- and Family-Centered Care. Changing hospital "visiting" and policies and practices: supporting family presence and participation. 2010. Retrieved from http://www.ipfcc.org.
25. Carlson B, Riegel B, Thomason T. Visitation: policy versus practice. Dimens Crit Care Nurs. 1998;17(1):40.
26. Hoonakker PL, Carayon P, McGuire K, Khunlertkit A, Wiegmann DA, Alyousef B, et al. Motivation and job satisfaction of tele-ICU nurses. J Crit Care. 2013;28(3):315–e13.
27. Mullen-Fortino M, DiMartino J, Entrikin L, Mulliner S, Hanson CW, Kahn JM. Bedside nurses' perceptions of intensive care unit telemedicine. Am J Crit Care. 2012;21(1):24–32.
28. Jahrsdoerfer M, Goran S. Voices of family members and significant others in the tele–intensive care unit. Crit Care Nurse. 2013;33(1):57–67.
29. Kauffmann D, Carmi G. How team leaders can use ICT to improve trust among virtual teams to increase collaboration. Int J Eng Innov Technol. 2014;3(9):204–21.
30. Nicholas B. Televisitation: virtual transportation of family to the bedside in an acute care setting. Perm J. 2013;17(1):50.
31. Yang NH, Dharmar M, Hojman NM, Sadorra CK, Sundberg D, Wold GL, et al. Videoconferencing to reduce stress among hospitalized children. Pediatrics. 2014;134(1):e169–75.
32. Stelson EA, Carr BG, Golden KE, Martin N, Richmond TS, Delgado MK, Holena DN. Perceptions of family participation in intensive care unit rounds and telemedicine: a qualitative assessment. Am J Crit Care. 2016;25(5):440–7.
33. Parsapour K, Kon AA, Dharmar M, McCarthy AK, Yang HH, Smith AC, et al. Connecting hospitalized patients with their families: case series and commentary. Int J Telemed Appl. 2011;2011:10.
34. Chi NC, Demiris G. A systematic review of telehealth tools and interventions to support family caregivers. J Telemed Telecare. 2015;21(1):37–44.

35. Eisdorfer C, Czaja SJ, Loewenstein DA, Rubert MP, Argüelles S, Mitrani VB, Szapocznik J. The effect of a family therapy and technology-based intervention on caregiver depression. The Gerontologist. 2003;43(4):521–31.
36. Dang S, Remon N, Harris J, Malphurs J, Sandals L, Cabrera AL, Nedd N. Care coordination assisted by technology for multiethnic caregivers of persons with dementia: a pilot clinical demonstration project on caregiver burden and depression. J Telemed Telecare. 2008;14(8):443–7.
37. Chih MY, DuBenske LL, Hawkins RP, Brown RL, Dinauer SK, Cleary JF, Gustafson DH. Communicating advanced cancer patients' symptoms via the internet: a pooled analysis of two randomized trials examining caregiver preparedness, physical burden, and negative mood. Palliat Med. 2013;27(6):533–43.
38. Taylor DM, Cameron JI, Walsh L, McEwen S, Kagan A, Streiner DL, Huijbregts MP. Exploring the feasibility of videoconference delivery of a self-management program to rural participants with stroke. Telemed e-Health. 2009;15(7):646–54.
39. Schwarz KA, Mion LC, Hudock D, Litman G. Telemonitoring of heart failure patients and their caregivers: a pilot randomized controlled trial. Prog Cardiovasc Nurs. 2008;23(1):18–26.
40. Elliott TR, Brossart D, Berry JW, Fine PR. Problem-solving training via videoconferencing for family caregivers of persons with spinal cord injuries: a randomized controlled trial. Behav Res Ther. 2008;46(11):1220–9.
41. Hauber RP, Jones ML. Telerehabilitation support for families at home caring for individuals in prolonged states of reduced consciousness. J Head Trauma Rehabil. 2002;17(6):535–41.
42. Vincent C, Reinharz D, Deaudelin I, Garceau M, Talbot LR. Public telesurveillance service for frail elderly living at home, outcomes and cost evolution: a quasi experimental design with two follow-ups. Health Qual Life Outcomes. 2006;4(1):41.
43. Ozkan B, Erdem E, Ozsoy SD, Zararsiz G. Effect of psychoeducation and telepsychiatric follow up given to the caregiver of the schizophrenic patient on family burden, depression and expression of emotion. Pak J Med Sci. 2013;29(5):1122.
44. Oliver DP, Demiris G. Comparing face-to-face and telehealth-mediated delivery of a psychoeducational intervention: a case comparison study in hospice. Telemed e-Health. 2010;16(6):751–3.
45. Stapleton RD, Engelberg RA, Wenrich MD, Goss CH, Curtis JR. Clinician statements and family satisfaction with family conferences in the intensive care unit. Crit Care Med. 2006;34(6):1679–85.
46. Mair F, Whitten P. Systematic review of studies of patient satisfaction with telemedicine. BMJ. 2000;320(7248):1517–20.
47. Ellison LM, Nguyen M, Fabrizio MD, Soh A, Permpongkosol S, Kavoussi LR. Postoperative robotic telerounding: a multicenter randomized assessment of patient outcomes and satisfaction. Arch Surg. 2007;142(12):1177–81.
48. Low JA, Beins G, Lee KK, Koh E. Last moments of life: can telemedicine play a role? Palliat Support Care. 2013;11(4):353–5.
49. Cook D, Rocker G. Dying with dignity in the intensive care unit. N Engl J Med. 2014;370(26):2506–14.
50. Johnson BH. Family-centered care: four decades of progress. Fam Syst Health. 2000;18(2):137.
51. Hennemann-Krause L, Lopes AJ, Araújo JA, Petersen EM, Nunes RA. The assessment of telemedicine to support outpatient palliative care in advanced cancer. Palliat Support Care. 2015;13(4):1025–30.
52. Bramstedt K. The use of telemedicine for clinical ethics consults pertaining to donation and transplant: abstract# B837. Transplantation. 2014;98:819.
53. Whitten P, Cook DJ, Doolittle G. An analysis of provider perceptions for telehospice™. Am J Hosp Palliat Med. 1998;15(5):267–74.
54. Smith B. Mission and leadership – details of encounter are key in telespiritual care. 2015. Retrieved https://www.chausa.org/.
55. Torke AM, Wocial LD, Johns SA, Sachs GA, Callahan CM, Bosslet GT, et al. The family navigator: a pilot intervention to support intensive care unit family surrogates. Am J Crit Care. 2016;25(6):498–507.

56. Lilly CM, Thomas EJ. Tele-ICU experience to date. J Intensive Care Med. 2010;25(1):16–22.
57. Rincon TA, Manos EL, Pierce JD. Telehealth intensive care unit nurse surveillance of Sepsis. CIN Comput Inform Nurs. 2017;35(9):459–64.
58. Goedken CC, Moeckli J, Cram PM, Reisinger HS. Introduction of Tele-ICU in rural hospitals: changing organizational culture to harness benefits. Intensive Crit Care Nurs. 2017;40:51–6.
59. Voigt LP, Reynolds K, Mehryar M, Chan WS, Kostelecky N, Pastores SM, Halpern NA. Monitoring sound and light continuously in an intensive care unit patient room: a pilot study. J Crit Care. 2017;39:36–9.
60. Reynolds HN, Bander JJ. Options for tele-intensive care unit design centralized versus decentralized and other considerations it is not just a another black sedan. Crit Care Clin. 2015;31(2):335–50.
61. Ryan E. Language use in the United States: 2011. American community survey reports. 2013. Retrieved from https://www.census.gov.
62. Scamman K. Telehealth: the importance of medical interpreters in telemedicine. 2018. Retrieved via https://telelanguage.com.
63. Wilkes MS, Marcin JP, Ritter LA, Pruitt S. Organizational and teamwork factors of tele–intensive care units. Am J Crit Care. 2016;25(5):431–9.
64. McGuire K, Carayon P, Hoonakker P, Khunlertkit A, Wiegmann D. Communication in the tele-ICU. In: Proceedings of the human factors and ergonomics society annual meeting (Vol 54, no 19, pp 1586–90). Los Angeles: Sage Publications; 2010
65. Goran SF. A new view: tele–intensive care unit competencies. Crit Care Nurse. 2011;31(5):17–29.
66. Hoonakker PL, Pecanac KE, Brown RL, Carayon P. Virtual collaboration, satisfaction, and trust between nurses in the tele-ICU and ICUs: results of a multilevel analysis. J Crit Care. 2017;37:224–9.
67. Moeckli J, Cram P, Cunningham C, Reisinger HS. Staff acceptance of a telemedicine intensive care unit program a qualitative study. J Crit Care. 2013;28(6):890–901.
68. Khunlertkit A, Carayon P. Contributions of tele–intensive care unit (TeleICU) technology to quality of care and patient safety. J Crit Care. 2013;28(3):315–e1. https://doi.org/10.1016/j.jcrc.2012.10.005.
69. Sapirstein A, Lone N, Latif A, Fackler J, Pronovost PJ. Tele ICU: paradox or panacea? Best Pract Res Clin Anaesthesiol. 2009;23(1):115–26. https://doi.org/10.1016/j.bpa.2009.02.001.
70. American Association of Critical Care. TeleICU nursing practice guidelines. 2018. Retrieved from http://www.aacn.org.
71. Garcia R, Olayele A, Han W. Defining dimensions of patient satisfaction with telemedicine an analysis of existing measurement instruments. In: Proceedings of the 50th Hawaii international conference on system sciences; 2017, January.

Chapter 11
Cost-Benefit Analysis of Implementing Telemedicine in the ICU

Sanjay Subramanian and Christopher M. Palmer

What Is the Cost of Implementing a New Tele-ICU Program?

Implementing any technology solution entails added cost for the healthcare system. Hospitals looking to implement such solutions should carefully review the features and functionalities of all hardware, software, and associated costs and factor that into the use cases prior to purchasing decisions. Although the models of tele-ICU vary, fundamentally, costs can be broken down into the major components outlined below.

Costs related to technology equipment include the hardware and software installation associated with the operation. The hardware costs can vary widely depending on the choice of equipment and the operational structure of the tele-ICU. In one of the most commonly used tele-ICU systems (Philips eICU®), the hardware costs include fixed mounted high-definition cameras in patient rooms, cabling costs for the cameras, desktop computers for the remote physician/nursing workstations, multiple monitors for each workstation, and T1 lines for assured connectivity. The core audio-video technology component in the Philips system is a non-negotiable cost since it is tightly integrated with their proprietary software on the back end. Upgrades for the audio-video service may be required periodically and will result in additional costs.

S. Subramanian (✉)
Division of Critical Care, Department of Anesthesiology, Washington University School of Medicine in St. Louis, St. Louis, MO, USA
e-mail: sanjay.subramanian@wustl.edu

C. M. Palmer
Department of Anesthesiology, Division of Critical Care, Division of Emergency Medicine, Washington University School of Medicine in St. Louis, St. Louis, MO, USA
e-mail: cmpalmer@wustl.edu

M. A. Koenig (ed.), *Telemedicine in the ICU*,
https://doi.org/10.1007/978-3-030-11569-2_11

Additionally, some tele-ICU programs may use robots (e.g., InTouch Systems®) or other commercial mobile carts to facilitate care deliver in non-ICU locations. These carts consist of audio-video interfaces, interfaces for diagnostic equipment like stethoscopes, and software interface to integrate into the parent tele-ICU software (such as Philips eCARE® software). Programs which utilize devices such as tablets/iPad (Apple Corp®, Samsung Corp®) in lieu of fixed cameras and desktop workstations will likely incur lower costs than the above fixed camera "eICU" model. Software costs depend on the type of system used. The commonly used Philips eCARE® software is a bundled product which includes licensing fees for a fixed number of beds, software integration costs associated with data extraction from the EMR, bedside patient monitoring devices, costs for utilizing proprietary risk adjustment software (APACHE® Cerner Corp), and server costs.

In addition, technology costs may also include commercial software solutions to facilitate communication (video/text/audio) between care professionals for ongoing workflow and operational issues. Examples of such solutions include Cisco Jabber®, Vidyo®, etc. An illustrative cost example for some of the IT/IS components of setting up a Philips eICU is given below:

- Virtual servers for eCare: $250,000
- Charter Internet: $26,000 per year (as of 2016)
- In room audio-video equipment: $7500 per room, installation at additional cost
- Mobile carts: $12,000 each
- Sit/stand desk, electronic: $5000 each
- Computer workstations: $1300 each
- Monitors: $ 280 each
- UPS for workstations: $300 per desk

Staffing costs typically depend on the structure of the tele-ICU care delivery model. The predominant model in the marketplace currently consists of a "hub" or a "core" which consists of nurses and physicians assisted by support staff who are involved in remote care delivery. The number of nursing staff varies based on the number of patients within that tele-ICU system. Typically, ratios are one nurse for every 30–50 patients. The number of physicians employed at the core again is based on the number of beds covered by the system. On average, the physician to patient ratio is 1:100, with the physician being a highly leveraged resource. This staffing ratio will of course depend on the acuity of the ICUs being covered, and high acuity patients can be expected to have lower provider-to-patient ratios. Nursing wages are determined locally and subject to organizational wage standards and incentives. Additionally, nursing supervisors or charge nurses may be needed to assist with administrative tasks, nursing schedules, and assignments. In specific cases, additional nurses may be employed to assist with specialized tasks such sepsis surveillance, best practice audits, or APACHE scoring.

Support staff may consist of staff to assist with answering calls for the remote location and helping triage incoming calls from various locations and information technology staff to assist with software/hardware maintenance, support, and troubleshooting. The wages for the support staff vary and are determined by local wage standards. Additionally, database analysts and administrators may be employed by tele-ICUs to assist with data collection, analysis, creation of a database, database server setup, and maintenance. Administrative personnel may be hired by tele-ICU systems to assist with staff management, physician licensure, finance and accounting, contract negotiations, strategy, and business development.

Physicians who provide tele-ICU care are most commonly paid an hourly salary rate between $180 and $225 per hour. If a physician is solely employed to provide tele-ICU services, additional costs would include usual benefits such as healthcare plan funding, retirement plan funding, disability and life insurance premiums, etc. It may be noted that current market forces favor at least a 25% additional incentive for tele-ICU services compared to bedside ICU services for physicians. In addition, nighttime coverage is paid out at a premium rate compared to daytime services. Over the last few years, given the concerns over sustainability of nighttime coverage models, tele-ICU nighttime coverage is sometimes outsourced to overseas physician staffing agencies located in Israel, India, Eastern Europe, or Africa where the time difference allows those physicians to work during daylight hours. The staffing costs for these outsourced models are dependent on prevailing wages for the country.

Other costs include contractual costs for vendors and licensing for applications and broadband coverage. Contractual relationships with technology vendors represent a common ongoing cost for tele-ICUs. The ongoing costs related to technology consist of support and maintenance costs for hardware and software platforms associated with the tele-ICU system. Contractual relationships with provider networks may be another source of ongoing cost, depending on the staffing model. Some tele-ICU systems may occasionally need to outsource providers such as physicians. Broadband, licensing, and IT-related costs represent yet another cost for tele-ICU systems. In the commonly used eICU model, dedicated T1 lines and broadband Internet access are required to keep all computer systems operational, and the yearly cost for this is roughly $26,000.

What Are the Financial Benefits of Implementing a New Tele-ICU Program?

In the absence of a defined insurer reimbursement model for care delivery, revenue sources for a tele-ICU system depend entirely on the organizational structure of the system/network and variable contractual relationships between entities. A few different revenue models appear to currently exist.

Fee-for-service remains the most common type of revenue model where recipients of the tele-ICU care delivery enter into a fee-for-service contract which is either based on the number of ICU beds being serviced or the number of ICU admissions. In the former, the tele-ICU provider charges an annual fee per bed to which the service is provided. The fee is essentially a pass-through cost incurred by the tele-ICU service provider for the expense of setting up the technology infrastructure to enable care delivery and other operational expenses, with an added markup to maintain profitability. These costs are reportedly between $20 and $30,000 per ICU bed for services provided using the Philips platform.

Shared savings models represent an alternative payment model. Conceptually, a shared savings model can be implemented wherein the tele-ICU provider would be paid a percentage of any demonstrated cost savings due to reduction in complications and reduction in ICU length of stay. It is unclear how prevalent this model currently is among tele-ICU providers, however.

In pay-for-value arrangements, tele-ICU providers may also enter into at-risk contracts, where payment is tied to achieving defined operational targets. While this model is theoretically attractive, there are many variables that may determine the outcome of interest, not all of which directly fall under the purview of the tele-ICU provider. Such a model is likely to be most successful when the tele-ICU functions as the sole provider for comprehensive ICU services with full control of upstream and downstream ICU care processes.

Payment can also be tied to increased ICU bed occupancy. As reported in various studies below, a reduction in ICU length of stay following implementation of tele-ICU creates added capacity for ICU patients, thus reducing the number of patients who may be getting transferred to outside facilities due to lack of ICU beds. The added ICU occupancy can elevate the case mix index for the hospital which in turn has a positive effect on reimbursement. Reducing ICU length of stay through tight management of care processes and efficient throughput driven by the tele-ICU system can lead to a reduction in ICU length of stay [1]. Given that ICU charges are not reimbursed fully (e.g., Medicare reimburses about 83% of ICU charges), a reduction in length of stay can reduce the losses incurred from ICU stays for hospitals.

Reduction in ICU harm and medical errors that incur financial penalties can also be a source of shared savings arrangements. Cost avoidance due to reduction in ICU complications, reduction in length of stay due to appropriate bed utilization, and improved decision support could justify the investment in tele-ICU [2, 3]. As reviewed below, these benefits are contingent upon a very deliberate integration of tele-ICU services with bedside services, allowing both to function cohesively to achieve strategic goals. An example is the "logistics center" approach by Lilly et al. which allowed for greater ICU bed utilization, driving up revenues and contribution margin [4]. The cost avoidance reported in the literature has varied and to a large extent will depend on the baseline performance of the units across which tele-ICU is implemented. High-performance institutions which already operate on the far end of the performance spectrum may see less benefits. Furthermore, once the processes that help drive down complications and improve compliance with best practices are hardwired, the incremental benefit will be expected to decrease over time.

Review of Published Studies on Cost-Benefit Analysis in Tele-ICU Programs

Cost-benefit analysis of ICU telemedicine implementation is not straightforward, as will be highlighted in the studies to follow. A few recurring issues in methodology should be considered whenever analyzing published results, whether they are pro/

con tele-ICU cost-effectiveness. The first revolves around the heterogeneity of case definitions of ICU telemedicine in the literature. Currently there is no standard definition for ICU telemedicine. There are many different models (centralized vs. decentralized being the most common), and within those models, there are a plethora of remote monitoring capabilities that will impact the effectiveness of tele-ICU care. This is an important consideration to keep in mind when evaluating the literature and applying the results to your institution. The second involves transparent, accurate, and comprehensive cost reporting. Many published studies lack all three of these elements, making it challenging to draw strong conclusions. Additional points to consider are tele-ICU monitoring of academic versus community hospitals or a mixture of both. Variability in acuity and volume of ICU patients monitored can bias results related to mortality and length of stay. Cost projections based off these models will then need to be accounted for across different health systems if their patient population is not similar.

One of the first published studies to analyze ICU telemedicine implementation reported on cost analysis in addition to patient care outcomes. The study was conducted by Rosenfeld et al. and published in *Critical Care Medicine* in 2000 [5]. The design of the study was an observational time series triple cohort study. The purpose of this study was to compare the prospective 16-week intervention period with two retrospective baseline periods of equal duration. One baseline was used to account for seasonal variations in critical care, and the other was used to account for any time-related, unit-based process improvement changes. The study site was a ten-bed surgical ICU in a large academic hospital. General medical patients, cardiac surgery, and transplant surgery patients were not included. Exclusion criteria were as follows: age <16, ICU stay <4 hours, transfer from ICU to another hospital, and missing APACHE data. The study ICU was an open unit without onsite ICU intensivist coverage. Daily ICU care was provided by house staff in addition to a surgical attending.

The intervention involved four intensivists providing patient care exclusively from their homes 24/7 for a 16-week period. Necessary equipment including cameras for remote care were installed in each ICU room and in the homes of the four intensivists. The intensivists rounded on "select patients," either as a consultant or a physician providing management services. Daily virtual rounds and frequent patient reviews were performed by the ICU physicians. Urgent and emergent communication with the bedside team was carried out as needed. The results of the study showed lower ICU mortality and ICU length of stay during the intervention period compared to the two baseline periods. In addition, the APACHE III observed/predicted ICU mortality and length of stay ratios were lower for the intervention period. Cost data are outlined in Table 11.1. Compared to both baselines, ICU-based costs were reduced by roughly 25–30%. Total hospital costs were also less, but this was not found to reach statistical significance. A large portion of the cost reduction was related to the decrease in complications noted in the intervention period.

Although the cost data certainly was significant in favor of ICU telemedicine, several factors should be considered in this study. First, given this study was published nearly 20 years ago, it was mostly a proof of concept design for ICU

Table 11.1 ICU cost data

	Baseline 1 ($)	Baseline 2 ($)	Intervention ($)	Intervention vs. baseline	Intervention vs. baseline 2
ICU-based					
Inpatient costs	7965 ± 8669	8922 ± 19,936	6273 ± 6330	0.79 (0.0255)	0.70 (0.0777)
Professional fees	3192 ± 2228	3317 ± 4349	2133 ± 1746	0.67 (0.0001)	0.64 (0.0005)
Total costs	11,157 ± 10,168	12,239 ± 23,448	8417 ± 7554	0.75 (0.0022)	0.69 (0.0308)
Hospital-based					
Inpatient costs	13,692 ± 13,688	15,211 ± 25,294	12,690 ± 13,023	0.93 (0.4438)	0.83 (0.2147)
Professional fees	4457 ± 3265	4577 ± 5129	3244 ± 2536	0.73 (0.0001)	0.71 (0.0012)
Total costs	18,149 ± 16,102	19,788 ± 29,809	15,935 ± 15,033	0.88 (0.1513)	0.81 (0.1077)

ICU = intensive care unit
Values are mean dollars (entire ICU and hospital stay) ± SD. Comparisons between intervention and baseline periods show ratio of costs, with *p* values in parentheses

telemedicine. Commercial technology and electronic medical records that are widely used today were not available at that time. The design of the study was not to prove cost-effectiveness given the limited scale of developed ICU telemedicine technology. Second, although the authors mentioned in the methods section that technology costs were accounted for, it is not readily apparent in the cost data tables or supplement sections, making conclusions on cost savings challenging. Results would also have to be taken into context given this was a single center study in a small, surgical ICU, in an academic environment where select patients were monitored by the tele-intensivists without specific mention of selection criteria.

A follow-up by Breslow et al. was published in *Critical Care Medicine* in 2004 [6]. The authors instituted an ICU telemedicine program with commercial technology in part to address some of the flaws in the initial study and build on the proof of concept established previously. The study design was a before-and-after trial comparing a 6-month intervention period to randomly selected patients from the year prior. Risk adjustment using APACHE scoring was used to compare the groups across the different time periods. An off-site, centralized model for patient monitoring was established (referred to as the eICU), and monitored patients were located in two ICUs (one medical ICU and one surgical ICU) at a large tertiary care teaching hospital. The bedside coverage model was slightly different between the two units. Nearly all medical ICU patients were staffed by an intensivist, while roughly 35% of surgical ICU patients had an intensivist consulting. The ICU telemedicine service monitored all patients admitted to these units during the intervention period, and the eICU was staffed 19 hours/day (noon–7 AM) when the bedside intensivist was often not present. The level of intervention of the eICU was determined a priori (categories 1–4 of involvement), but bedside teams could not completely "opt out."

This centralized eICU was similar to many tele-ICU models currently in use, with advanced audio-video equipment, access to real-time patient data, and computerized decision support tools. Like the previous study, overall ICU mortality and ICU length of stay decreased during the intervention period. ICU mortality was down approximately 25%, and ICU length of stay decreased by nearly 16%. More robust financial data were captured and are illustrated in Table 11.2. This financial analysis was performed by an independent firm using financial data provided by the hospital. ICU variable costs per case decreased by $2500 or roughly 25%. A significant increase in monthly contribution margin was seen, totaling nearly $525,000. Over a 6-month time period, this equated to $3.14 million of financial benefit. ICU telemedicine hardware/software costs and eICU physician staffing cost roughly $600,000 over the same 6-month period.

Although it was not completely clear from the data presented if this amount was factored into the variable costs, a sizeable financial gain is still apparent even if it was not. How exactly this ICU telemedicine program generated a large financial impact is likely multifactorial. One theory is that variable costs were reduced secondary to a decrease in length of stay, and lower daily ICU ancillary costs were also achieved. Factored into this equation would also be a reduction in complications observed which would decrease costs and length of stay. Furthermore, with increased bed availability, there was an increase in case volume, increasing the total contribution margin. This study was a significant step toward a better understanding of

Table 11.2 Cost and revenue data

	All patients		MICU		SICU	
	Base	Intervention	Base	Intervention	Base	Intervention
Average ICU daily cost	$1648	$1411	$1303	$1041	$1933	$1756
Average floor daily cost	$389	$366	$387	$394	$390	$340
Average case cost[a]	$10,444	$7871	$10,926	$8494	$9698	$6528
Average case revenue	$17,276	$18,510	$17,281	$16,950	$17,272	$19,964
Average case contribution margin	$6832	$10,639	$6355	$8456	$7574	$13,436
Cases per month	116.4[b]	124	52.6	59.8	63.8[b]	64.2
Contribution margin per month	$795,245	$1,319,236	$334,273	$505,669	$483,221	$862,591

MICU medical intensive care unit, *SICU* surgical intensive care unit, *ICU* intensive care unit
[a]Calculated from average daily ICU and floor costs and average ICU and floor lengths of stay
[b]SICU during the baseline period had ten beds

modern-day ICU telemedicine program capabilities and cost-effectiveness. Although there were considerable strengths to this study, weaknesses related to vendor funding, as well as author affiliation with the vendor as a conflict of interest, should be noted. Similarly, as is problematic with all ICU telemedicine studies, a causal relationship is challenging to prove given before-and-after study designs. However, conducting a randomized controlled trial of tele-ICU implementation would be challenging given the culture change in each ICU required and the variability that exists between different hospitals and ICUs.

Given the limited quantity of ICU telemedicine cost-effectiveness studies to date, Yoo et al. published an intriguing article in *Critical Care Medicine* in 2016 using a simulation model to perform a cost-effectiveness analysis [7]. Recognizing that capital startup costs for ICU telemedicine can be exorbitant (up to $75–100,000 per ICU bed), it is understandable that hospital administrators may be reluctant to institute such a program without predictive financial tools. The purpose of this study was to provide an economic evaluation using a hypothetical model of patients monitored with ICU telemedicine and those without. Their primary objectives were to determine incremental cost-effectiveness in dollars and incremental cost-benefit (in quality-adjusted life-years [QALYs]). Using QALYs supports the theory that an ICU telemedicine program can impact more than just patient survival but also enhance their quality of life post ICU discharge [8]. These hypothetical results could potentially impact both policy decision-makers (federal and state payers) and hospital systems exploring the financial impact of starting an ICU telemedicine program.

In order to perform a simulation analysis, data based on prior published literature was used to construct parameters to run the simulation model. Two separate analyses were run: a cost-effectiveness analysis and a break-even analysis. The cost-effectiveness analysis examined whether the incremental cost-effectiveness ratio (ICER) of ICU telemedicine exceeded a $100,000 threshold (not cost-effective) or was less than zero (indicating cost savings). This threshold is often cited in the medical literature as a reasonable target for determining the cost-effectiveness of an intervention, albeit it is a subjective determination [7]. The break-even analysis then analyzed the threshold values for key predetermined parameters. Their simulation model results estimated that tele-ICU had an approximate ICER of $45–50,000 per QALY compared to an ICU without telemedicine. In simplified terms, the hypothetical model estimated that tele-ICU extends life with a perfect health status by 1 year to a single ICU patient at a cost of $45–50,000 [7]. Running nearly 1000 simulations resulted in wide confidence intervals, but nearly 67% of all iterations resulted in an ICER below $100,000, indicating cost-effectiveness.

The break-even analysis reported several parameters where ICU telemedicine would be considered cost-effective. Examples included per-patient per-hospital stay tele-ICU operation cost <$1560 and baseline ICU mortality without telemedicine that was greater than 6.3%. This hypothetical simulation model adds value to the existing literature regarding tangible figures and endpoints to which interested parties in ICU telemedicine can consider during the decision-making process. Limitations of this study include the assumptions that are made from secondary data. The model utilized the few existing ICU telemedicine cost reporting studies to create cost estimations, some of which are of questionable quality and applicability. This in turn makes interpreting and applying the simulated cost-effectiveness analysis more challenging. Furthermore, the model was based on a centralized system of ICU telemedicine using data extracted from telemedicine programs using Philips eICU technology. Any hospital system with plans to operate under a different model or use non-Philips software technology would not be able to apply these projections, albeit costs would likely be lower and favor tele-ICU implementation. Finally, this simulation model cannot account for all variables that a tele-ICU program may experience, such as changes in case volume or patient transfers. These are critical elements that any healthcare leader would need to consider during the evaluation process.

One particular study that focused exclusively on ICU telemedicine cost-effectiveness was published in 2017 by Lilly et al. [4]. This publication was a detailed financial analysis of a tele-ICU program over time. In addition, a description of a logistics center operated by the tele-ICU and the impact on financial outcomes were detailed along with a series of care-standardization projects. The logistics center was phased in over many years, functioning essentially as a bed 'czar' to coordinate effective patient placement due to limited ICU availability year-round. The financial analysis was a before-and-after study examining a consecutive case cohort of roughly 50,000 ICU patients over a period of 9 years. It was conducted in a large academic medical center covering seven adult ICUs. The primary outcome was change in the annual direct contribution margin. Secondary outcomes were changes in case volume, annual per-case revenue, and hospital length of stay, among others. Finances from three separate time periods were compared: pre-ICU telemedicine group, ICU telemedicine group, and logistic center group.

The total annual direct contribution margin, total annual revenue, revenue per case, and annual case volume increased significantly from the pre-ICU telemedicine implementation period to the ICU telemedicine period. The contribution margin increase was roughly $30 million. When the logistic center time period was compared to the ICU telemedicine group, a further increase in total annual direct contribution margin of nearly $25 million was observed after adjustment for inflation. The capital costs of implementing a tele-ICU program (~$7 million) were recuperated in roughly 3 months based on the improved net contribution margin of $30 million seen with the tele-ICU program. In addition to improved clinical outcomes, this study showed improved financial outcomes with an ICU telemedicine program. The cause of this is likely multifactorial and includes increased case volume and increased per-case net revenue with a tele-ICU program and further enhancements with the addition of a logistics center (Fig. 11.1).

Creating a centralized command center for bed allocation helped decrease ICU length of stay, which in turn allowed for increased case volume. This concept may not pertain to all hospital systems that do not run at maximum ICU bed capacity but is a potential key benefit of ICU telemedicine implementation. Potential limitations to the impressive financial outcomes documented in this study may relate to the single center, before-and-after design. Similar outcomes may not be seen in hospi-

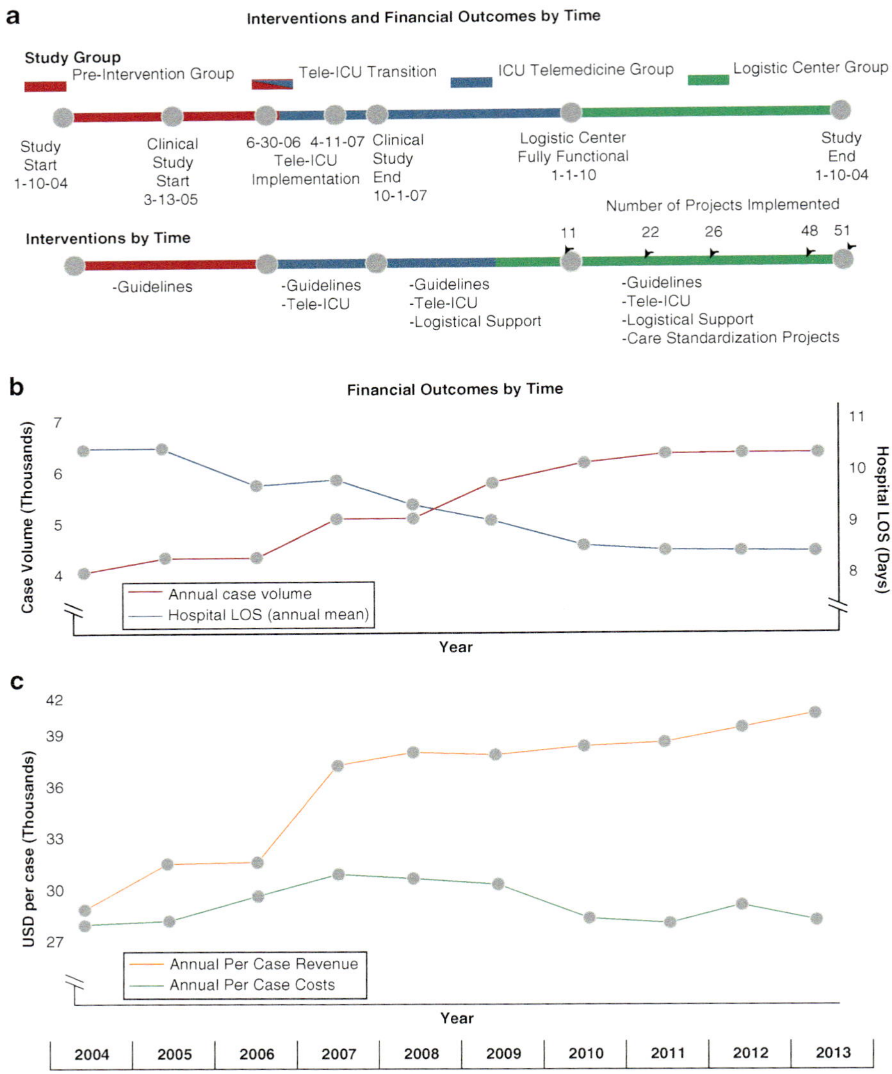

Fig. 11.1 Relation of study interventions to financial outcomes. (**a**) The study groups are indicated by color on the top bar. The pre-ICU telemedicine group is indicated by the red bar, the ICU telemedicine group by the blue bar, and the logistic center group by the green bar. The time in which some ICUs had telemedicine support, whereas others did not, is represented by the blue-red bar. The bar below presents the times of the interventions. The pre-ICU telemedicine group task forces are represented by the red bar, and the period in logistic center function that was added in a graded manner is represented by the blue bar. The green bar defines the times in which care-standardization projects were implemented. The cumulative numbers of implemented care-standardization projects are presented at the time designated by the arrows. (**b**) Case volume is plotted in red, and mean annual hospital LOS is plotted in red as a function of time and in relation to intervention bundle elements. (**c**) Inflation-adjusted annual case revenue is plotted in orange as a function of time, and annual direct costs are plotted in green as a function of time. The difference between annual per-care direct costs and revenue is per-case direct margin. Direct cost and revenue plots are presented in relation to intervention bundle elements. LOS = length of stay

tals with different ICU bed availability or patient acuity. Regarding the temporal changes related to the before-and-after trial design, the tele-ICU and logistic center time period utilized a more efficient and effective documentation system for coding compared to the pre-tele-ICU timeframe. This may have led to increases in case revenue separate from any ICU telemedicine influence.

Future studies and unanswered questions for cost-benefit of tele-ICU programs are needed. As the pressure for cost containment and more efficient care delivery grows, reimbursement models are expected to shift more toward value-based payments and shared risk contracts and away from traditional fee-for-service models. The ability of tele-ICU and telemedicine in general to facilitate efficient care delivery and manage population health will likely lead to more reimbursement for telemedicine-based services, but how this component of reimbursement will evolve remains unknown.

Answering the Question for Yourself: How to Measure Costs and Benefits of Your Hospital's Tele-ICU Program?

Depending on choice of vendor, the adoption of tele-ICU may require a substantial up-front capital investment with ongoing costs of operation and maintenance. The dominant product in this domain is provided by Philips Corporation (eICU), and in general, \$2–\$5 million is the estimated cost to set up a command center and install a centralized tele-ICU system, with operating costs ranging from \$600,000 to \$1.5 million per year, according to costs reported by various adopters. These costs may impede the adoption of this technology, especially with the lack of fee-for-service reimbursement for many tele-ICU services and uncertainties about return-on-investment calculations. Moreover, the return on investment is merely calculated using indirect clinical effects and the expected length of stay reduction. We recommend that hospitals perform an exhaustive cost-benefit analysis customized to their unique situation rather than extrapolating data from other institutions for the reasons mentioned earlier. Payback period or net present value (NPV) is a commonly used indicator to calculate return on investment. More specifically, the financial equation related to tele-ICU is desired to be the following [5]:

$$\left[\text{Capital cost} + \text{Operating cost}\right] \leq \begin{bmatrix} \text{Revenue from reimbursement} \\ + \text{ Cost savings attained} \end{bmatrix}$$

As discussed above, the cost of tele-ICU varies depending on the setting, hardware, software, training, and compatibility with other systems. Institutions should, therefore, create a detailed itemized list with associated costs. One study reported a cost of more than \$2 million to set up a command center and its components [8]. In general, \$2–\$5 million is the estimated cost to set up a command center and install a tele-ICU system, with operating costs ranging from \$600,000 to \$1.5 million per year, according to costs reported by various adopters (unpublished communications). On the revenue side, one study found a 10% reduction in ICU length of stay, creating the ability to care for one new ICU patient per day, which could result in a positive $2.5 million NPV.

Most studies reviewed above used length of stay and mortality to determine cost savings. For example, according to Rosenfeld et al., ICU costs decreased between 25% and 31% during the intervention period, and hospital costs decreased by 12–19% [5]. Breslow et al. hired an independent consulting firm to determine the financial outcome of a tele-ICU program [6]. They determined the cost of care per day of service and also included equipment costs, staff costs, and other costs associated with having a tele-ICU system. The report showed a 24.6% decrease in variable costs per patient. This decrease is probably due to a shorter length of stay in the ICU and improved clinical outcomes [5, 9].

The impact of an ICU telemedicine program has the potential to be far reaching, both clinically and financially, if it is well planned and operated with calculated intentions. Healthcare leaders must have a vision for their organization's strategic goals and decide if telemedicine technology can affect those goals and if the additional cost is warranted [8]. The up-front capital investment in a tele-ICU program may be substantial, but through cost-effective care, the return on investment can be significant and realized quickly. It has been repeatedly shown that when ICU telemedicine can assist in driving down ICU mortality and shortening length of stay, there is a tremendous opportunity for financial gain. While the question of technology versus human factors being responsible for these gains is debatable, the creation of a coordinated ICU care delivery system has the clear potential for significant financial gains [10]. Furthermore, not only can an ICU telemedicine program potentially improve ICU patient outcomes, but it can facilitate outreach and growth of a hospital system into the community, if desired. This can be a cost-effective means for community hospitals to provide high-level care closer to the patient's home while simultaneously off-loading the receiving hospital of lower acuity patients that can be safely managed elsewhere.

A detailed and careful analysis of the current ICU must be considered when doing a cost-effectiveness analysis pre-implementation. Not only must administrators evaluate ICU mortality, length of stay, acuity scores, best practice compliance, and opportunities for intervening on common ICU medical errors, but they also should consider factors such as nursing competency, staff burnout, and the current culture of the ICU. Each of these entities can have indirect effects on cost-effectiveness and is variable between different hospitals and ICUs.

Further cost-effectiveness research is needed to continue to evaluate the complex and rapidly growing ICU telemedicine venture. Studies with decentralized models, comprehensive financial data, community hospital focus, and a more current timeframe would be helpful. It is likely that, as technology evolves and patient care moves from the bedside to the digital world, ICU telemedicine will grow with it. Efficient, cost-effective, and improved patient care is the goal for healthcare systems, and ICU telemedicine may prove to be a pivotal and transformative link if instituted wisely.

References

1. Wilcox M, et al. Do intensivist staffing patterns influence hospital mortality following ICU admission? A systematic review and meta-analysis. Crit Care Med. 2013;41(10):2253–74.
2. Lilly CM, et al. Hospital mortality, length of stay, preventable complications among critically ill patients before and after tele-ICU re-engineering of critical care processes. JAMA. 2011;202:2175–83.
3. Wilcox ME, et al. The effect of telemedicine in critically ill patients: systematic review and meta-analysis. Crit Care. 2012;16:R127.
4. Lilly CM, et al. ICU telemedicine program financial outcomes. Chest. 2017;151(2):286–97.
5. Rosenfeld BA, et al. Intensive care unit telemedicine: alternate paradigm for providing continuous intensivist care. Crit Care Med. 2000;28(12):3925–31.
6. Breslow MJ, et al. Effect of a multiple – site intensive care unit telemedicine program on clinical and economic outcomes: an alternative paradigm for intensivist staffing. Crit Care Med. 2004;32(1):31–8.
7. Yoo B-K, et al. Economic evaluation of telemedicine for patients in ICUs. Crit Care Med. 2016;44:265–74.
8. Ries M. Evaluating tele-ICU cost – an imperfect science. Crit Care Med. 2016;44(2):441–2.
9. Celi LA, Hassan E, Marquardt C, Breslow M, Rosenfeld B. The eICU: it's not just telemedicine. Crit Care Med. 2001;29:N183–9.
10. Castlight Leapfrog Group – ICU physician staffing survey. 2016.

Part III
Clinical Applications of Tele-ICU

Chapter 12
Telestroke and Neurocritical Care

Bart M. Demaerschalk

Introduction

Telemedicine is defined as the use of medical information exchanged from one site to another using electronic communications in an effort to improve consumer health status [1] and to deliver medical and educational services [2], in hospital and clinic settings. Teleneurology is an emerging subspecialty in neurology [3], developed to improve access to neurological expertise in underserved areas.

Increasing world burden of stroke-related morbidity and mortality [4] is partly due to low numbers of healthcare providers and insufficient resources in rural, remote, and low socioeconomic areas. Telestroke is the most rapidly evolving and best studied application of teleneurology in the USA, with proven clinical benefits to provide prompt expert evaluation and treatment, thus overcoming geographical and temporal obstacles to access to appropriate stroke services [5, 6].

Clinical Uses

The 2018 guidelines for acute ischemic stroke care [7] underscored the importance of telemedicine for the immediate assessment of patients with stroke using synchronous audio-video clinical evaluations and diagnostic neuroimaging reviews to make quick diagnostic decisions and determinations of intravenous alteplase candidacy, for guidance over thrombolysis administration and for triaging patients who may be eligible for inter-facility transfer for mechanical thrombectomy. Similarly, telestroke can be used to support specialized care in telemedicine-enabled ambulances and in more sophisticated mobile stroke units.

B. M. Demaerschalk (✉)
Mayo Clinic College of Medicine and Science, Rochester, MN, USA
e-mail: demaerschalk.bart@mayo.edu

M. A. Koenig (ed.), *Telemedicine in the ICU*,
https://doi.org/10.1007/978-3-030-11569-2_12

Telestroke services have been demonstrated to be valuable for deciding on patient suitability for intravenous alteplase treatment [8], clinical diagnostic accuracy [9], interpretation of brain computed tomography [10], improved stroke care delivery times [11], and determination of transfers to stroke centers for routine post-alteplase intensive care ("drip & ship") or for intensive care management directed at patients with hemorrhagic stroke and transfers to a higher level of stroke center care for neurosurgical treatment and neurocritical care for patients with intracranial hemorrhage requiring hematoma evacuation or with malignant cerebral infarction in need of decompressive hemicraniectomy [12]. These examples of various telestroke services have each exhibited high quality and outcomes compared to standard in-person assessments.

Telestroke in the Emergency Department Setting

When patients present to remote hospital EDs with acute stroke syndromes, the telestroke service responsibilities include determining a correct diagnosis, quickly deciding on alteplase therapy eligibility and administration, and guiding transfers to appropriate destination stroke centers for a higher level of care or continuation of care.

Multiple clinical research studies have evaluated the feasibility, benefits, and risks of telestroke services to facilitate delivery of acute stroke treatments in EDs without local around-the-clock neurology coverage, when the time to intravenous alteplase administration is critical for improving stroke outcomes [11, 13–15]. The American Heart Association/American Stroke Association recommends the use of high-quality video teleconferencing technologies to provide a medical opinion for or against the use of intravenous alteplase in patients with suspected acute ischemic stroke when on-site stroke expertise is not immediately available [7, 16]. After telestroke network implementation, standard of care for acute stroke treatment with intravenous alteplase became more broadly available and was more frequently administered to eligible patients [6]. Functional outcomes and mortality are similar between specialized stroke center hubs and telestroke-served spoke hospitals [17, 17B].

Telestroke consultations are optimally performed using synchronous two-way audio-video technology supplemented by additional laboratory and teleradiology review. Participating sites' ED personnel are trained to complete National Institutes of Health Stroke Scale (NIHSS) assessments in conjunction with the remote telemedicine examiner. Remote NIHSS evaluations were determined to be similar to on-site examinations for patients with acute and subacute stroke [18], including those acquired with mobile devices such as smartphones and tablets [19].

Emergency medicine provider to neurology provider telephone-only consultations can be a useful backup if technical difficulties are encountered or in instances and hospital environments without audio-video telestroke network connectivity [7]. The National Institutes of Health-funded Stroke Team Remote Evaluation Using a Digital Observation Camera (STRokE DOC) trial was a randomized controlled trial that compared telestroke using video telecommunications technologies and remote review of imaging with telephone-only consultation [8]. The study was terminated early because telephone-only medical decision-making was determined to be inferior when compared to the telestroke arm, although the rates of post-thrombolysis intracerebral hemorrhage were similar in the two groups [8].

Teleradiological trials have demonstrated that remote emergency viewing and interpretation of CT scans by telestroke physicians is reliable [20, 21]. The Alberta Stroke Program Early CT Score (ASPECTS) is a semiquantitative score to measure the volume of early ischemic changes in acute stroke. Fair inter-rater agreement between neurologists and neuroradiologists in ASPECTS [22] interpretation has been reported in telestroke programs, without significant implications on outcomes [20]. Imaging workflow now frequently includes more advanced multimodal neurovascular imaging, if it can be completed rapidly and not increase the door-to-groin puncture time or delay transfers to a destination thrombectomy-capable center or comprehensive stroke center for endovascular therapy.

Endovascular reperfusion therapy is now recognized as a standard of care after large clinical trials demonstrated its value incremental to intravenous alteplase, in a subset of patients with large vessel occlusions [23]. Telestroke physicians may play a critical role in screening, triaging, and selecting patients as candidates for endovascular treatment [7, 24]. Published studies reported improved triage, faster intervention times, and superior outcomes in patients evaluated via telestroke prior to endovascular procedures [25, 26]. Telestroke networks may assist in the delivery of endovascular treatment to candidate ischemic stroke patients transferred from remote hospitals with outcomes similar to patients admitted directly to tertiary hospitals [27].

If the originating site lacks post-intravenous alteplase care or vascular neurosurgical capabilities in selected clinical scenarios, the telestroke patients can also be transferred to the nearest most capable stroke center with the necessary personnel and resources. A priori transfer agreements and plans for patients should be established, with careful consideration of the destination center's capabilities for intervention and monitoring, treatment time windows, and the distance and time via ground and air [28], so that all aspects of acute stroke care are covered in a timely, coordinated, and seamless manner.

For patients with hemorrhagic stroke (e.g., intracerebral hemorrhage and subarachnoid hemorrhage) presenting to a rural hospital lacking neurosurgical expertise, telestroke specialists may help to identify patients who are candidates for stabilization and emergency transport to comprehensive stroke centers for prompt neurosurgical and neurocritical care [29]. Despite the high mortality rates, early aggressive medical, surgical, and endovascular surgical interventions may improve outcomes for patients with hemorrhagic stroke.

Telestroke consultations are also effective for individuals who may not be candidates for acute stroke therapies or who may present with a stroke mimic syndrome [14, 30]. Approximately twenty percent of acute telestroke consultations are reported to be for patients ultimately diagnosed with a stroke mimic at discharge [31], and nearly twenty percent of them were treated with intravenous alteplase in the emergency department setting [30]. Using several tools that were developed for bedside determination [32] in adults and children, telestroke physicians aim to reduce the unnecessary treatment with intravenous alteplase in patients presenting with a diagnosis other than ischemic stroke [33]. Their diagnostic impression, management, and disposition recommendations should be discussed with the referring emergency physician in order to assure effective communication and high-quality neurological care and to prevent unnecessary hospital admissions.

A consultation note documented by the consulting telestroke physician should be made available to the originating site. A discharge summary including a definitive diagnosis should be transmitted to the telestroke physician. The hospital documentation is used for monitoring important quality measures concerning telestroke practice.

Telestroke in Settings Spanning the Continuum of Stroke Care

In prehospital stroke care, telemedicine applications are more variable and present new challenges. An unassisted telestroke examination scale was evaluated with healthy volunteers mimicking stroke syndromes during ambulance transportation, and sufficiently reliable evaluations were demonstrated in a moving ground ambulance using 4G connectivity [34]. Stroke expert assessments in mobile stroke units (MSUs) versus regular ambulances transporting patients to the closest ED have proven value in reducing time to IV alteplase [35, 36].

In an MSU, stroke patient examination and CT angiogram interpretation via telestroke open the opportunity for fast clinical decision-making for IV alteplase administration in the field, which is of critical importance considering that the reduced assessment and treatment times in the prehospital setting are associated with better outcomes [37]. Satisfactory connectivity (98%) and agreement on the alteplase decision (88%) were demonstrated in a study of simultaneous and independent assessment by a stroke specialist in the MSU and a remote telestroke physician [38]. Decisions for subsequent transfers to either the nearest center with neurocritical care monitoring or the closest thrombectomy-capable center are made immediately after alteplase administration in the MSU.

Telemedicine for patients in the neuro-intensive care unit plays an important role beyond the hyperacute phase of stroke. Teleneurocritical care is valuable for prevention, diagnosis, and timely management of primary neurovascular emergencies and secondary neurologic injuries [39]. Teleneurocritical care has demonstrated reliability and improvement in patient-related outcomes [40].

The concept of an electronic stroke unit [2] refers to remote tele-neurovascular services for patients admitted to stroke units without continuous neurology or stroke coverage. This concept has somewhat limited applicability currently; however, it shows promise for the future.

The domain of virtual poststroke rehabilitation was studied in home and ambulatory settings for serial assessments, monitoring, and timely adjustment of therapies. The limited quality evidence showed that tele-rehabilitation approaches were similar to conventional rehabilitation in improving activities of daily living and motor function for stroke survivors [41, 42]. Perceived obstacles were patients and caregivers potentially lacking understanding of the technology and variable resources for virtual tele-rehabilitation networks.

Secondary stroke prevention and monitoring through telestroke services (i.e., virtual neurovascular clinic) is another potential application of telestroke that is growing in rural areas and long-term care units for patients without feasible transportation options [2]. The virtual applications of transcranial Doppler ultrasound and carotid duplex ultrasound via teleneurosonology have also demonstrated technical feasibility in a proof-of-concept study [43]; however, its routine applicability in acute care or ambulatory settings warrants further investigation.

Telestroke for Clinical Research

Telestroke encounters may assist with screening and identifying patients who may be potentially eligible for participation in clinical trials of novel treatments for ischemic and hemorrhagic stroke, neuroprotective agents, or innovative diagnostic tests. The subjects' consent and randomization can occur at the originating sites immediately before transfer to a stroke center [44] or in an MSU or virtual stroke clinic [45]. The tele-investigators should be familiar with the eligibility criteria and research protocols and, when appropriate, offer the patient the opportunity to participate in clinical trials without regard to geographical constraints. These projects need to comply with approved research policies, and increasingly, Institutional Review Boards are familiar with the adoption of digital health in clinical research.

Telestroke for Teaching

Tele-mentoring for neurology trainees' medical education using virtual supervision has emerged in numerous training programs [3]. In-person faculty supervision was preferred over robotic telepresence and telephone-only consultations in a study conducted at Mayo Clinic [46]. Various different training methodologies are applicable for medical students, residents, and fellows, respectively. Different models of formal incorporation of telestroke training during vascular neurology fellowship training have also been proposed [47], without any specific recommendations existing currently to guide training program accreditation agencies. Similarly, simulation training for emergency teams [48] and nursing staff [49] has been demonstrated as successful approaches to virtual stroke management.

Technological Considerations

Telestroke networks are designed as a combination of primary, secondary, and tertiary care settings [1] working together to provide comprehensive in-person and virtual stroke care. Currently, there are two fundamental telestroke models: the distributed model and hub-and-spoke model. They include distant sites (where the telemedicine physician is located) and originating sites (where the patients are located). The services at all sites for acute stroke evaluation are generally available 365 days a year, 24 hours a day, and 7 days a week.

In the hub-and-spoke model, a comprehensive stroke center or academic medical center provides consultative expert services at remote "spoke" sites. Sub-hubs can also be integrated in this model, mainly consisting of small community hospitals that can serve as an intermediate to some spokes and are linked to the main hub [50]. The telestroke physicians are licensed in each state and credentialed at each of the hubs and at all of the spoke sites. Their services consist of time-sensitive emergency evaluations and clinical decisions for acute therapies and subsequent management in the most appropriate setting, including transfer decisions and involvement in clinical trials, if applicable.

In the distributive model, an independent corporation or an affiliated network of telestroke physicians provides services at various originating sites.

Some networks include virtual telestroke units, allowing patients to remain in the original hospital with access to higher-quality stroke care by providing additional resources like therapists and ongoing telestroke consultations [51].

Decentralized telestroke thrombolysis services have been shown to achieve similar treatment rates and time delays for a rural population as a centralized system can achieve for an urban population [15].

Irrespective of the model or network, well-delineated workflow protocols and agreements for inter-facility transfers whenever a higher level of care is indicated need to be established. Training and maintenance of continuous education should be provided to all telestroke providers and referring services (physicians, nurses, and ancillary staff), at both the distant and originating sites. Clinical and technical roles and responsibilities need to be acknowledged.

Telestroke Quality and Outcome Metrics

An external accreditation body should conduct the telestroke network certification based on a review of performance, processes, and outcomes. Measures of quality performance should be collected in a standardized fashion and shared across the network, according to an agreement between telestroke sites and either a coordinating stroke center or distributed partner [28]. Every telestroke network hospital should participate in the collection of stroke quality measures [52].

Current American Heart Association guidelines make suggestions for different telestroke metrics [28], such as process and performance, outcomes, patient and provider satisfaction, and technological quality. Administrative, technical, and clinical quality indicators should be systematically and regularly reviewed by telestroke leadership in order to assure quality and improvement.

Telestroke Network Operational Considerations

Policies and procedures for telestroke network operation and administration must be developed and followed to assure good quality clinical care and organizational success. The key stakeholders include hub and distant site physician directors, program manager, ED stroke champions, EMS personnel, IT administrators, laboratory and radiology personnel, and human resources, legal, and finance personnel. Personalized algorithms and workflows for each setting of the telestroke consultation (ED, MSU, ICU, medical-surgical floor, outpatient) should be created and available to the personnel. Oversight, timely feedback, and personnel development are indicated to assure a telestroke program maintains competency. Patient records' storage, retrieval, privacy, and confidentiality should follow HIPAA and applicable state laws. The American Telemedicine Association has published technical requirements for operation of telestroke networks [1].

Physician licensing and credentialing rules [53], infrastructure development, staffing, training, partnership development, fragmentation of care, limited coordination [5], and poor internet access for people living in rural areas have all been reported as obstacles to telestroke implementation. Different states have adopted a variety of policies to facilitate the adoption of telestroke services and overcome licensing, liability, and reimbursement challenges [54].

Health Economic Evaluations of Telestroke

Analysis of several telestroke networks demonstrated an increase in the number of patients discharged home independently and reduced costs for the network hospitals [55], with the highest cost-effectiveness revealed in the most severe strokes cases [56]. Societal perspectives have similarly indicated cost utility for hub-and-spoke networks [57]. In resource-limited developing countries, affordable smartphone-based technology has been pioneered and is associated with improved outcomes [58]. Mobile telestroke assessment was also demonstrated to be feasible using low-cost components and commercial available wireless connectivity in rural settings [59]. Likewise, tele-neurological ICUs are described as safe and cost-saving strategies that improve the timely response to neurological emergencies and decrease hospital length of stay [40]. While prehospital stroke care has demonstrated cost-effectiveness [60], the cost-benefit analysis of MSUs remains to be determined. Teleneurology for patients in ambulances (in-transit telestroke) was demonstrated to be a scalable and affordable alternative to MSUs, with similar efficacy in diagnosis and treatment [61].

Comprehensive Virtual Stroke Centers of the Future

The majority of current telestroke providers are vascular neurologists, general neurologists, and neurocritical care specialists. Virtual assessment and management of more complex neurovascular emergencies is likely to be associated with improved outcomes if patients could have prompt, seamless, and integrated neuroradiological, neurocritical care, and neurosurgical expertise available, in addition to the vascular neurology opinion and coordination of care [62].

From the introduction of portable CT scanners in rural EDs [63] to multimodal CT imaging [64] and CT angiography in MSUs that improves patients selection, quality control of teleradiology interpretation is recommended in order to provide the best medical care to individual stroke patients [65]. Therefore, the addition of a tele-neuroradiologist to the virtual stroke team is commendable, especially in the view of more advanced neuroimaging techniques for complex neurovascular cases. Complex cerebrovascular conditions require emergency neurosurgical and neurocritical care management [40]. Early rehabilitation poststroke is also critical to improving patient outcomes [66]. Tele-rehabilitation starting with early dysphagia assessment and ending with virtual visits in long-term care facilities for therapy adjustments are resourceful [67, 68].

The recommendations for comprehensive stroke centers delivery of specialized stroke care include healthcare providers with expertise in neurosurgery and vascular neurology, access to advanced neuroimaging capabilities, surgical and endovascular techniques, ICU care, and a stroke registry [69]. Correspondingly, virtual comprehensive stroke networks should be multidisciplinary and follow key accreditation guidelines in an organized, systematic, and efficient manner. National registries that collect and monitor telestroke outcome measures should assure standardization of best telestroke practices.

Summary

With the evolution of comprehensive stroke care, telestroke applications have also expanded. Virtual stroke assessments in rural and underserved urban areas have largely overcome the historically limited access to expeditious stroke expertise and currently represent the standard practice nationally and internationally.

References

1. Demaerschalk BM, Berg J, Chong BW, Gross H, Nystrom K, Adeoye O, et al. American Telemedicine Association: Telestroke Guidelines. Telemed J E Health. 2017;23(5):376–89.
2. Blacquiere D, Lindsay MP, Foley N, Taralson C, Alcock S, Balg C, et al. Canadian Stroke Best Practice Recommendations: Telestroke Best Practice Guidelines Update 2017. Int J Stroke. 2017;12(8):886–95.
3. Mutgi SA, Zha AM, Behrouz R. Emerging Subspecialties in Neurology: Telestroke and teleneurology. Neurology. 2015;84(22):e191–3.
4. Krishnamurthi RV, Moran AE, Feigin VL, Barker-Collo S, Norrving B, Mensah GA, et al. Stroke prevalence, mortality and disability-adjusted life years in adults aged 20–64 years in 1990-2013: data from the Global Burden of Disease 2013 Study. Neuroepidemiology. 2015;45(3):190–202.
5. Dorsey ER, Topol EJ. State of Telehealth. N Engl J Med. 2016;375(2):154–61.
6. Amorim E, Shih MM, Koehler SA, Massaro LL, Zaidi SF, Jumaa MA, et al. Impact of telemedicine implementation in thrombolytic use for acute ischemic stroke: the University of Pittsburgh Medical Center telestroke network experience. J Stroke Cerebrovasc Dis. 2013;22(4):527–31.
7. Powers WJ, Rabinstein AA, Ackerson T, Opeolu MA, Bambakidis NC, Becker K, et al. Guidelines for the early management of patients with acute ischemic stroke: a guideline for healthcare professionals from the American Heart Association/American Stroke Association. Stroke. 2018;49:e46–99.
8. Meyer BC, Raman R, Hemmen T, Obler R, Zivin JA, Rao R, et al. Efficacy of site-independent telemedicine in the STRokE DOC trial: a randomised, blinded, prospective study. Lancet Neurol. 2008;7(9):787–95.
9. Agrawal K, Raman R, Ernstrom K, Claycomb RJ, Meyer DM, Hemmen TM, et al. Accuracy of Stroke Diagnosis in Telestroke-Guided Tissue Plasminogen Activator Patients. J Stroke Cerebrovasc Dis. 2016;25(12):2942–6.
10. Demaerschalk BM, Bobrow BJ, Raman R, Ernstrom K, Hoxworth JM, Patel AC, et al. CT interpretation in a telestroke network: agreement among a spoke radiologist, hub vascular neurologist, and hub neuroradiologist. Stroke. 2012;43(11):3095–7.
11. Muller-Barna P, Hubert GJ, Boy S, Bogdahn U, Wiedmann S, Heuschmann PU, et al. TeleStroke units serving as a model of care in rural areas: 10-year experience of the TeleMedical project for integrative stroke care. Stroke. 2014;45(9):2739–44.
12. Audebert HJ, Wimmer ML, Hahn R, Schenkel J, Bogdahn U, Horn M, et al. Can telemedicine contribute to fulfill WHO Helsingborg Declaration of specialized stroke care? Cerebrovasc Dis. 2005;20(5):362–9.
13. Sanders KA, Patel R, Kiely JM, Gwynn MW, Johnston LH. Improving Telestroke Treatment Times in an Expanding Network of Hospitals. J Stroke Cerebrovasc Dis. 2016;25(2):288–91.
14. Audebert HJ, Kukla C, Clarmann von Claranau S, Kuhn J, Vatankhah B, Schenkel J, et al. Telemedicine for safe and extended use of thrombolysis in stroke: the Telemedic Pilot Project for Integrative Stroke Care (TEMPiS) in Bavaria. Stroke. 2005;36(2):287–91.
15. Hubert GJ, Meretoja A, Audebert HJ, Tatlisumak T, Zeman F, Boy S, et al. Stroke Thrombolysis in a Centralized and a Decentralized System (Helsinki and Telemedical Project for Integrative Stroke Care Network). Stroke. 2016;47(12):2999–3004.
16. Schwamm LH, Holloway RG, Amarenco P, Audebert HJ, Bakas T, Chumbler NR, et al. A review of the evidence for the use of telemedicine within stroke systems of care: a scientific statement from the American Heart Association/American Stroke Association. Stroke. 2009;40(7):2616–34.
17. Schwab S, Vatankhah B, Kukla C, Hauchwitz M, Bogdahn U, Furst A, et al. Long-term outcome after thrombolysis in telemedical stroke care. Neurology. 2007;69(9):898–903.

17B. Demaerschalk BM, Boyd EL, Barrett KM, Gamble DM, Sonchik S, Comer MM, et al. Comparison of stroke outcomes of hub and spoke hospital treated patients in mayo clinic telestroke program. J Stroke Cerebrovasc Dis. 2018;27(11):2940–2.

18. Wang S, Lee SB, Pardue C, Ramsingh D, Waller J, Gross H, et al. Remote evaluation of acute ischemic stroke: reliability of National Institutes of Health Stroke Scale via telestroke. Stroke. 2003;34(10):e188–91.
19. Demaerschalk BM, Vegunta S, Vargas BB, Wu Q, Channer DD, Hentz JG. Reliability of real-time video smartphone for assessing National Institutes of Health Stroke Scale scores in acute stroke patients. Stroke. 2012;43(12):3271–7.
20. Puetz V, Bodechtel U, Gerber JC, Dzialowski I, Kunz A, Wolz M, et al. Reliability of brain CT evaluation by stroke neurologists in telemedicine. Neurology. 2013;80(4):332–8.
21. Mitchell JR, Sharma P, Modi J, Simpson M, Thomas M, Hill MD, et al. A smartphone client-server teleradiology system for primary diagnosis of acute stroke. J Med Internet Res. 2011;13(2):e31.
22. Pexman JH, Barber PA, Hill MD, Sevick RJ, Demchuk AM, Hudon ME, et al. Use of the Alberta Stroke Program Early CT Score (ASPECTS) for assessing CT scans in patients with acute stroke. AJNR Am J Neuroradiol. 2001;22(8):1534–42.
23. Goyal M, Menon BK, van Zwam WH, Dippel DW, Mitchell PJ, Demchuk AM, et al. Endovascular thrombectomy after large-vessel ischaemic stroke: a meta-analysis of individual patient data from five randomised trials. Lancet. 2016;387(10029):1723–31.
24. Smith EE, Schwamm LH. Endovascular clot retrieval therapy: implications for the organization of stroke systems of care in North America. Stroke. 2015;46(6):1462–7.
25. Pedragosa A, Alvarez-Sabin J, Rubiera M, Rodriguez-Luna D, Maisterra O, Molina C, et al. Impact of telemedicine on acute management of stroke patients undergoing endovascular procedures. Cerebrovasc Dis. 2012;34(5–6):436–42.
26. Kepplinger J, Dzialowski I, Barlinn K, Puetz V, Wojciechowski C, Schneider H, et al. Emergency transfer of acute stroke patients within the East Saxony telemedicine stroke network: a descriptive analysis. Int J Stroke. 2014;9(2):160–5.
27. Barlinn J, Gerber J, Barlinn K, Pallesen LP, Siepmann T, Zerna C, et al. Acute endovascular treatment delivery to ischemic stroke patients transferred within a telestroke network: a retrospective observational study. Int J Stroke. 2016;12(5):502–9.
28. Wechsler LR, Demaerschalk BM, Schwamm LH, Adeoye OM, Audebert HJ, Fanale CV, et al. Telemedicine Quality and Outcomes in Stroke: a Scientific Statement for Healthcare Professionals From the American Heart Association/American Stroke Association. Stroke. 2017;48(1):e3–e25.
29. Backhaus R, Schlachetzki F, Rackl W, Baldaranov D, Leitzmann M, Hubert GJ, et al. Intracranial hemorrhage: frequency, location, and risk factors identified in a TeleStroke network. Neuroreport. 2015;26(2):81–7.
30. Yaghi S, Rayaz S, Bianchi N, Hall-Barrow JC, Hinduja A. Thrombolysis to stroke mimics in telestroke. J Telemed Telecare. 2012.
31. Ali SF, Viswanathan A, Singhal AB, Rost NS, Forducey PG, Davis LW, et al. The TeleStroke mimic (TM)-score: a prediction rule for identifying stroke mimics evaluated in a Telestroke Network. J Am Heart Assoc. 2014;3(3):e000838.
32. Mackay MT, Churilov L, Donnan GA, Babl FE, Monagle P. Performance of bedside stroke recognition tools in discriminating childhood stroke from mimics. Neurology. 2016;86(23):2154–61.
33. Demaerschalk BM, Kleindorfer DO, Adeoye OM, Demchuk AM, Fugate JE, Grotta JC, et al. Scientific Rationale for the Inclusion and Exclusion Criteria for Intravenous Alteplase in Acute Ischemic Stroke: a Statement for Healthcare Professionals From the American Heart Association/American Stroke Association. Stroke. 2016;47(2):581–641.
34. Van Hooff RJ, Cambron M, Van Dyck R, De Smedt A, Moens M, Espinoza AV, et al. Prehospital unassisted assessment of stroke severity using telemedicine: a feasibility study. Stroke. 2013;44(10):2907–9.
35. Walter S, Kostopoulos P, Haass A, Keller I, Lesmeister M, Schlechtriemen T, et al. Diagnosis and treatment of patients with stroke in a mobile stroke unit versus in hospital: a randomised controlled trial. Lancet Neurol. 2012;11(5):397–404.

36. Kunz A, Ebinger M, Geisler F, Rozanski M, Waldschmidt C, Weber JE, et al. Functional outcomes of pre-hospital thrombolysis in a mobile stroke treatment unit compared with conventional care: an observational registry study. Lancet Neurol. 2016;15(10):1035–43.
37. Ebinger M, Kunz A, Wendt M, Rozanski M, Winter B, Waldschmidt C, et al. Effects of golden hour thrombolysis: a Prehospital Acute Neurological Treatment and Optimization of Medical Care in Stroke (PHANTOM-S) substudy. JAMA Neurol. 2015;72(1):25–30.
38. Wu TC, Parker SA, Jagolino A, Yamal JM, Bowry R, Thomas A, et al. Telemedicine Can Replace the Neurologist on a Mobile Stroke Unit. Stroke. 2017;48(2):493–6.
39. Vespa PM, Miller C, Hu X, Nenov V, Buxey F, Martin NA. Intensive care unit robotic telepresence facilitates rapid physician response to unstable patients and decreased cost in neurointensive care. Surg Neurol. 2007;67(4):331–7.
40. Klein KE, Rasmussen PA, Winners SL, Frontera JA. Teleneurocritical care and telestroke. Crit Care Clin. 2015;31(2):197–224.
41. Laver KE, Schoene D, Crotty M, George S, Lannin NA, Sherrington C. Telerehabilitation services for stroke. Cochrane Database Syst Rev. 2013;12:CD010255.
42. Chen J, Jin W, Zhang XX, Xu W, Liu XN, Ren CC. Telerehabilitation Approaches for Stroke Patients: Systematic Review and Meta-analysis of Randomized Controlled Trials. J Stroke Cerebrovasc Dis. 2015;24(12):2660–8.
43. Rubin MN, Barrett KM, Freeman WD, Lee Iannotti JK, Channer DD, Rabinstein AA, et al. Teleneurosonology: a novel application of transcranial and carotid ultrasound. J Stroke Cerebrovasc Dis. 2015;24(3):562–5.
44. Switzer JA, Hall CE, Close B, Nichols FT, Gross H, Bruno A, et al. A telestroke network enhances recruitment into acute stroke clinical trials. Stroke. 2010;41(3):566–9.
45. Lin MP, Sanossian N, Liebeskind DS. Imaging of prehospital stroke therapeutics. Expert Rev Cardiovasc Ther. 2015;13(9):1001–15.
46. Kramer NM, Demaerschalk BM. A novel application of teleneurology: robotic telepresence in supervision of neurology trainees. Telemed J E Health. 2014;20(12):1087–92.
47. Jagolino AL, Jia J, Gildersleeve K, Ankrom C, Cai C, Rahbar M, et al. A call for formal telemedicine training during stroke fellowship. Neurology. 2016;86(19):1827–33.
48. Richard S, Mione G, Varoqui C, Vezain A, Brunner A, Bracard S, et al. Simulation training for emergency teams to manage acute ischemic stroke by telemedicine. Medicine (Baltimore). 2016;95(24):e3924.
49. Rafter RH, Kelly TM. Nursing implementation of a telestroke programme in a community hospital in the US. J Nurs Manag. 2011;19(2):193–200.
50. Hess DC, Audebert HJ. The history and future of telestroke. Nat Rev Neurol. 2013;9(6):340–50.
51. Audebert H. Telestroke: effective networking. Lancet Neurol. 2006;5(3):279–82.
52. Schwamm LH, Audebert HJ, Amarenco P, Chumbler NR, Frankel MR, George MG, et al. Recommendations for the implementation of telemedicine within stroke systems of care: a policy statement from the American Heart Association. Stroke. 2009;40(7):2635–60.
53. Rogove HJ, McArthur D, Demaerschalk BM, Vespa PM. Barriers to telemedicine: survey of current users in acute care units. Telemed J E Health. 2012;18(1):48–53.
54. Kulcsar M, Gilchrist S, George MG. Improving stroke outcomes in rural areas through telestroke programs: an examination of barriers, facilitators, and state policies. Telemed J E Health. 2014;20(1):3–10.
55. Switzer JA, Demaerschalk BM, Xie J, Fan L, Villa KF, Wu EQ. Cost-effectiveness of hub-and-spoke telestroke networks for the management of acute ischemic stroke from the hospitals' perspectives. Circ Cardiovasc Qual Outcomes. 2013;6(1):18–26.
56. Nelson RE, Okon N, Lesko AC, Majersik JJ, Bhatt A, Baraban E. The cost-effectiveness of telestroke in the Pacific Northwest region of the USA. J Telemed Telecare. 2016;22(7):413–21.
57. Demaerschalk BM, Switzer JA, Xie J, Fan L, Villa KF, Wu EQ. Cost utility of hub-and-spoke telestroke networks from societal perspective. Am J Manag Care. 2013;19(12):976–85.
58. Sharma S, Padma MV, Bhardwaj A, Sharma A, Sawal N, Thakur S. Telestroke in resource-poor developing country model. Neurol India. 2016;64(5):934–40.

59. Lippman JM, Smith SN, McMurry TL, Sutton ZG, Gunnell BS, Cote J, et al. Mobile Telestroke During Ambulance Transport Is Feasible in a Rural EMS Setting: the iTREAT Study. Telemed J E Health. 2016;22(6):507–13.
60. Gyrd-Hansen D, Olsen KR, Bollweg K, Kronborg C, Ebinger M, Audebert HJ. Cost-effectiveness estimate of prehospital thrombolysis: results of the PHANTOM-S study. Neurology. 2015;84(11):1090–7.
61. Belt GH, Felberg RA, Rubin J, Halperin JJ. In-Transit Telemedicine Speeds Ischemic Stroke Treatment: Preliminary Results. Stroke. 2016;47(9):2413–5.
62. Demaerschalk BM. Seamless integrated stroke telemedicine systems of care: a potential solution for acute stroke care delivery delays and inefficiencies. Stroke. 2011;42(6):1507–8.
63. Shuaib A, Khan K, Whittaker T, Amlani S, Crumley P. Introduction of portable computed tomography scanners, in the treatment of acute stroke patients via telemedicine in remote communities. Int J Stroke. 2010;5(2):62–6.
64. Demeestere J, Sewell C, Rudd J, Ang T, Jordan L, Wills J, et al. The establishment of a telestroke service using multimodal CT imaging decision assistance: "Turning on the fog lights". J Clin Neurosci. 2017;37:1–5.
65. Muller-Barna P, Audebert HJ. High-standard TeleStroke: need for experienced stroke experts trained in imaging interpretation. Neurology. 2013;80(4):326–7.
66. Winstein CJ, Stein J, Arena R, Bates B, Cherney LR, Cramer SC, et al. Guidelines for Adult Stroke Rehabilitation and Recovery: a Guideline for Healthcare Professionals From the American Heart Association/American Stroke Association. Stroke. 2016;47(6):e98–e169.
67. Malandraki GA, McCullough G, He X, McWeeny E, Perlman AL. Teledynamic evaluation of oropharyngeal swallowing. J Speech Lang Hear Res. 2011;54(6):1497–505.
68. Rubin MN, Wellik KE, Channer DD, Demaerschalk BM. Systematic review of telestroke for post-stroke care and rehabilitation. Curr Atheroscler Rep. 2013;15(8):343.
69. Alberts MJ, Latchaw RE, Selman WR, Shephard T, Hadley MN, Brass LM, et al. Recommendations for comprehensive stroke centers: a consensus statement from the Brain Attack Coalition. Stroke. 2005;36(7):1597–616.

Chapter 13
Advances in Tele-Cardiology

Jayashree Raikhelkar and Jayant K. Raikhelkar

Advances in Tele-Cardiology

Telemedicine is recognized as the application of modern information and communications technologies for the delivery of health services [1]. Telemedicine has become increasingly adopted over the past 50 years and successfully applied in a variety of subspecialties. Telemedicine in the field of cardiology has been continuously evolving and is considered an extremely important application, allowing for the rapid transmission of relevant cardiovascular data such as the electrocardiogram (ECG) and echocardiogram (ECHO) as well as remote tele-consultation. Its earliest reference in the field of cardiology can be traced back to early twentieth century when electrocardiographic data was first transmitted over telephonic wires [2].

Progressive research in cardiac care has led to a profound decline in cardiac morbidity and mortality over the last 50 years. In spite of this, cardiovascular diseases are still the leading cause of death in the USA with over 2000 Americans dying of cardiovascular causes on a daily basis [3]. With the baby boomer generation well into retirement, there has been a significant increase in the prevalence of coronary artery disease and chronic heart failure. It is hoped that research in the field of tele-cardiology will benefit this aging population and help bring the latest diagnostic modalities and therapies in cardiovascular medicine to the most geographically isolated patients [4].

This chapter will illustrate the current advancements and sphere of tele-cardiology within the realm of telemedicine and its growing number of applications to patients with cardiovascular disease. Tele-cardiology can be divided somewhat arbitrarily

J. Raikhelkar (✉)
Emory University School of Medicine, Atlanta, GA, USA

J. K. Raikhelkar
Department of Medicine, Division of Cardiovascular Medicine, University of Chicago School of Medicine, Chicago, IL, USA
e-mail: jraikhelkar1@medicine.bsd.uchicago.edu

M. A. Koenig (ed.), *Telemedicine in the ICU*,
https://doi.org/10.1007/978-3-030-11569-2_13

Table 13.1 Classification of tele-cardiology supports

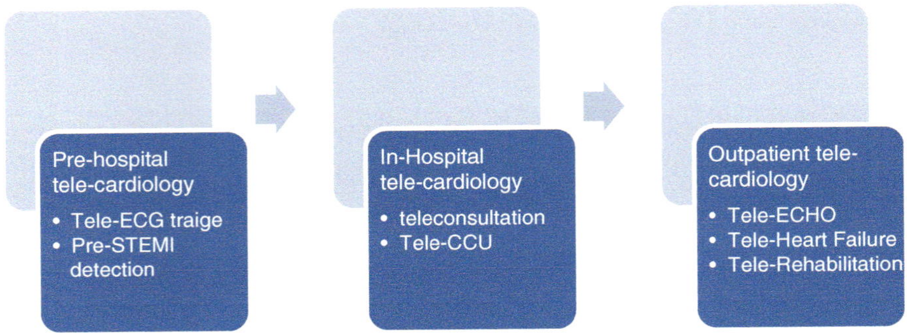

into the following classification (Table 13.1) based on the location of telemedicine support:

Pre-hospital Tele-cardiology:

(a) Tele-ECG triage
(b) Pre-STEMI detection

In-Hospital tele-cardiology:

(a) Tele-consultation
(b) Tele-CCU

Outpatient tele-cardiology:

(a) Tele-ECHO
(b) Tele-heart failure
(c) Tele-rehabilitation

ECG Transmission

The ability to the accurately transmit recorded ECG in real time to a cardiologist for evaluation is one of the most crucial applications of tele-cardiology today. This is the critical first step in triaging patients requiring potential interventions. With wireless technology, ECG transmission can occur with the use of mobile phones/tablets at home via Bluetooth to the hospital [5]. ECG transmission can occur with or without Internet access as well. Technology has been developed to record ECG signals as audio inputs which are then transmitted to a hospital with a landline or mobile phone. This allows patients without access to the Internet to have the ability to record and transmit data to specialized centers [6, 7].

Since the time to reperfusion is crucial to improving prognosis in patients with acute myocardial infarction, many studies have looked at implementation of

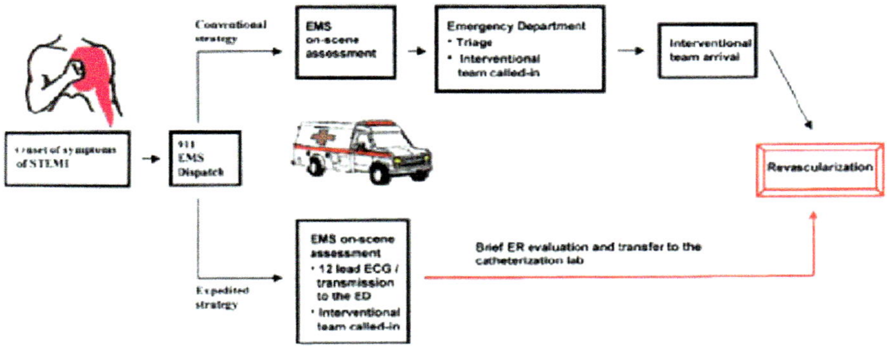

Fig. 13.1 Conventional versus expedited strategy for STEMI revascularization. (Used with permission. Rao et al. [80])

tele-cardiology applications in this limited period of time. Numerous studies have shown remote ECG transmission, such as within a moving vehicle, is achievable [8–10]. Tele-ECG consultation has allowed for expedited triage and abbreviated in-hospital times in STEMI patients when compared to control groups [8–10]. Figure 13.1 demonstrates how an expediated strategy with EMS 12-lead ECG transmission and communication with cardiac catheterization teams prior to transfer to hospital abbreviates emergency room consultation times and improves revascularization times.

Brunetti's study demonstrated that STEMI patients in rural areas with tele-cardiology evaluation had evaluation and treatment times that were comparable to patients living close to a PCI center [10]. The Acute Cardiac Care Association of the European Society of Cardiology guidelines on the pre-hospital management of chest pain and dyspnea have mandated the use of pre-hospital ECG with telemedicine when a skilled physician is absent for ECG interpretation [11].

Early Identification of STEMI

One of the most established roles for telemedicine in cardiology is early triage and management of ST segment elevation MI (STEMI), which is defined as the syndrome of persistent ECG ST elevation and subsequent release of biomarkers of myocardial necrosis [12]. In the USA, there are estimated to be over 250,000 STEMIs presenting to the emergency department per year [13]. Although the outcomes for patients with STEMI are improving, the 30-day case fatality rate remains 11.4%. Thus, it remains an important public health concern [14]. Minimizing the time from diagnosis of STEMI to reperfusion therapy either by thrombolysis or percutaneous coronary intervention (PCI) has been shown to be associated with decreased mortality [15]. Modern healthcare systems have thus identified pre-hospital 12-lead ECG transmission as the standard of care documented in both European and American guidelines [12, 15].

Brunetti [16] reported preliminary data regarding pre-hospital transmission of ECG data and triage in STEMI patients. Patients with STEMI transferred by regional emergency services were enrolled in the study. Patients were randomized to receive pre-hospital ECG triage by tele-cardiology and, if required, direct transfer to cardiac catheterization for PCI or transfer to the emergency department where the diagnosis would be made. Time-to-balloon with PCI treatment within 60 minutes occurred much more frequently in patients triaged with tele-cardiology ECG, in both short- and long-distance groups versus controls (85% vs. 35%, $p < 0.001$, +141%). One of the major limitations of this study was that it carried out at a single center [16].

In the MonAMI study [17], the performance of pre-hospital 12-lead ECG triage and emergency room activation of an infarct team significantly improved door-to-balloon times. The proportion of patients achieving a door-to-balloon time of ≤90 minutes increased from 39% to 93% in the tele-cardiology supported group leading to a greater proportion of patients achieving guideline recommendations.

Rasmussen and colleagues demonstrated that the use of telemedicine in diagnosis and triage of patients to direct cardiac intervention is feasible in close to 90% of patients living up to 95 km or less. Patients with pre-hospital diagnosis and triage of STEMI could be treated with primary PCI within 120 minutes [18]. A retrospective study of 673 patients by Tanguay in Quebec, Canada, recently showed the pre-hospital 12-lead ECG use and activation of the cardiac catheterization lab preemptively led to a first medical contact-to-start of PCI time of approximately 47 minutes and with a false-positive activation rate of only 14% [19]. Thus, the current literature supports the use of pre-hospital ECG transmission and transfer of STEMI patients for treatment. This technology has expedited the treatment of a significant number of patients with the most serious form of acute coronary syndrome.

Sivagangabalan examined the efficacy of pre-hospital triage and early activation of cardiac catheterization teams on revascularization times and left ventricular (LV) ejection fractions. STEMI patients were triaged in the ambulance, in community hospital emergency departments, or tertiary hospital emergency departments. Those triaged in an ambulance had significantly decreased door-to-balloon times and higher LV ejection fractions compared to the other groups. In addition, this group has a significant long-term survival advantage [20]. Chan demonstrated that pre-hospital triage of patients with STEMI was an independent predictor of survival. Patients who were diagnosed in the ambulance instead of in the hospital more frequently achieved a 90-minute door-to-balloon time benchmark (80.4% vs. 8.7%, $p < 0.001$) and lower 30-day and 1-year mortality [21].

Currently, healthcare systems in the USA are not organized in a way to encourage the adoption of pre-hospital ECG within their regional emergency medical services. The one-size-fits-all approach is impractical. Before implementation of an organized pre-hospital ECG program into regional transport systems, it is reasonable to explore specific community limitations and question the following concepts listed in Table 13.2.

Table 13.2 Top questions to ask before implementing pre-hospital ECG in your system workflow for acute coronary syndromes

1. What are the benefits of using pre-hospital ECG in patients with STEMI?
2. What model will be used for interpreting pre-hospital ECG (computer algorithm vs. paramedic interpretation vs. wireless physician interpretation)?
3. Can EMS providers reliably acquire and interpret pre-hospital ECGs?
4. What training and maintenance of competency do EMS providers need?
5. What would be the systems workflow once the patient arrives to the hospital?
6. What additional costs are expected to have pre-hospital ECG incorporated into existing systems of care?
7. How can the pre-hospital ECG workflow be incorporated into our research and quality assurance process, and what type of regulatory oversight is necessary?

Tele-ECG has been shown to improve quality of healthcare delivery. The greater emphasis on tele-ECG in the STEMI diagnosis has led to the question of its cost-effectiveness. An observational study done by Brunetti [22] explored this issue in their cost analysis based in the Apulia region in Italy. Included were patients who called the local emergency medical services during 2012 and underwent pre-hospital triage with telemedicine ECG in the case of suspected acute cardiac disease. The ECGs were read by a cardiologist remotely. The cost of conventional hospital triage versus pre-hospital triage was calculated. There was a potential savings in presumed lives per year saved and cost per quality-adjusted life year gained [22].

Currently, there are no cost-effectiveness models to evaluate this technology. Davis reported the total cost to upgrade pre-hospital ECG equipment was more than $16,000 [23]. This included funding for a receiving station, cellular phones, and data cables. Other collateral costs to consider include training personnel, quality assurance, and the actual organization and integration of EMS and hospital systems [24].

Key Points

- The use of pre-hospital ECG for the diagnosis of STEMI is recommended and, if properly implemented, results in shortening reperfusion time and lowering mortality rates.
- The preferred model of interpretation of pre-hospital ECG is wireless cardiologist interpretation.

Tele-Coronary Care Unit

Tele-coronary care units (CCU) are an exciting subset of tele-cardiology. The contemporary CCU includes patients with complicated myocardial infarction, decompensated heart failure, cardiogenic shock, and refractory ventricular arrhythmias. The literature to date has numerous clinical trials examining the effects of tele-ICU support on the ICU care team model. If implemented appropriately, tele-ICU has the potential to significantly reduce the mortality rate, length of stay, and complication rates and while improving best practice adherence [25, 26]. Some tele-ICU software platforms allow for continuous, real-time transmission of patients' vital signs. In addition, smart and sentry alert prompts use a combination of averages and medians to evaluate vital sign values over time to detect changes in heart rate, blood pressure, oxygen saturation, and respiratory rate [27]. These prompts notify clinicians early, allowing for timely intervention by monitoring staff. In this way, tele-ICU monitoring can provide tele-consultation and support to bedside physicians and nurses by continuous surveillance. Tele-ICU consultation in the CCU allows for continuous monitoring of vital signs, ECG, blood pressure waveforms, oxygen saturation (SpO_2), pulmonary artery catheter (PAC) waveforms, as well as respirations and body temperature. The feasibility of remote surveillance was studied by Nikus [28]. In this Finnish study, remote monitoring of the CCU and cardiology ward was carried out by a cardiologist who had access to electronic medical records and digitally stored 12-lead ECGs. The telecardiologist role was supportive and he/she was available for consultation and emergencies. The remote access to the hospital intranet and server applications proved reliable, secure, and technically feasible. The study indicated a potential for reducing the delay for diagnostic and therapeutic interventions. The study was limited by the fact that the cardiologist played a somewhat passive role [28].

Prompt diagnosis of acute myocardial infarction and reperfusion by interventions, either PCI or thrombolysis, has been shown to reduce morbidity and mortality, especially in the setting of STEMI [29, 30]. The 2013 American Heart Association/American College of Cardiology STEMI guidelines have stressed the need for integrated regional medical systems to provide reperfusion therapy in rural areas [31].

As seen in Fig. 13.2, pre-hospital thrombolysis in route to the CCU with telemedicine support has become an important modality in achieving timely reperfu-

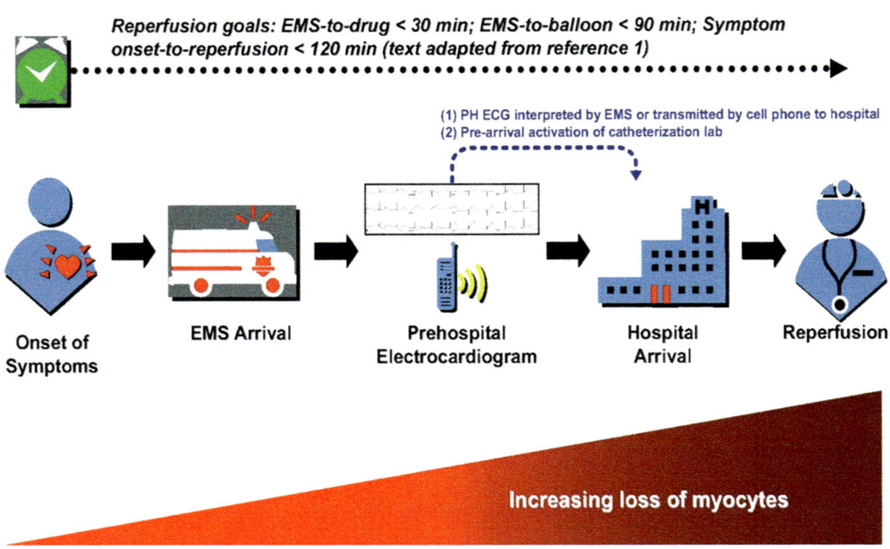

Fig. 13.2 Reperfusion time goals for patients after STEMI. (Used with permission. Ting, et al. [82]

sion [32, 33]. Tele-consultation and remote interaction with emergency medical transport staff with a cardiologist available in the CCU have been shown to reduce door-to-needle and door-to-balloon time delay. This may in turn increase patients' chances of survival and decrease the risks of postinfarction sequelae [34]. Tele-consultation with the support of wireless and mobile technology during transport has also been shown to be feasible [35, 36]. Integrated smartphone technology is now allowing for accurate interpretation of angiographic lesions and effortless communication between emergency medical services and the cardiologist [7].

Tele-Echocardiography

Cardiologists rely on echocardiography for the evaluation ventricular function, valvular disease, and physiological functions. Tele-echocardiography is a widely applied and accepted tool used between rural hospitals and tertiary care centers. With the advancement of telemedicine technologies, there is improved access to specialists capable of echocardiography interpretation. This has enabled cardiologists to guide sonographers remotely to make the correct diagnosis and formulate treatment plans.

Finley was the first to mention the interpretation of echocardiography by telemedicine support in the 1980s [37]. By 1990, there was mention of the establishment of a real-time pediatric echocardiography service at a tertiary care center which serviced regional hospitals. The system of transmission used in this case was dial-up broadband video transmission. Most studies were urgent in nature. A comparison between transmitted images and bedside "in person" images showed little differences in diagnoses and the rate of unnecessary transfers.

In 1996, Trippi studied the utilization of tele-echocardiography consultation in emergency telemedicine [38]. In their prospective study, urgent echocardiograms were performed during off-peak hours (nights, weekends, and holidays) to assess for ventricular function, ischemia, and valvular disease. Interpretation of the echocardiograms was compared to interpretation made by reviewing videotapes in a blinded manner. Off-site echocardiographers reviewed the images at home. Abnormalities were identified in more than 80% of the studies, including wall motion abnormalities, pulmonary hypertension, aortic dissection, valvular dysfunction, and tamponade. Telemedicine and videotape interpretations correlated 99% of the time and the time needed to generate official echocardiogram reports were reduced significantly as well. In the same year, Trippi [39, 40] also studied dobutamine stress tele-echocardiography (DSTE) in a small number of low-risk patients in the emergency room admitted for chest pain. The echocardiogram was performed by nurses and sonographers. All study images (DSTEs and ECGs) were interpreted by a remote cardiologist. The sensitivity and specificity of dobutamine stress tele-echocardiography versus clinical and cardiac catheterization findings were 89.5% and 88.9%, respectively, with a negative predictive value for DSTE of 98.5%. The use of DSTE as a screening tool in the evaluation of patients presenting with chest pain in the emergency department is reasonable when a skilled clinician is unavailable on site [39, 40].

Stress tele-echocardiography has also been used in the arena of heart transplantation. The Adonhers (Aged Donor Heart Rescue by Stress Echo) project created a network for second-opinion stress-echocardiography [41]. The project aimed to expand the heart donor pool by shifting upward the donor age cutoff limit (from 55 to 65 years). If older donor hearts had negative stress tele-echocardiogram for coronary heart disease and cardiomyopathy, they were included. The involved cardiologist sent digitized images to a central core echo lab in Pisa, Italy, for a second opinion. In the early years, the program to its credit provided second opinions to safely transplant six donor hearts in marginal patients. The authors suggested that second-opinion stress tele-echocardiography for aged donor heart selection can be done safely and may potentially extend the donor criteria for heart transplantation [41].

The field of pediatric cardiology has benefited greatly from the concept and implementation of tele-echocardiography. Neonates in smaller towns and rural areas have a scarcity of pediatric sonographers and cardiologists. The shortage of specialists in the field has preempted the early development of telemedicine services and led to a dramatic rise in pediatric tele-echocardiography in recent years [42]. Accurate remote diagnosis and the exclusion of congenital heart disease may avoid unnecessary patient transport and expedited care of sick neonates, thereby lowering mortality and cost [43–45].

Tele-echocardiography is limited by the fact that it requires a skilled operator for proper ultrasound image acquisition and exam quality. In an attempt to overcome this limitation, Courreges [46] developed and studied a robotic tele-ultrasound system (OTELO). The equipment consisted of two stations, an expert station where the remote sonographer controls a virtual probe and a patient station where a real probe is held by a robot and positioned on the patient. More than 50 patients at 2 different hospitals underwent virtual ultrasound examinations. The diagnosis made with this remote scanning system concurred in at least 80% of cases with the diagnosis made by bedside scanning. Disagreements with the final diagnosis occurred with lesions due to suboptimal and inadequate image acquisition.

Recent technology enables for video communication between families and their physicians and simultaneous live streaming of echocardiographic imaging. The "EchoCart" by StatVideo [47] streams over the web thereby negating the need for costly leased lines. It streams high definition and high frame rate echo images and also supports patient-to-physician interaction remotely. It is currently used in select tertiary centers in the USA.

In spite of inherent limitations of real-time tele-echocardiography, this modality has been effective in assisting with diagnostically challenging patients requiring complex management. For example, Otto described a case of a patient with pericarditis which required tele-ultrasound consultation between cardiologists at the University of Texas at Galveston and staff in a research center in Antarctica [48]. The use of this technology prevented unwarranted medical evacuation and transfer, allowing the patient to receive treatment at the local center. This case highlighted the importance of remote tools in the delivery of healthcare to geographically isolated populations. Other exciting and interesting research applications of tele-echocardiography have been demonstrated on the International Space Station [49].

Role of Telemedicine in Chronic Heart Failure Monitoring

There are currently over 5.7 million Americans with heart failure, and about 650,000 new diagnoses are made yearly [50]. By the year 2030, there will be a projected increase in heart failure diagnoses by 46%, with over 8 million patients living with the disease [51]. This epidemic is a significant driver of healthcare expenditure. The cost related to healthcare services, medications, and sick days due to heart failure was estimated to exceed $30 billion in 2013, with the average cost of a heart failure admission averaging about $23,000 [52]. And notably, the Center for Medicare and Medicaid Services (CMS) began public reporting of all-cause readmission rates after a heart failure admission in 2009 [53]. In 2010, the Patient Protection and Affordable Care Act enacted financial penalties to hospitals with the high readmission rates within 30 days of discharge for heart failure [54]. Thus, there is a drive to develop new strategies to improve heart failure care overall and focus to reduce readmission rates.

A reported 19–25% of heart failure patients admitted to US hospitals are admitted to a CCU; thus, it is vital to understand current strategies of heart failure telemonitoring and its impact on critical care utilization [55].

New drug therapies and remote monitoring of heart failure patients have become the cornerstone in heart failure management. Due to the complex nature of heart failure management, intermittent remote monitoring has become very appealing and potentially a cost-effective way of management at home. This intermittent remote support includes telephone communication with advanced practice providers and electronic monitoring with peripheral devices along with video consultation [56].

The initial experience with remote monitoring in heart failure did not show promising results and the data was somewhat conflicting. Rich demonstrated that nursing-directed, multidisciplinary inventions including family education, medication review, and social service consultation with outpatient follow-up (individualized home visits and telephone contact) reduced the rate of readmission, reduced cost per patient, and increased quality of life scores [57]. A clinical trial by Reigel in 2002, indicated that standardized nurse case management provided to sick heart failure patients by telephone in the first 6 months after discharge can reduce hospitalizations and costs and improve resource utilization and patient satisfaction [58]. Reigel placed a heavy emphasis on patient education. In this study, the patients' clinical status was followed by registered nurses for the first 6 months after discharge. The nurses were instructed to educate patients regarding their disease process and emphasize deterioration of illness with the help of decision support software [58]. A report of clinical status was sent to the patient's physician, who in turn chose appropriate interventions and therapies. Hospitalization rates were lowered by close to 50%, thus lowering inpatient costs.

In DeBusk's study in 2004 [59], low-risk heart failure patients in a single healthcare system were randomized to nursing interventions (i.e., telephone surveillance) with regular care or regular care alone. The intervention group received symptom monitoring, education, and medications for heart failure with the help of a study protocol. Their care was coordinated with the patients' primary care physician. Patients were contacted via telephone intermittently. The authors demonstrated telesupported nursing care management in low-risk heart failure patients did not significantly reduce hospitalization rates between the two groups and thus was not beneficial [59]. The DIAL trial was a trial comparing frequent centralized telephone interventions by a nurse trained in the management of chronic heart failure with usual care in 51 centers in Argentina [60]. The aim was to educate, counsel, and monitor patients through frequent telephone follow-up. The focus was adherence to diet, drug treatments, fluid status, and symptom monitoring. Software was used to determine the frequency of calls, and algorithms were used to adjust diuretic doses. With these interventions, there was a significant reduction in admissions for heart failure in the intervention group (relative risk reduction = 29%, $p = 0.005$), and better quality of life was noted in this group (mean total score on Minnesota living with heart failure questionnaire 30.6 vs. 35, $p = 0.001$) as compared to the nonintervention group.

A trial by Dunagan [61] randomized patients to usual care or scheduled telephone calls by nurses emphasizing self-care and guideline-based therapy as prescribed by primary physicians. The nurses screened for heart failure decompensation and changed diuretic dosing accordingly. Only structured telephone calls and telemonitoring were effective in reducing the risk of all-cause mortality. The intervention patients experienced a delay to encounter (hazard ratio (HR) = 0.67; 95% confidence interval (CI) 0.47–0.96; $p = 0.29$) and reduced frequency of hospital and heart failure-specific readmission. Hospital costs, hospital days, and admissions were significantly lower in the first 6 months, but this difference was not seen at 1 year. There was minimal impact on quality of life, functional status, or mortality.

In the TELE-HF trial (Tele-monitoring to Improve Heart Failure Outcomes), tele-monitoring by an interactive voice system collecting daily information regarding symptoms and weights was compared to standard care [62]. In this trial of over 1600 patients, there was no difference in the combined primary endpoint of readmission or death. The BEAT-HF (Better Effectiveness After Transition-Heart Failure) trial enrolled patients who were 50 years of age or older and recently admitted with heart failure [63]. In this trial of over 1400 patients, tele-monitoring using a comprehensive daily electronic collection of blood pressure, heart rate symptoms, and weights, targeted nurse phone calls and health coaching phone calls, was found to be no better than usual care.

Remote monitoring in chronic heart failure currently encompasses various technologies, including structured telephone calls, videophone, interactive voice response devices, and tele-monitoring consultation. But no one technology has been proven to be consistently superior to others. In Conway's sub-analysis and meta-analysis [64], two of the four modalities – structured telephone calls and tele-monitoring – were found to be effective in reducing the risk of all-cause mortality (relative risk (RR) 0.87, 95% confidence interval (CI) 0.75–1.01, $p = 0.06$ and RR 0.62, 95% CI 0.50–0.77, $p < 0.0001$, respectively) as well as heart failure-related hospitalizations (RR 0.77, 95% CI 0.68–0.87, $p < 0.001$ and RR 0.75, 95% CI 0.3–0.91, $p = 0.0003$, respectively). More randomized studies need to be done to focus on the effectiveness of remote monitoring in heart failure. Inglis looked at the efficacy of tele-monitoring (TM) and structured telephone support (STS) in a meta-analysis in 2011. The aim was to review randomized controlled trials for all-cause mortality and CHF-related hospitalizations. Tele-monitoring reduced all-cause mortality (RR 0.66, $p < 0.0001$). Both TM (RR 0.79, $p = 0.008$) and STS (RR 0.77, $p < 0.0001$) reduced CHR-related hospitalizations and cost, as well as improved quality of life scores [65].

A review looking at both telephone support and monitoring of vital signs and data by Schmidt concluded that vital sign monitoring may lower mortality, but improvements in patient-related outcomes have yet to be demonstrated [66]. Both modalities appear to be effective, but there is no evidence that one modality is superior to the other. Koehler [67] performed a study to determine whether physician-led remote telemedical management (RTM) would reduce mortality in outpatient chronic heart failure patients (New York Heart Association class II or III). A wireless Bluetooth device was connected to an ECG, blood pressure cuff, and weighing scale in the patient's home. Patients performed daily self-assessment with the devices and data was transmitted to the telemedicine center. Physicians in the center were available at any time for consultation and instituted treatments that they deemed necessary. The median follow-up was 26 months. Compared with usual care, there was no significant effect on all-cause mortality (RR 0.97, 95% CI 0.67–0.41, $p = 0.87$), cardiovascular death, or HF hospitalization.

A Japanese study by Kotooka aimed to investigate whether an automated physiological monitoring system HOMES-HF (body weight, blood pressure, and pulse rate) in a heart failure treatment program could reduce mortality and readmission rates after acute decompensated heart failure [68]. The primary endpoint was a composite of all-cause death or rehospitalization due to worsening heart failure. Patients were randomized into either the tele-monitoring group or usual care. The mean follow-up period was 15 months. There was no significant difference in the primary endpoint, and beneficial effects of tele-monitoring were not demonstrated.

The rate of implantation of cardiac implantable electronic devices (CIEDs) has been on the rise. These devices are able to record patient-specific variables like intrathoracic impedance that can serve as surrogate markers of fluid overload. Unfortunately, clinical trials using these technologies have not been shown to change clinical outcomes to date [69, 70]. The greatest advance in remote monitoring has been in the form of implantable pressure sensors as seen in Fig. 13.3. This is a monitoring system where information is provided by an implantable or noninvasive device is transmitted to a secure server. Clinicians can access the server via the Internet. The clinicians can then review data, respond to overall data trends or alerts, and communicate medical interventions directly to the patient.

The CardioMEMS HF system (Abbott, Sylmar, California) is a wireless pulmonary arterial pressure monitoring system that is implanted into a branch of the pul-

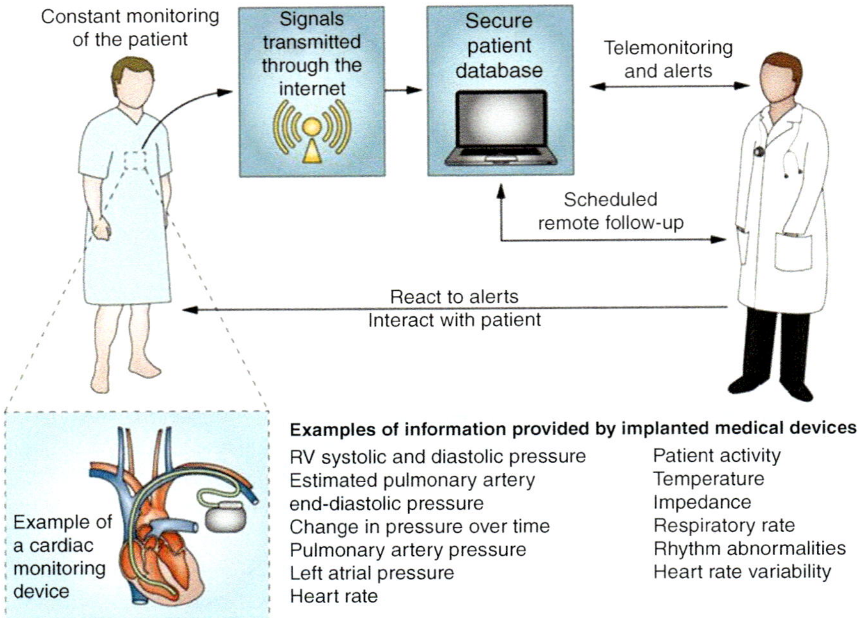

Fig. 13.3 Cardiac remote monitoring systems. (Used with permission. Abraham et al. [81])

monary artery. In the CHAMPION trial, 550 HF patients with both reduced ejection fraction as well as preserved ejection fraction were randomized to two groups. In the first group, physicians used daily monitoring of pulmonary arterial pressure in addition to standard care, while the second group consisted of standard care alone [71]. There was a 28% RR reduction in the primary endpoint of heart failure admissions at 6 months. In a pre-specified analysis of patients in the CHAMPION trial with HF with reduced EF, patients on two guideline-directed medications showed a 57% reduction in mortality [72]. A retrospective analysis of over 1100 patients who received the CardioMEMS device in a "real-world" setting showed a 45% lower rate of heart failure admissions 6 months after device implantation with a HF cost reduction of $7433 per patient [73]. There is great enthusiasm within the cardiology community for further developments in the field of pressure-guided remote heart failure management [74].

Key Points

- Remote telemedicine monitoring of chronic heart failure patients is recommended to reduce readmission rates.
- Home monitoring of cardiac implantable electronic devices is feasible and is associated with the early detection of medical and technical events.

Tele-Cardiology Prevention

The impact of telemedicine on preventative cardiac events was not been established. Since telemedicine has the capability of reaching people who would otherwise be isolated, the possibility of obtaining epidemiological data and controlling disease and other factors related to health is within reach. The CAPITAL study assessed cardiovascular risk and status of prevention in a Mediterranean region. This Italian study obtained the history and demographic information of patients and used screening ECG with remote telemedicine support at local pharmacies in Apulia, Italy. It concluded that awareness, therapy, and control of cardiovascular risk factors remain unsatisfactory in this particular geographical region and there remains a large scope for improvement in the control of cardiovascular risk factors with telemedicine support [75].

Tele-Cardiology for Rehabilitation

Support with the use of tele-cardiology has been demonstrated in the field of rehabilitation medicine after a cardiac event (acute coronary syndrome and cardiac surgery). Remote rehabilitation after cardiac surgery has been demonstrated to be effective and safe when compared with conventional rehabilitation [76]. Supervised home rehabilitation programs with nurses and physiotherapists have been shown to increase six-minute walking distance when compared to baseline [77]. After acute myocardial infarction, patients followed by telemedicine had significantly higher rates of survival at 1 year compared to usual care (4.4% vs. 9.7%, $p < 0.0001$) [78]. When compared directly with conventional therapy, telemedicine-supported rehabilitation was feasible for risk-factor modification and exercise monitoring of patients who would otherwise have had no access to these therapies [79].

Conclusion

Telemedicine continues to have a broadening impact in the field of cardiology with many applications in acute coronary syndrome, valvular disease, and chronic heart failure with positive implications on admission rates, morbidity, and mortality. The impact is being experienced in the pre-hospital, CCU, and post-discharge environments. More research is required to evaluate the potential benefits and cost-effectiveness of tele-cardiology support services.

Key Point
- The use of telemedicine support is effective in healthcare delivery in patients with cardiovascular disease.

Disclosure Statement The authors have nothing to disclose.

References

1. Strehle EM, Shabde N. One hundred years of telemedicine: does this technology have a place in paediatrics? Achiv Dis Child. 2006;91(12):956–9.
2. Einthoven W. Le telecardiogramme (the telecardiogram). Arch Int Physiol. 1906;4:132–64.
3. Go AS, Mozaffarian D, Roger VL, Benjamin EJ, Berry JD, Blaha MJ, Dai S, Ford ES, Fox CS, Franco S, Fullerton HJ, Gillespie C, Hailpern SM, Heit JA, Howard VJ, Huffman MD, Judd SE, Kissela BM, Kittner SJ, Lackland DT, Lichtman JH, Lisabeth LD, Mackey RH, Magid DJ, Marcus GM, Marelli A, Matchar DB, DK MG, Mohler ER 3rd, Moy CS, Mussolino ME, Neumar RW, Nichol G, Pandey DK, Paynter NP, Reeves MJ, Sorlie PD, Stein J, Towfighi A, Turan TN, Virani SS, Wong ND, Woo D, Turner MB. Executive summary: heart disease and stroke statistics--2014 update: a report from the American Heart Association. Circulation. 2014;129:399–410.
4. Morrow DA, Fang JC, Fintel DJ, Granger CB, Katz JN, Kushner FG, Kuvin JT, Lopez-Sendon J, McAreavey D, Nallamothu B, Page RL 2nd, Parrillo JE, Peterson PN, Winkelman C. Evolution of critical care cardiology: transformation of the cardiovascular intensive care unit and the emerging need for new medical staffing and training models: a scientific statement from the American Heart Association. Circulation. 2012;126:1408–28.
5. Yousef J, Lars A. Validation of a real-time wireless telemedicine system, using Bluetooth protocol and mobile phone, for remote monitoring patient in medical practice. Eur J Med Res. 2005;10:254–62.
6. Giannakakis G, Buliev I. ECG signal recording, processing and transmission using a mobile phone. Proceedings of the 1st international conference on pervasive technologies related to assistive environments; 2008 July 15–19; Athens, Greece. New York: ACM Digital Library; 2008.
7. Hsieh J, Li A, Yang C. Mobile, cloud, and big data computing: contributions, challenges, and new directions in tele-cardiology. Int J Environ Res Public Health. 2013;10:6131–615.
8. Giovas P, Papadoyannis D, Thomakos D, et al. Transmission of electrocardiograms from a moving ambulance. J Telemed Telecare. 1998;4:S5–7.
9. Carmody BJ. A novel approach to transmission of the out-of-hospital EKG in patients with ST segment elevation myocardial infarction. Ann Emerg Med. 2008;52:183–4.
10. Brunetti ND, De Gennaro L, Amodio G, et al. Tele-cardiology improves quality of diagnosis and reduces delay to treatment in elderly patients with acute myocardial infarction and atypical presentation. Eur J Cardiovasc Prev Rehabil. 2010;17:615–20.
11. Beygui F, Castren M, Brunetti ND, et al. ACCA Study Group on Pre-hospital Care. Pre-hospital management of patients with chest pain and/or dyspnoea of cardiac origin. A position paper of the Acute Cardiovascular Care Association (ACCA) of the ESC. Eur Heart J Acute Cardiovasc Care. Epub ahead of print 27 Aug 2015.
12. O'Gara PT, Kushner FG, Ascheim DD, Casey DE Jr, Chung MK, de Lemos JA, et al. 2013 ACCF/AHA guideline for the management of ST-elevation myocardial infarction: a report of the American College of Cardiology Foundation/American Heart Association Task Force on Practice Guidelines. Circulation. 2013;127(4):e362–425.
13. Ward MJ, Kripalani S, Zhu Y, Storrow AB, Dittus RS, Harrell FE Jr, et al. Incidence of emergency department visits for ST-elevation myocardial infarction in a recent six-year period in the United States. Am J Cardiol. 2015;115(2):167–70.
14. McManus DD, Gore J, Yarzebski J, Spencer F, Lessard D, Goldberg RJ. Recent trends in the incidence, treatment, and outcomes of patients with STEMI and NSTEMI. Am J Med. 2011;124(1):40–7.

15. Ibanez B, James S, Agewall S, Antunes MJ, Bucciarelli-Ducci C, Bueno H, et al. 2017 ESC Guidelines for the management of acute myocardial infarction in patients presenting with ST-segment elevation: The Task Force for the management of acute myocardial infarction in patients presenting with ST-segment elevation of the European Society of Cardiology (ESC). Eur Heart J. 2018;39(2):119–77.
16. Brunetti ND, Di Pietro G, Aquilino A, Bruno AI, et al. Pre-hospital electrocardiogram triage with tele-cardiology support is associated with shorter time-to-balloon and higher rates of timely reperfusion even in rural areas: data from the Bari-Barletta/Andria/Trani public emergency medical service 118 registry on primary angioplasty in ST-elevation myocardial infarction. Eur Heart J Acute Cardiovasc Care. 2014;3(3):204–13.
17. Hutchison AW, Malaiapan Y, Jarvie I, et al. PreHospital and emergency department activation of the infarct team significantly improves door-to-door times: ambulance Vistoria and MonashHEART Acute Myocardial Infarction (MonAMI) 12-lead ECG project. Circ Cardiovasc Interv. 2009;2:528–34.
18. Rasmussen MB, Frost L, Stengaard C, Brorholt-Petersen JU, et al. Diagnostic performance and system delay using telemedicine for prehospital diagnosis in triage and treatment of STEMI. Heart. 2014;100(9):711–5.
19. Tanguay A, Brassard E, Lebon J, Begin F, Hebert D, Paradis JM. Effectiveness of a prehospital wireless 12-Lead electrocardiogram and cardiac catheterization laboratory activation for ST-elevation myocardial infarction. Am J Cardiol. 2017;119(4):553–9.
20. Sivagangabalan G, Ong AT, Narayan A, Sadick N, et al. Effect of prehospital triage on revascularization times, left ventricular function, and survival in patients with ST-elevation myocardial infarction. Am J Cardiol. 2009;103(7):907–12.
21. Chan AW, Kornder J, Elliott H, Brown RI, et al. Improved survival associated with pre-hospital strategy in a large regional ST-segment elevation myocardial infarction program. JACC Cardiovasc Interv. 2012;5(12):1239–46.
22. Brunetti ND, Dellegrottaglie G, Lopriore C, Di Giuseppe G, et al. Prehospital telemedicine electrocardiogram triage for a regional public emergency medical service: is it worth it? a preliminary cost analysis. Clin Cardiol. 2014;37(3):140–5.
23. Davis DP, Graydon C, Stein R, Wilson S, Buesch B, Berthiaume S, Lee DM, Rivas J, Vilke GM, Leahy DR. The positive predictive value of paramedic versus emergency physician interpretation of the prehospital 12-lead electrocardiogram. Prehosp Emerg Care. 2007;11:399–402.
24. Aufderheide TP, Kereiakes DJ, Weaver WD, Gibler WB, Simoons ML. Planning, implementation, and process monitoring for prehospital 12-lead ECG diagnostic programs. Prehosp Disaster Med. 1996;11:162–71.
25. Lilly CM, Cody S, Zhao H, Landry K, Baker SP, et al. Hospital mortality, length of stay and preventable complications among critically ill patients before and after tele-ICU reengineering of critical care processes. JAMA. 2011;305(21):2175–83.
26. Sadaka F, Palagiri A, Trottier S, Deibert W, et al. Telemedicine intervention improves ICU outcomes. Crit Care Res Pract. 2013;2013:456389.
27. 3.9 eCareManager User guide. https://www.usa.philips.com/healthcare/product/HC865325CM/ecaremanager-enterprise-tele-health-software.
28. Nikus K, Lahteenmaki J, Lehto P, Eskola M. The role of continuous monitoring in a 24/7 telecardiology consultation service- a feasibility study. J Electrocardiol. 2009;42(6):473–80.
29. Keeley EC, Boura JA, Grines CL. Primary angioplasty versus intravenous thrombolytic therapy for acute myocardial infarction: a quantitative review of 23 randomised trials. Lancet. 2003;361:13–20.
30. Dalby M, Bouzamondo A, Lechat P, Montalescot G. Transfer for primary angioplasty versus immediate thrombolysis in acute myocardial infarction: a meta-analysis. Circulation. 2003;108:1809–14.
31. O'Gara PT, Kushner FG, Ascheim DD, Casey DE Jr, Chung MK, de Lemos JA, Ettinger SM, Fang JC, Fesmire FM, Franklin BA, Granger CB, Krumholz HM, Linderbaum JA, Morrow DA, Newby LK, Ornato JP, Ou N, Radford MJ, Tamis-Holland JE, Tommaso CL, Tracy CM, Woo

YJ, Zhao DX, Anderson JL, Jacobs AK, Halperin JL, Albert NM, Brindis RG, Creager MA, DeMets D, Guyton RA, Hochman JS, Kovacs RJ, Kushner FG, Ohman EM, Stevenson WG, Yancy CW. 2013 accf/aha guideline for the management of st-elevation myocardial infarction: a report of the American College of Cardiology Foundation/American Heart Association task force on practice guidelines. Circulation. 2013;127:e362–425.
32. Danchin A, Durand E, Blanchard D. Pre-hospital thrombolysis in perspective. Eur Heart J. 2008;29(23):2835–42.
33. Danchin N, Blanchard P, Steg PG, et al. Impact of prehospital thrombolysis for acute myocardial infarction on 1 year outcome: results from the French nationwide USIC 2000 registry. Circulation. 2004;110(14):1909–15.
34. McLean S, Wild S, Connor P, Flapan AD. Treating ST elevation myocardial infarction by primary percutaneous coronary intervention, in-hospital thrombolysis and prehospital thrombolysis. An observational study of timelines and outcomes in 625 patients. Emerg Med J. 2011;28(3):230–6.
35. Correa BS, Goncalves B, Teixeira IM, Gomes AT, Ziviani A. AToMS: a Ubiquitous teleconsultation system for supporting AMI patients with prehospital thrombolysis. Int J Telemed Appl. 2011;2011:560209.
36. Bilgi M, Erol T, Gullu H, Sezgin AT, Hamad S, Bilgel ZG, Muderrisoglu H. Teleconsultation of coronary angiograms using smartphones and an audio/video conferencing application. Technol Health Care. 2013;21(4):407–14.
37. Finley JP, Sharratt GP, Nanton MA, Chen RP, et al. Paediatric echocardiography by telemedicine—nine years' experience. J Telemed Telecare. 1997;3(4):200–4.
38. Trippi JA, Lee KS, Kopp G, et al. Emergency echocardiography telemedicine: an efficient method to provide 24-hour consultative echocardiography. J Am Coll Cardiol. 1996;27:1748–52.
39. Trippi JA, Kopp A, Lee KS, Morrison H, Risk G, et al. The feasibility of dobutamine stress echocardiography in the emergency department with telemedicine interpretation. J Am Soc Echocardiogr. 1996;9(2):113–8.
40. Trippi JA, Lee KS, Kopp G, et al. Dobutamine stress tele-cardiography for evaluation of emergency department patients with chest pain. J Am Coll Cardiol. 1997;30:627–32.
41. Franchi D, Cini D, Arpesella G, et al. Second-opinion stress tele-echocardiography for the Adonhers (aged donor heart rescue by stress echo) project. Cardiovasc Ultrasound. 2010;1:20.
42. Krishnan A, Fuska M, Dixon R, et al. The evolution of pediatric tele-echocardiography: 15-year experience of over 10,000 transmissions. Telemed J E Health. 2014;20:681–6.
43. Grant B, Morgan GJ, McCrossan BA, Crealey GE, Sands AJ, et al. Remote diagnosis of congenital heart disease: the impact of telemedicine. Arch Dis Child. 2010;95:270–80.
44. Dowie R, Mistry H, Yound TA, Franklin RC, Gardiner HM. Cost implications of introducing a tele-cardiology service to support fetal ultrasound screening. J Telemed Telecare. 2008;14:412–22.
45. Haley JE, Klewer SE, Barber BJ, Meaney FJ, Donnerstein RL, et al. Remote diagnosis of congenital heart disease in southern Arizona: comparison between tele-cardiography and videotapes. Telemed J E Health. 2012;18(10):736–42.
46. Fabien C, Vieyres P, Istepanian R, Arbeille P, Bru C. Clinical trials and evaluation of a mobile, robotic tele-ultrasound system. J Telemed Telecare. 2005;11(Suppl. 1):46–9.
47. http://www.itnonline.com/article/statvideos-echocart-streams-tele-echocardiography-images-babies'-hearts-duke-childrens-hospital.
48. Otto CA, Shemenski R, Drudi L. Real-time tele-echocardiography: diagnosis and management of a pericardial effusion secondary to pericarditis at Antarctic research station. Telemed J E Health. 2012 Sep;18(7):521–4.
49. Hamilton DR, Sargsyyan AE, Martin DS, Garcia KM, Melton SL, et al. On-orbit prospective echocardiography on International Space Station crew. Echocardiography. 2011;28(5):491–501.
50. Yancy CW, Jessup M, Bozkurt B, et al. 2013 ACCF/AHA guideline for the management of heart failure: a report of the American College of Cardiology Foundation/American Heart Association Task Force on Practice Guidelines. J Am Coll Cardiol. 2013;62:e147–239.

51. Benjamin EJ, Virani SS, Callaway CW, Chamberlain AM, Chang AR, Cheng S, et al. Heart disease and stroke statistics-2018 update: a report from the American Heart Association. Circulation. 2018;137(12):e67–e492.
52. Vigen R, Maddox TM, Allen LA. Aging of the United States population: impact on heart failure. Curr Heart Fail Rep. 2012;9:369–74.
53. Desai AS, Stevenson LW. Rehospitalization for heart failure: predict or prevent? Circulation. 2012;126:501–6.
54. http://housedocs.house.gov/energycommerce/ppacacon.pdf.
55. van Diepen S, Podder M, Hernandez AF, Westerhout CM, Armstong PW, McMurray JJ, et al. Acute decompensated heart failure patients admitted to critical care units: insights from ASCEND-HF. Int J Cardiol. 2014;177(3):840–6.
56. Riley JP, Cowie MR. Telemonitoring in heart failure. Heart. 2009;95:1964–8.
57. Rich MW, Beckham V, Wittenberg C, Leven CL, Freeland KE, Carney RM. A multidisciplinary intervention to prevent the readmission of elderly patients with congestive heart failure. N Engl J Med. 1995;333:1190–5.
58. Riegel B, Carlson B, Kopp Z, LePetri B, Glaser D, Unger A. Effect of a standardized nurse case-management telephone intervention on resource use in patients with chronic heart failure. Arch Intern Med. 2002;162(6):705–12.
59. DeBusk RF, Miller NH, Parker KM, Bandura A, et al. Care management for low-risk patients with heart failure, a randomized, control trial. Ann Intern Med. 2004;141:606–13.
60. GESICA Inventigators. Randomised trial of telephone intervention in chronic heart failure: DIAL trial. BMJ. 2005;331(7514):425.
61. Dunagan WC, Littenberg B, Ewald GA, Jones CA, et al. Randomized trial of a nurse-administered, telephone-based disease management for patients with heart failure. J Card Fail. 2005;11(5):358–65.
62. Chaudhry SI, Mattera JA, Curtis JP, Spertus JA, Herrin J, Lin Z, et al. Telemonitoring in patients with heart failure. N Engl J Med. 2010;363(24):2301–9.
63. Ong MK, Romano PS, Edgington S, Aronow HU, Auerbach AD, Black JT, et al. Effectiveness of remote patient monitoring after discharge of hospitalized patients with heart failure: the better effectiveness after transition – heart failure (BEAT-HF) randomized clinical trial. JAMA Intern Med. 2016;176(3):310–8.
64. Conway A, Inglis SC, Clark RA. Effective technologies for noninvasive remote monitoring in heart failure. Telemed J E Health. 2014;20:531–8.
65. Inglis SC, Clack RA, McAlister FA, Stewart S, Cleland JG. Which components of heart failure programmes are effective? a systematic review and meta-analysis of the outcome of structures telephone support or telemonitoring as the primary component of chronic heart failure management in 8323 patients: abridged cochrane review. Eur J Heart Fail. 2011;13(9):1028–40.
66. Schmidt S, Schuchert A, Krieg T, Oeff M. Home telemonitoring in patients with chronic heart failure: a chance to improve care? Dtsch Arztebl Int. 2010;107(8):131–8.
67. Koehler F, Winkler S, Scheiber M, Sechtem U, Stangl K, et al. Impact of remote telemedicine management on mortality and hospitalizations in ambulatory patients with chronic heart failure. Circulation. 2011;123:1873–80.
68. Kotooka N, Kitakaze M, Nagashima K, Asaka M, et al. The first multicenter, randomized, controlled trial of home telemonitoring for Japanese patients with heart failure: home telemonitoring study for patients with heart failure [HOMES-HF]. Heart Vessels. 2018;33(8):866–76.
69. van Veldhuisen DJ, Braunschweig F, Conraads V, Ford I, Cowie MR, Jondeau G, et al. Intrathoracic impedance monitoring, audible patient alerts, and outcome in patients with heart failure. Circulation. 2011;124(16):1719–26.
70. Morgan JM, Dimitrov BD, Gill J, Kitt S, Ng GA, McComb JM, et al. Rationale and study design of the REM-HF study: remote management of heart failure using implanted devices and formalized follow-up procedures. Eur J Heart Fail. 2014;16(9):1039–45.
71. Abraham WT, Adamson PB, Bourge RC, Aaron MF, Costanzo MR, Stevenson LW, et al. Wireless pulmonary artery haemodynamic monitoring in chronic heart failure: a randomised controlled trial. Lancet (London, England). 2011;377(9766):658–66.

72. Givertz MM, Stevenson LW, Costanzo MR, Bourge RC, Bauman JG, Ginn G, et al. Pulmonary artery pressure-guided management of patients with heart failure and reduced ejection fraction. J Am Coll Cardiol. 2017;70(15):1875–86.
73. Desai AS, Bhimaraj A, Bharmi R, Jermyn R, Bhatt K, Shavelle D, et al. Ambulatory hemodynamic monitoring reduces heart failure hospitalizations in "real-world" clinical practice. J Am Coll Cardiol. 2017;69(19):2357–65.
74. Abraham WT, Perl L. Implantable hemodynamic monitoring for heart failure patients. J Am Coll Cardiol. 2017;70(3):389–98.
75. Brunetti ND, Lanzone S, Dellegrottaglie G, Di Giuseppe G, De Gennaro L, Novielli V, Straziota E, Loiacone T, Di Biase M. The CAPITAL study {CArdiovascular prevention with tele-cardiology in ApuLia}: preliminary results. J Cardiovasc Med(Hagerstown). 2016;17(7):455–61.
76. Scalvini S, Zanelli E, Comini L, Dalla Tomba M, Troise G, Febo O, Giordano A. Home-based versus in-hospital cardiac rehabilitation after cardiac surgery: a nonrandomized controlled study. Phys Ther. 2013;93(8):1073–83.
77. Scalvini S, Zanelli E, Comini L, et al. Home-based exercise rehabilitation with telemedicine following cardiac surgery. J Telemed Telecare. 2009;15:297–301.
78. Roth A, Malov N, Steinberg DM, et al. Telemedicine for post-myocardial infarction patients: an observational study. Telemed J E Health. 2009;15:24–30.
79. Dalleck LC, Schmidt LK, Lueker R. Cardiac rehabilitation outcomes in a conventional versus telemedicine-based programme. J Telemed Telecare. 2011;17:217–21.
80. Rao A, Kardouh Y, Darda S, Desai D, Devireddy L, Lalonde T, Rosman H, David S. Impact of the pre-hospital ECG on door-to-balloon time in STEMI. Catheter Cardiovasc Interv. 2010;75(2):174–8.
81. Abraham WT, Stough WG, Pina IL, Linde C, Borer JS, De Ferrari GM, Mehran R, Stein KM, Vincent A, Yadav JS, Anker SD, Zannad F. Trials of implantable monitoring devices in heart failure: which design is optimal? Nat Rev Cardiol. 2014;11(10):576–85.
82. Ting HH, Krumholz HM, Bradley EH, Cone DC, Curtis JP, Drew BJ, Field JM, French WJ, Gibler WB, Goff DC, Jacobs AK, Nallamothu BK, O'Connor RE, Schuur JD, American Heart Association Interdisciplinary Council on Quality of Care and Outcomes Research, Emergency Cardiovascular Care Committee; American Heart Association Council on Cardiovascular Nursing; American Heart Association Council on Clinical Cardiology. Implementation and integration of prehospital ECGs into systems of care for acute coronary syndrome: a scientific statement from the American Heart Association Interdisciplinary Council on Quality of Care and Outcomes Research, Emergency Cardiovascular Care Committee, Council on Cardiovascular Nursing, and Council on Clinical Cardiology. Circulation. 2008;118(10):1066–79. https://doi.org/10.1161/CIRCULATIONAHA.108.190402. Epub 2008 Aug 13.

Chapter 14
Telemedicine in the Pediatric ICU

S. David McSwain, John Chuo, Carley M. Howard Draddy, and Dana Schinasi

History and Early Programs

Just as pediatric practice encompasses the full array of healthcare services, pediatric telemedicine encompasses a broad and diverse array of primary care, specialty, and interprofessional services [1]. This variety also extends to the areas of pediatric critical care, emergency medicine, and neonatology. While specialists in these areas often face emergent, critical, and time-sensitive situations, their expertise also extends to chronic conditions such as asthma, chronic lung disease, diabetes, and pulmonary hypertension and encompasses the full spectrum of disease severity, from minor skin conditions to life-threatening organ failure. As such, telemedicine has been applied successfully in numerous ways to complement, extend, and coordinate the care by these providers.

Early programs for pediatric critical care, emergency medicine, and neonatology focused on the on-demand, emergent management of children presenting to (or born

S. D. McSwain (✉)
Pediatric Critical Care Medicine, Telehealth Optimization, Medical University of South Carolina, Charleston, SC, USA
e-mail: mcswains@musc.edu

J. Chuo
Clinical Pediatrics, Children's Hospital of Philadelphia, Philadelphia, PA, USA
e-mail: chuoj@email.chop.edu

C. M. Howard Draddy
Pediatric Telehealth and Special Projects, Children's Hospital of Greenville Health System, Greenville, SC, USA
e-mail: choward@ghs.org

D. Schinasi
Pediatric Emergency Medicine, Telehealth Programs, Ann & Robert H. Lurie Children's Hospital of Chicago, Chicago, IL, USA
e-mail: DSchinasi@luriechildrens.org

M. A. Koenig (ed.), *Telemedicine in the ICU*,
https://doi.org/10.1007/978-3-030-11569-2_14

into) remote facilities that did not have pediatric specialists available on staff [2, 3]. Programs in Arkansas, California, Oregon, and Vermont pioneered this approach, which has subsequently been successfully deployed in many other locations in the USA and across the globe [4–8]. The use of telemedicine also expanded beyond the ad hoc emergency encounter, to address a variety of other clinical and care coordination scenarios: home management and care coordination for medically complex children [9–12], pediatric critical care consultation to adult ICUs [13, 14], telemedicine provision during critical care transport [15, 16], family involvement in critical care team rounds [17], family connections with their hospitalized children, healthcare education for remote providers, and more.

The use cases for pediatric critical care telemedicine-based consultation can be categorized based on the following characteristics: patient location, provider location, acuity of consult, and chronicity of the condition. Patients receiving pediatric critical care consultation are most often located in rural community emergency departments (ED), where pediatric critical care telemedicine consultation is utilized to assist in acute management, triage, and transfer decisions. However, services can be provided to patients in any location, including rural community hospital inpatient wards, outpatient clinics, patient homes, remote pediatric and adult ICUs, and various locations within the consulting physician's home institution. Home consultations and outpatient clinic consultations may be offered for children with chronic conditions or as follow-up to an acute inpatient admission. Consultation to rural community hospital inpatient wards is often an extension of an existing consultation program to community EDs at the same location. Consultation to adult ICUs has been provided as a means of keeping older pediatric patients in their own communities, while consultation to remote pediatric ICUs can be used as a means of assessing patients in need of transfer for specialized care not available at the referring PICU, such as extracorporeal life support (ECLS) or transplant services. Consultation within the consultant's home institution may be provided for quicker response to acute clinical situations (rapid response and/or codes) occurring in patients admitted to the floor, as well as for assessment of patients admitted to the home PICU when providers are taking call from home [6].

Pediatric Critical Care Teleconsultation to Remote EDs and Hospital Floors

The best studied example of pediatric critical care telemedicine is pediatric critical care teleconsultation to remote EDs and hospital floors. Early examples of such programs [2, 18] demonstrated both the feasibility and the high level of provider satisfaction with such services. The rationale for these programs is simple to understand: pediatric critical care providers practice almost exclusively in metropolitan and suburban areas, and yet the majority of pediatric ED visits occur at sites that do not have pediatric critical care expertise [19]. In a critical clinical situation, in which time is of the essence and community providers often do not have the training, experience, resources, or equipment to deal effectively with critically ill or severely injured pediatric patients, the provision of emergent remote consultative services by subspecialty trained pediatric critical care physicians can have dramatic impacts on a variety of factors surrounding the encounter.

These programs typically involve a mobile cart-based videoconferencing endpoint on the patient side, which often includes multiple peripheral examination devices, most often a tele-stethoscope. Consultants connect to the patient endpoint using a variety of devices, including similar cart-based solutions, computers loaded with videoconferencing software, or mobile devices with videoconferencing applications. Providers consult from a variety of locations, depending on the predetermined workflow of the service and the existing clinical practice patterns for the providers, including the consulting institution PICU, provider offices, dedicated teleconsultation rooms or stations, provider homes, or even using mobile devices with cellular data services to consult from anywhere.

Pediatric Critical Care Teleconsultation to Remote ICUs

Patients in pediatric intensive care units often have conditions that require multiple subspecialists to consult – not only in pediatric intensive care but also pediatric cardiology, pulmonology, infectious disease, rheumatology, nephrology, neurology, and surgery, to name a few. The availability of such consultants may not be readily accessible in community hospital PICUs and therefore result in over-triage or transfer to quaternary pediatric centers [20]. A tele-ICU care model (episodic consultative and/or continuous monitoring) that allows a regional children's hospital pediatric team to be immediately available via telemedicine and remote monitoring enables lower acuity children to stay in their community safely and have high patient satisfaction [21]. Meta-analyses studies on continuous monitoring models show a reduction in ICU mortality and length of stay, while there is at least a trend toward reduction in overall hospital mortality and length of stay [22, 23] .

Pediatric Emergency Medicine Teleconsultation to Remote EDs

In 2010, patients under 18 years of age accounted for one-fifth of all ED visits nationally, with over 25 million unique visits [24, 25] Many community EDs do not have the capacity to support staffing subspecialty trained pediatric emergency medicine (PEM) providers around the clock, with the expertise to evaluate, treat, and direct disposition decisions for acutely ill and injured children [19]. Children are often transferred to academic pediatric EDs for conditions that could be addressed in a community setting [26], such as orthopedic problems, bronchiolitis, and acute gastroenteritis. With telemedicine, many of these patients can receive the same quality of care without transferring. PEM providers at academic institutions are increasingly connecting with community hospital EDs to provide virtual support for the care of these children, with the goal of keeping children with common pediatric conditions in their local communities, supporting the real-time management of children with rare or complex pediatric conditions, and improving access to pediatric subspecialists. As the ED is often the point of entry for children requiring hospitalization, ED-based pediatric telemedicine has the added benefit of providing additional data to inform disposition decisions, directing admissions, and often replacing the need for ED evaluation prior to transfer to the inpatient unit.

Family-Centered Care

Children do best when they are surrounded by their parents/guardians/caregivers, who in turn are best equipped to cope with the stress of an acutely ill or injured child when their support system is intact. Telemedicine technologies enable the reinforcement of family-centered care in three main ways: avoiding inter-facility transfers thereby keeping children in their local communities whenever safe and feasible, improving communication between families and the consulting care team during remote consultations, and connecting caregivers with their hospitalized child and/or care team when circumstances do not allow a caregiver to stay at the child's bedside throughout the hospitalization.

The burden of inter-facility transfer of a child away from his or her local community on family-centered care extends beyond the emotional and psychological impact. There are costs of transportation (e.g., personal vehicle, gas, ambulance fees), opportunity costs (e.g., reallocation of transport services for other patients), family costs of being transported away from their community, and redundant care at the accepting institution [26, 27]. A downstream effect of critically ill children hospitalized away from their local communities is that parents are not consistently able to be present during family-centered PICU rounds. Telemedicine allows for remote parent participation in rounds when parents are unable to be physically present at the bedside, thereby enhancing parent-provider communication and offering parental reassurance [17].

Pediatric Telemedicine Guidelines and Operating Procedures

Regardless of the clinical setting, there are unique considerations related to provision of telemedicine in the pediatric population. Guidance on the safe and effective practice of pediatric telemedicine was published in 2017 by the American Telemedicine Association [28] and endorsed by multiple professional societies including the American Academy of Pediatrics. Clinical practice guidelines for specific pediatric conditions and diagnoses have yet to be developed due to a lack of adequate evidence base to make specific recommendations. However, much of the guidance available is relevant to pediatric critical care, emergency care, and neonatology telemedicine services. Notable considerations in pediatrics are highlighted in this section.

Standard of Care

Telemedicine providers must comply with the established standard of care for any clinical situation as they would during an in-person encounter. A key factor in telemedicine evaluation is recognizing the limitations of the telemedicine encounter which may prevent adherence to the standard of care and referring to an appropriate clinical location in that event. In emergency and critical care situations, it should be noted, however, that an evaluation by a trained pediatric specialist which is limited by technical constraints may still provide a higher level of care than an in-person examination by a provider without the same level of pediatric expertise. As such, a limited telemedicine evaluation in a critical situation may actually represent an improvement over the standard of care in comparison to the lack of evaluation by a pediatric specialist. A thorough understanding of the expertise, resources, and capabilities of the referring site is crucial to determining the benefits that telemedicine evaluation can provide. Consulting providers must also understand the constraints on their physical exam imposed by the use of technology and have a plan in place for how to address these constraints without sacrificing the standard of care. Since most critical care consultation services occur with the assistance of another trained healthcare professional at the patient location, the consulting provider can often leverage the physical exam findings of the on-site providers to supplement their own exam and aid in decision-making.

Informed Consent

Consent procedures for pediatric telemedicine services should address potential privacy and security issues inherent in a virtual encounter, including the risks of transmitting and/or storing private patient health information and images electronically. Informed consent should also include information on billing procedures, record sharing, and the relevant credentials of the telemedicine provider. While telemedicine-specific consent is recommended for pediatric telemedicine encounters, many emergency and critical care encounters represent a situation in which obtaining consent in a timely manner is either impractical or could result in a delay in potentially lifesaving care. Therefore, consent requirements may be waived for emergency encounters or may be included within the general ED consent form. However, in the event that written informed consent is not obtained, providers should introduce themselves and any other team members participating from the consulting site, including their relevant credentials, and describe the purpose of the telemedicine encounter to the patient or patient family as appropriate at the initiation of the encounter.

Child Abuse

The evaluation of children suspected of having suffered child abuse or nonaccidental trauma is common in critical care and emergency environments. In these situations, state child protective rules supersede individual HIPAA regulations for consent. Additionally, given the risk of disrupting the legal chain of evidence, the acquisition and storage of any images related to the evaluation of suspected or potential child abuse must follow strict, prospectively determined procedures for safety, security, privacy, storage, and transmission.

Expected Areas of Growth for Telemedicine in Pediatric Intensive Care

Neonatal ICU

The neonatal intensive care unit is a unique type of intensive care environment treating patients as young as 23 weeks of gestation to 1-year-old, with length of stay averaging much longer than typical pediatric ICU stays. Similar to PICUs, NICUs present opportunities for tele-transport, tele-resuscitation [29], pretransfer teleconsultation before the ICU admission [30], teleconsultation, and family engagement during the admission. Interestingly, post-discharge tele-visits may have more application for NICUs since most NICU patients are discharged directly from the intensive care unit to their primary care physicians – therefore, presenting a unique opportunity for post-discharge tele-visits as well as tele-signouts for medically complex infants [31].

Acute Resuscitation Guidance

Per the Neonatal Resuscitation Program (NRP), approximately 10% of all newborns will need some assistance at delivery, and approximately 1% will need significant resuscitation [32]. The American Academy of Pediatrics Committee on Fetus and Newborn has defined Levels of Neonatal Care, recognizing that the availability of neonatal intensive care has improved outcomes of high-risk infants born either preterm or with serious medical or surgical conditions. Nationally, there has been a move toward the concept and implementation of regionalized systems of perinatal care [33]. Despite these advancements and the best risk stratifications and predictions, complications during labor and delivery still arise unexpectedly and can and will occur in level 1 facilities. Telemedicine offers a unique solution to support the on-site team in the care of these infants. Telemedicine provided by neonatal nurse practitioners and neonatologists to outlying delivery centers during acute neonatal resuscitation has been shown to significantly reduce the time to establish effective ventilation and improve provider adherence to NRP guidelines [34]. This leads to improved outcomes including prevention of unnecessary transfers to a higher level of care [29], decreasing the time interval for transport when necessary including streamlining the entire transport process and handoff, and shortening the time to initiation of passive cooling for neuroprotection when indicated [35].

Patient Handoffs and Provider Communication

Clinicians have suggested the potential benefits of using telemedicine to improve the transition of care among providing teams (which includes the family provider role), especially for children with medical complexity that involve many subspecialists, care facilities, and home caregivers. Examples include transitioning from hospital to ambulatory care, pediatric to adult subspecialists, and between facilities where procedures and diagnostic testing are often done. A telemedicine conversation provides a better, more effective way to transmit such information. A judicious approach to identifying clinical situations that can most benefit from telemedicine is critical, both to guide implementation and reimbursement.

Children who are discharged from ICU stays often are medically complex and/or technology-dependent and at high risk for readmission within the first 2 weeks following hospital discharge [36]. Therefore, connecting the intensive care team with the families and/or their pediatricians shortly after leaving the hospital may uncover gaps in practice and knowledge, evolving medical complications, and reinforce education. A recent report of 93 post-discharge tele-visits showed that at least 50% of parents reported that the tele-visits prevented them from either making a call to their pediatrician or visiting an urgent care facility or ED. Conversely, approximately 12% of the telemedicine encounters prompted additional medical evaluation and treatment – some were addressed to avoid an ED visit [31].

Pediatric Urgent Care

It is estimated that 40–60% of all ED visits for children are considered non-emergent [37]. Stand-alone urgent care centers, which succeed by appealing to consumer demand and convenience, may be the most at risk of being disrupted by telemedicine [38]. Convenience is a key driver for consumer interest in telemedicine, which has shown to be safe and effective for evaluation of uncomplicated conditions in the urgent care setting [39]. As urgent care centers target the care of such low acuity patients, subspecialty consultation at these facilities is occasionally needed. While staffing in-person subspecialists may be too expensive, "on-call" availability of such subspecialists by telemedicine can be more cost effective. Given the challenges in feasibility of on-demand telemedicine consultation by pediatric subspecialists, organizations have explored implementation of a PICU telemedicine provider as the initial point of contact in these settings.

In-Home Management of Medically Complex Children

Children discharged from neonatal or pediatric ICUs with chronic conditions such as bronchopulmonary dysplasia (BPD), congenital heart disease, severe asthma, and chronic respiratory failure requiring home ventilation are at very high risk of unplanned hospital readmission, high ED utilization, and carry increased rates of morbidity and mortality [40]. In addition, given the frequent comorbidities and complex social situations often associated with these conditions, these patients typically benefit greatly from a coordinated, multidisciplinary care team approach utilizing multiple medical specialists, care coordinators, and other allied health professionals to optimize their care [41]. Home telemedicine provides a very promising means of facilitating the improved management of these complex children in their home environment, with the goal of reducing unnecessary ED visits and hospitalizations, reducing risk of iatrogenic infections introduced by visiting healthcare facilities, improving overall care and care coordination, and reducing the burden on families to manage repeated visits to multiple different clinics and other sites of care. Several programs across the country have implemented or are in the process of implementing such services [9–12]. Key barriers to such program implementation include a lack of reimbursement for home telemedicine services in many states, a lack of reimbursement for multidisciplinary care team approaches, and the challenge of integrating the workflow for such encounters into the daily routine of multiple healthcare team members.

Key Considerations Prior to Implementing Pediatric Telemedicine Programs

As hospital systems proceed with implementation of telemedicine in the pediatric ICU, they will encounter key questions related to cost, staffing, change management, technology, regulatory requirements, state and federal policies, impact, and effectiveness evaluation in terms of operations and clinical services. The ICU implementation is also influenced by how leadership plans to implement telemedicine across the entire organization. A recent publication on the pediatric telemedicine landscape highlights key process and staffing characteristics associated with the number of services in telemedicine programs, such as presence of a telemedicine director, manager, technical staff, clinical champions at remote sites, and overall steering committee [1]. Additionally, pediatric telemedicine programs require formal processes to manage technical problems, regulatory compliance, finances, provider competency, evaluation, legal counsel, contracting, and quality improvement. Of these factors, the presence of clinical champions and processes to manage technical problems, finances, compliance, and contracts had the highest correlation with success. Funding sources for these programs vary, ranging from direct institutional investment, philanthropy, grant funding support, subscription-based payments, and fee-for-service models. Key barriers include provider engagement, licensing, reimbursement, and business model sustainability. Generally, stakeholders should be engaged early and often throughout the program development and implementation to develop workflows and maximize program acceptability by frontline providers. In the case of pediatric telemedicine programs, organizations should also consider including children and caregivers in an advisory role. It must be emphasized that the delivery of healthcare via telemedicine – particularly in the critically ill child – carries a risk of care fragmentation, a concern which is acutely relevant in the pediatric population [42]. Therefore, any telemedicine program must establish a connection with the medical home.

References

1. Olson CA, McSwain SD, Curfman AL, Chuo J. The Current Pediatric Telehealth Landscape. Pediatrics. 2018;141(3). PubMed PMID: 29487164.
2. Heath B, Salerno R, Hopkins A, Hertzig J, Caputo M. Pediatric critical care telemedicine in rural underserved emergency departments. Pediatr Crit Care Med. 2009;10(5):588–91.
3. Marcin JP, Nesbitt TS, Kallas HJ, Struve SN, Traugott CA, Dimand RJ. Use of telemedicine to provide pediatric critical care inpatient consultations to underserved rural Northern California. J Pediatr. 2004;144(3):375–80.
4. Harvey JB, Yeager BE, Cramer C, Wheeler D, McSwain SD. The Impact of Telemedicine on Pediatric Critical Care Triage. Pediatr Crit Care Med. 2017;18(11):e555–60. PubMed PMID: 28922271. eng.
5. Bell RC, Yager PH, Clark ME, Roumiantsev S, Venancio HL, Chipman DW, et al. Telemedicine Versus Face-to-Face Evaluations by Respiratory Therapists of Mechanically Ventilated Neonates and Children: A Pilot Study. Respir Care. 2016;61(2):149–54. PubMed PMID: 26647456. Epub 2015/12/08. eng.
6. Yager PH, Cummings BM, Whalen MJ, Noviski N. Nighttime telecommunication between remote staff intensivists and bedside personnel in a pediatric intensive care unit: a retrospective study. Crit Care Med. 2012;40(9):2700–3.
7. Yager PH, Clark ME, Dapul HR, Murphy S, Zheng H, Noviski N. Reliability of Circulatory and Neurologic Examination by Telemedicine in a Pediatric Intensive Care Unit. J Pediatr. 2014;165:962–966.e5.
8. Ellenby MS, Marcin JP. The role of telemedicine in pediatric critical care. Crit Care Clin. 2015;31(2):275–90. PubMed PMID: 25814454.
9. Cady R, Kelly A, Finkelstein S. Home telehealth for children with special health-care needs. J Telemed Telecare. 2008;14(4):173–7.

10. Cady R, Finkelstein S, Kelly A. A telehealth nursing intervention reduces hospitalizations in children with complex health conditions. J Telemed Telecare. 2009;15(6):317–20.
11. Casavant DW, McManus ML, Parsons SK, Zurakowski D, Graham RJ. Trial of telemedicine for patients on home ventilator support: feasibility, confidence in clinical management and use in medical decision-making. J Telemed Telecare. 2014;20:441.
12. Graham RJ, McManus ML, Rodday AM, Weidner RA, Parsons SK. Pediatric specialty care model for management of chronic respiratory failure: cost and savings implications and misalignment with payment models. Pediatr Crit Care Med. 2018;19(5):412–20. PubMed PMID: 29406371. eng.
13. Marcin JP, Nesbitt TS, Struve S, Traugott C, Dimand RJ. Financial benefits of a pediatric intensive care unit-based telemedicine program to a rural adult intensive care unit: impact of keeping acutely ill and injured children in their local community. Telemed J E Health. 2004;10 Suppl 2:S-1-5.
14. Marcin JP, Schepps DE, Page KA, Struve SN, Nagrampa E, Dimand RJ. The use of telemedicine to provide pediatric critical care consultations to pediatric trauma patients admitted to a remote trauma intensive care unit: a preliminary report. Pediatr Crit Care Med. 2004;5(3):251–6.
15. Jackson EM, Costabile PM, Tekes A, Steffen KM, Ahn ES, Scafidi S, et al. Use of Telemedicine During Interhospital Transport of Children With Operative Intracranial Hemorrhage. Pediatr Crit Care Med. 2018;19(11):1033–8. PubMed PMID: 30134361. Epub 2018/08/21. eng.
16. Fugok K, Slamon NB. The Effect of Telemedicine on Resource Utilization and Hospital Disposition in Critically Ill Pediatric Transport Patients. Telemed J E Health. 2018;24(5):367–74. PubMed PMID: 29028420. Epub 2017/10/13. eng.
17. Yager PH, Clark M, Cummings BM, Noviski N. Parent Participation in Pediatric Intensive Care Unit Rounds via Telemedicine: Feasibility and Impact. J Pediatr. 2017;185:181–6.e3. PubMed PMID: 28363361. Epub 2017/03/28. eng.
18. Dharmar M, Marcin JP. A picture is worth a thousand words: critical care consultations to emergency departments using telemedicine. Pediatr Crit Care Med. 2009;10(5):606–7. PubMed PMID: 19741451. Epub 2009/09/11. eng.
19. Schappert SM, Bhuiya F. Availability of pediatric services and equipment in emergency departments: United States. Natl Health Stat Report. 2006, 2012;(47):1–21. PubMed PMID: 22690535. eng.
20. Wakefield DS, Ward M, Miller T, Ohsfeldt R, Jaana M, Lei Y, et al. Intensive care unit utilization and interhospital transfers as potential indicators of rural hospital quality. J Rural Health 2004 Fall;20(4):394–400. PubMed PMID: 15551857.
21. Marcin J, Marcin M, Sadorra C, Dharmar M. The role of telemedicine in treating the critically ill. ICU Dir. 2012;3(2):70–4.
22. Young LB, Chan PS, Lu X, Nallamothu BK, Sasson C, Cram PM. Impact of telemedicine intensive care unit coverage on patient outcomes: a systematic review and meta-analysis. Arch Intern Med. 2011;171(6):498–506. PubMed PMID: 21444842. eng.
23. Wilcox ME, Adhikari NK. The effect of telemedicine in critically ill patients: systematic review and meta-analysis. Crit Care. 2012;16(4):R127. PubMed PMID: 22809335. PMCID: PMC3580710.
24. Wier LM, Yu H, Owens PL, Washington R. Overview of Children in the Emergency Department, 2010: Statistical Brief #157. Healthcare Cost and Utilization Project (HCUP) Statistical Briefs. Rockville. 2006.
25. Goto T, Hasegawa K, Faridi MK, Sullivan AF, Camargo CA, Jr. Emergency Department Utilization by Children in the USA, 2010–2011. West J Emerg Med. 2017;18(6):1042–6. PubMed PMID: 29085535. PMCID: PMC5654872 are required to disclose all affiliations, funding sources and financial or management relationships that could be perceived as potential sources of bias. Dr. Goto was supported by a grant from St. Luke's Life Science Institute and Uehara Kinen Memorial founding.
26. Li J, Monuteaux MC, Bachur RG. Interfacility transfers of noncritically ill children to academic pediatric emergency departments. Pediatrics. 2012;130(1):83–92. PubMed PMID: 22665410.

27. Mohr NM, Harland KK, Shane DM, Miller SL, Torner JC. Potentially Avoidable Pediatric Interfacility Transfer Is a Costly Burden for Rural Families: A Cohort Study. Acad Emerg Med. 2016;23(8):885–94. PubMed PMID: 27018337.
28. McSwain SD, Bernard J, Burke BL, Cole SL, Dharmar M, Hall-Barrow J, et al. American Telemedicine Association Operating Procedures for Pediatric Telehealth. Telemed J E Health. 2017;23(9):699–706. PubMed PMID: 28829680. Epub 2017/08/22. eng.
29. Fang JL, Collura CA, Johnson RV, Asay GF, Carey WA, Derleth DP, et al. Emergency Video Telemedicine Consultation for Newborn Resuscitations: The Mayo Clinic Experience. Mayo Clin Proc. 2016;91(12):1735–43. PubMed PMID: 27887680.
30. Makkar A, McCoy M, Hallford G, Escobedo M, Szyld E. A Hybrid Form of Telemedicine: A Unique Way to Extend Intensive Care Service to Neonates in Medically Underserved Areas. Telemed J E Health. 2018;24(9):717–21. PubMed PMID: 29298407.
31. Willard A, Brown E, Masten M, Brant M, Pouppirt N, Moran K, et al. Complex Surgical Infants Benefit From Postdischarge Telemedicine Visits. Adv Neonatal Care. 2018;18(1):22–30. PubMed PMID: 29373346.
32. Zaichkin JG. Neonatal Resuscitation: Neonatal Resuscitation Program 7th Edition Practice Integration. Crit Care Nurs Clin North Am. 2018;30(4):533–47. PubMed PMID: 30447812.
33. Rashidian A, Omidvari AH, Vali Y, Mortaz S, Yousefi-Nooraie R, Jafari M, et al. The effectiveness of regionalization of perinatal care services – a systematic review. Public Health. 2014;128(10):872–85. PubMed PMID: 25369352.
34. Fang JL, Carey WA, Lang TR, Lohse CM, Colby CE. Real-time video communication improves provider performance in a simulated neonatal resuscitation. Resuscitation. 2014;85(11):1518–22. PubMed PMID: 25132477.
35. Scheans P. Telemedicine for neonatal resuscitation. Neonatal Netw. 2014;33(5):283–7. PubMed PMID: 25161137.
36. Toly VB, Musil CM, Bieda A, Barnett K, Dowling DA, Sattar A. Neonates and Infants Discharged Home Dependent on Medical Technology: Characteristics and Outcomes. Adv Neonatal Care. 2016;16(5):379–89. PubMed PMID: 27275531.
37. Larson M. Specialty Urgent Care: What's the Best Option for Your Market? Sg2 Healthcare Intelligence;2015.Availablefrom:https://www.sg2.com/health-care-intelligence-blog/2015/10/specialty-urgent-care-whats-the-best-option-for-your-market/.
38. Raskas MDGK, Aronson Schinasi D, Vyas S. Telemedicine and Pediatric Urgent Care: A Vision into the Future. Clin Pediatr Emerg Med. 2017;18(1):24–31.
39. Mehrotra A. The convenience revolution for treatment of low-acuity conditions. JAMA. 2013;310(1):35–6. PubMed PMID: 23821082. PMCID: PMC3792718.
40. Patra K, Greene MM. Health Care Utilization after NICU Discharge and Neurodevelopmental Outcome in the First 2 Years of Life in Preterm Infants. Am J Perinatol. 2018;35(5):441–7. PubMed PMID: 29132180.
41. Zhang HNK, Dysart K, Fox W, Jensen E, Maschhoff K, Munson D, Stoller J, Kirpalani H. Caring for Infants with Severe Chronic Lung Disease – Five Year Experience of a Multidisciplinary Care Program. Pediatrics. 2018;141(1)
42. Committee On Pediatric W, Marcin JP, Rimsza ME, Moskowitz WB. The Use of Telemedicine to Address Access and Physician Workforce Shortages. Pediatrics. 2015;136(1):202–9. PubMed PMID: 26122802.

Chapter 15
Telemedicine for Early Treatment of Sepsis

Nicholas M. Mohr, Emily K. Hurst, A. Clinton MacKinney, Emma C. Nash, Brendan G. Carr, and Brian Skow

> Telemedicine is a tool, not a goal, and it needs to solve a real problem. Medicine is still about people, patients, quality of service, and processes. [1]

Introduction

Sepsis is a life-threatening condition that affects more than 1.6 million Americans annually and is now recognized as a leading cause of death in US hospitals [2, 3]. In the USA alone, sepsis care costs over $24 billion annually, making it among the

N. M. Mohr (✉)
Department of Emergency Medicine, University of Iowa Carver College of Medicine, Iowa City, IA, USA

Department of Anesthesia Division of Critical Care, University of Iowa Carver College of Medicine, Iowa City, IA, USA
e-mail: nicholas-mohr@uiowa.edu

E. K. Hurst
Avera eCARE, Sioux Falls, SD, USA

Henry Ford Health System, Detroit, MI, USA
e-mail: Emily.Hurst@avera.org

A. C. MacKinney
Department of Health Management and Policy, University of Iowa College of Public Health, Iowa City, IA, USA
e-mail: clintmack@cloudnet.com

E. C. Nash
Department of Emergency Medicine, University of Iowa Carver College of Medicine, Iowa City, IA, USA
e-mail: emma-nash@uiowa.edu

B. G. Carr
Department of Emergency Medicine, Thomas Jefferson University, Philadelphia, PA, USA
e-mail: Brendan.Carr@jefferson.edu

B. Skow
Avera eCARE, Sioux Falls, SD, USA
e-mail: Brian.Skow@avera.org

M. A. Koenig (ed.), *Telemedicine in the ICU*,
https://doi.org/10.1007/978-3-030-11569-2_15

Table 15.1 Surviving Sepsis Campaign guideline elements, incorporating recommendations of current guidelines for sepsis care [14]

To be completed within...	Surviving Sepsis Campaign guideline elements
3 hours of ED arrival	1. Measure lactate level 2. Obtain blood cultures prior to administration of antibiotics 3. Administer broad-spectrum antibiotics 4. Administer 30 mL/kg crystalloid fluid bolus
6 hours of ED arrival	1. Apply vasopressors for hypotension (mean arterial blood pressure < 65 mm Hg) 2. Reassess resuscitation and volume status (central venous pressure, clinical exam, S_cVO_2) 3. Re-measure lactate if initial lactate elevated

most expensive acute medical conditions and responsible for more than 40% of total ICU expenditures [4, 5]. Despite an 18% decline in case mortality over a 15-year period, sepsis remains responsible for 17% of all US in-hospital deaths and is the leading cause of hospital readmissions [6–8].

Timely and appropriate medical care, consisting of early sepsis recognition, early appropriate antibiotics, and early resuscitation, has been shown to improve survival from sepsis [9–13]. The *Surviving Sepsis Campaign* is a multispecialty sepsis collaborative that has published guidelines for sepsis care management since 2002 (Table 15.1) [14–17], and an updated Surviving Sepsis Bundle was published in 2018 [18]. A bundle related to those recommendations became a quality metric (*Early Management Bundle, Severe Sepsis/Septic* Shock, SEP-1) initially endorsed by the Centers for Medicare and Medicaid Services (CMS) in 2015 [19, 20]. Starting in July 2018, CMS began publicly reporting sepsis bundle adherence on *Hospital Compare*, the first time that these data have been publicly reported [21].

Adherence with *Surviving Sepsis Campaign* bundles have be associated with improved hospital-based mortality [22–25], but adherence with *Surviving Sepsis Campaign* recommendations remains less than 50% [26–29], potentially attributable to delays in sepsis recognition, provider education, and access to sepsis specialty care [30–32]. In 2013, New York enacted legislation requiring hospitals to have sepsis care protocols and report outcomes. Subsequently, Seymour showed that adherence with recommended care in New York was associated with 4% better survival for every hour earlier of bundle completion, with the greatest impact being observed with early appropriate antibiotics [33].

Unfortunately, hospitals continue to struggle to achieve high sepsis process adherence. Although sepsis management requires no specialized equipment or procedural capabilities, hospitals that treat more than 500 cases annually have 36% better survival than those with fewer than 50 cases [34]. The same relationship has been observed in emergency departments (EDs), with the highest volume quintile of EDs having 38% higher survival than the lowest quintile for sepsis patients [35]. In many low-volume and rural hospitals, sepsis patients are transferred to high-volume centers, but even patients who are transferred to higher volume centers have 9% higher mortality than their counterparts whose early resuscitation was completed in high-volume hospitals [36, 37]. Furthermore, patients living in rural areas have 6% higher mortality even if they bypass rural centers to seek care in high-volume hospitals, suggesting that delays may be partly responsible for sepsis outcome disparities [38].

Telemedicine has been one promising strategy adopted in some rural hospitals to improve quality and efficiency of care [39–45]. Telemedicine networks provide a real-time, high-definition, on-demand video connection between a provider and a patient for the purposes of monitoring hospitalized patients, identifying deterioration, and evaluating newly arrived patients. Telemedicine networks seek to make tertiary-level expertise available at the bedside where it would otherwise be inaccessible. These systems can be installed in low-volume hospitals without access to specialty care or in high-volume hospitals to extend the ability of a single clinician to provide real-time surveillance and monitoring of a large patient cohort. As sepsis care quality has been an increasing focus to improve acute care outcomes, providing sepsis care via telemedicine has been increasingly proposed as a vehicle for disseminating high-quality sepsis care in the ED, hospital floor, and intensive care unit (ICU).

Telemedicine-Supplemented Sepsis Care

Telemedicine-supplemented sepsis care is the provision of care to patients diagnosed with or suspected of having sepsis using real-time telemedicine. This care can be provided by telemedicine-enabled monitoring, telemedicine-enabled nursing care, or telemedicine-enabled physician consultation. Implementing a telemedicine sepsis program most effectively occurs in an established telemedicine program. Telemedicine programs for sepsis are similar to other telemedicine screening and treatment programs for acute care conditions (e.g., myocardial infarction, stroke) and are often implemented in the context of an ED-based or ICU-based telemedicine network.

Tele-monitoring

Detection of clinical deterioration can be challenging, and inpatient nurses frequently suffer from task switching, cognitive overload, and alarm fatigue [46–48]. Tele-ICU models can be integrated with artificial intelligence-based algorithms to identify patients experiencing subtle decline up to 12 hours prior to clinical recognition [49]. In these networks, tele-ICU nurses trained in early sepsis detection can continuously screen a group of up to 40 patients, decreasing time to identification and treatment [50]. Algorithms running in the background can utilize continuous physiologic data and laboratory notifications to notify tele-ICU providers of patients requiring detailed evaluation. Other algorithms use a more traditional medical record-based notification system that initiates telemedicine consultation [51]. In each of these models, the value of telemedicine-based monitoring resides in having a clinician not tasked with bedside nursing activities who assumes responsibility for identifying subtle changes that may reflect evolving sepsis.

Telemedicine-Enabled Protocolled Care

Sepsis identification is the first challenge in sepsis care. Once sepsis patients have been identified, though, implementing and monitoring protocol completion remains important. Many hospitals lack the resources needed for continuous monitoring to identify early sepsis. One hospital system has utilized telemedicine to screen patients, offer consultations, and implement established protocols for a variety of common emergencies including acute coronary events, stroke, and sepsis via a secure broadband connection. Using telemedicine-based protocols in this system led to a 30% decrease in sepsis mortality over 12 months [1]. Another program used trained ICU nurses to screen large numbers of patients admitted to ICUs over a 500-mile region. This program performed almost 90,000 sepsis screens over 3 years and was able to impact elements of sepsis bundle compliance by increasing antibiotic administration by 19%, lactate measurement by 16%, and fluid bolus appropriateness by 47% [52]. One health system in Texas uses a central location to remotely monitor 134 beds in 5 hospital ICUs to screen for sepsis and facilitate timely bundle implementation. This program helps not only with clinical care, but also it provides a central repository of data that a multidisciplinary sepsis team can use to continuously review and improve protocols within their health system [53].

Emergency Department-Based Telemedicine

The role of telemedicine in an ED differs from networks that continuously monitor admitted patients. These networks evaluate new patients as a discrete incident and provide specific care recommendations and disposition – even before a patient reaches the ICU. In most cases, ED-based telemedicine programs provide specific consultation by a sepsis specialist (either a critical care physician or an emergency physician) to aid in providing high quality and timely guideline-adherent care [51, 54]. These systems can be installed permanently in a specially equipped ED evaluation room, or they can reside on a portable cart that is wheeled into a qualifying patient's room. In one network that used a portable wheeled cart, a remote critical care physician provided consultation, reducing the time to antibiotics by 40 minutes, increasing the proportion who had lactate measured by 9%, and shortening the ED length-of-stay. This project was conducted in a tertiary center, perhaps highlighting that telehealth consultation may supplement care in both rural and urban hospitals [54].

Telemedicine resources must also be easily accessible and rapidly available. Another pilot program demonstrated that real-time telemedicine consultation was feasible for ED patients with both cardiac arrest and sepsis. In this program, telemedicine consultations were automatically triggered by certain criteria, but ultimately the choice to use this resource was left to the emergency physician. The results of this trial showed that telemedicine provided a feasible, fast, and effective way to bring real-time consultants to the bedside, a crucial objective in a disease entity that can evolve rapidly [51].

Cost-Effectiveness

Cost-effectiveness of telemedicine has been debated in the literature, and the cost-effectiveness of using telemedicine for sepsis care remains unanswered [54–57]. Because of the high costs and the strong association between high-quality early sepsis care and clinical outcomes, sepsis is one condition where early telemedicine use might be cost-effective. Most of the cost of telemedicine networks resides in high start-up costs, with ongoing incremental costs being offset in large networks with high usage [58]. If telemedicine-enabled care is able to reduce inpatient length-of-stay and shorten sepsis-associated organ failure, telemedicine may be a cost-effective intervention, but this effectiveness in improving clinical outcomes remains unproven. Likely, the impact of telemedicine will vary based on current staffing and pre-intervention sepsis performance [59].

Role of Telemedicine in Achieving Quality Metrics

As more data suggest that early protocolized sepsis care influences outcomes, the Centers for Medicare and Medicaid Services (CMS) has published quality metrics and started collecting bundle adherence data [20]. Many health systems have struggled to achieve sepsis metrics, with US national adherence estimated at 49% in 2017 [29]. Public reporting has driven health systems to identify strategies, such as telemedicine, to improve resuscitation performance. In addition to challenges with implementation, the CMS-endorsed sepsis quality measure, SEP-1, has evolved, with annual changes that have been challenging to disseminate to frontline clinical staff, especially in clinical environments where sepsis is infrequently managed [60].

The difficulty and time-sensitivity of applying SEP-1 are compounded by the manner in which it is measured. The SEP-1 bundle requires abstracting 78 data elements from the medical record to demonstrate adherence to 8 time-sensitive bundle elements [19]. Qualifying as "guideline-adherent care" requires meeting all of the elements of this bundle – there is no credit for partial adherence [61]. Thus, the SEP-1 bundle is a high-stakes measure that is particularly susceptible to communication barriers, incomplete documentation, and treatment in the face of early diagnostic uncertainty. The complexity of the SEP-1 bundle also highlights a potential benefit for telemedicine – focusing on documentation, communication, and quality metrics could dramatically improve bundle adherence.

Telemedicine networks can also leverage the impact of quality managers, who may be able to implement changes in documentation and bundle requirements rapidly in a small cohort of sepsis telemedicine nursing staff or clinicians. They can follow patients across transitions in care, reducing communication errors through handoffs. Additionally, operating a large network with a small cohort of providers can reduce variation, allowing for more consistent implementation of system-wide quality improvement initiatives.

How to Design and Implement a Telemedicine-Based Sepsis Program

Implementing a telemedicine-based sepsis program has the potential to improve sepsis clinical performance and outcomes, but program effectiveness is predicated on successful implementation. Using a robust quality improvement framework, such as the plan-do-study-act (PDSA) model, can maintain focus on clinical endpoints [62]. Telemedicine should be employed as a solution to an identified sepsis care problem. In most cases, a sepsis telemedicine program will use the infrastructure of other telemedicine networks (e.g., tele-ED, tele-stroke, tele-ICU, tele-hospitalist) to leverage previous investments with a new focus.

Define the Problem

The first step to building a sepsis telemedicine program is to define the extent of the problem. Sepsis programs could be designed to address any of the following problems:

- Inpatients are deteriorating and sepsis is recognized late, leading to medical emergency team activations after opportunities to intervene are missed.
- Completion of bundle-adherent care in rural emergency departments is low because nursing documentation of interventions is poor.
- Patients with sepsis eligible for transfer to a tertiary ICU have high mortality because the local tertiary care center is often full and transfers are delayed for 12–24 hours.
- Patients have sepsis recognized in a teaching hospital, but resident physicians are selecting inappropriate antibiotic coverage, leading to delays in appropriate antibiotic administration.

The solution for each of these problems might be very different, and if that solution incorporates telemedicine, staffing, technology, and implementation might vary significantly. As the problem is defined, it is important to select a specific measurable metric that can be tracked (e.g., bundle adherence, timeliness of transfer, delays in diagnosis). Ideally that metric is a process measure (such as antibiotic appropriateness) that is thought to influence a patient-relevant outcome (such as mortality).

Selecting and measuring the problem first allows the quality improvement team to identify optimal strategies that use all available resources, of which telemedicine might just be one. Implementing a telemedicine program modeled after another health system may be effective only in as much as the problem mirrors that being solved by the model system.

Select a Care Model

After the problem is defined and a tracking metric is selected, a care model should be designed. Sepsis telemedicine models could mirror any of the following systems or incorporate hybrid features of multiple systems:

- Nurse-based tele-ICU monitoring (with or without bedside clinical nursing documentation)
- Physician-based tele-ICU monitoring and consultation
- Emergency department-based tele-ED with emergency physician consultation
- Emergency department-based tele-ICU with critical care specialist consultation
- Dedicated consultative service (e.g., hospitalist program, tele-pharmacy)

Each of these systems offers different services, and those services will influence the process of care and outcomes that can be achieved. The structure of a sepsis telemedicine network should reflect the problem being addressed and the metrics being measured. For the purpose of the remainder of this chapter, we will assume that the sepsis system functions in a hub-and-spoke model, where telemedicine providers are centralized in a "hub" that provides services to many remote "spokes." While other models can be conceived, this model is common and is used in many ED-based and ICU-based telemedicine applications.

Staffing

The professional team needed for a sepsis telemedicine program includes physicians (or advanced practice providers), nurses, and support specialists (including technical support). Specific professional team members include the program director, telemedicine system hub clinicians, clinical educator, administrator, marketing specialist, data analyst, and user stakeholders (customers or telemedicine recipient users) (Table 15.2). Depending on the size of the program, individuals may fill multiple roles or additional team members may be required. Common to all team member roles is an understanding of the unique challenges of bedside health care

Table 15.2 Roles required to operate a sepsis telemedicine program

Role	Responsibilities
Program Director	Overall project leader of sepsis telemedicine program who sets the priorities and evaluation criteria and leads initiatives to improve sepsis quality of care and performance improvement
Hub Clinician	Provide reliable, evidence-based, and respectful clinical recommendations in the dual context of clinical care and education and contribute to protocol adherence and documentation to optimize institutional performance
Clinical Educator	Develop local or regional evidence-based treatment guidelines and provide ongoing training to both hub and spoke clinicians
Administrator	Provide managerial support to telemedicine program, including liaison activities, contracts, and strategic planning
Marketing Specialist	Develop marketing materials to promote sepsis telemedicine program
Data Analyst	Collect, analyze, and report data detailing program performance, clinical outcomes, and financial factors
User Stakeholder	Represent telemedicine spoke users in program development and ongoing quality improvement

in the setting where the telemedicine services will be provided. For example, a telemedicine sepsis intervention in a rural ED must include experts who understand the training, equipment, and experience available in the rural setting, and this baseline knowledge is different from what might be necessary in a teaching hospital ICU. Clinicians staffing rural hospitals often work alone with a small nursing team that may have additional responsibilities (such as working in a small inpatient unit and in the ED at the same time). These roles can make the treatment of high-risk cases even more challenging, and these specific institutional challenges may be used to define the problem that telemedicine might attempt to solve [63].

Program Director The telemedicine sepsis program director provides clinical leadership for the program, and in many cases this role will be filled by the telemedicine service medical director. Program director roles include:

- Engage and train hospital clinicians regarding telemedicine sepsis program and develop protocols as an administrative champion.
- Educate and serve as role model for telemedicine system hub clinicians – clinically current, professional, helpful, and respectful.
- Develop and administer a performance review process and quality monitoring system for telemedicine system hub clinicians.
- Develop sepsis quality assurance and performance improvement metrics, report these metrics to clinicians, and work to improve system performance.
- Support the telemedicine program clinical educator and nurse manager.
- Serve as the liaison between hub and spoke clinicians, understanding the unique practice environment and serving to maintain organizational customer focus.

Hub Clinician The telemedicine system hub clinician provides real-time, audio-video, telemedicine consultations. The hub clinician interfaces directly with the spoke hospital clinicians caring for patients with suspected sepsis. Telemedicine system hub clinician roles include:

- Provide clinically current, helpful, and respectful telemedicine consultations.
- Navigate the dual role of health-care provider and local clinician educator, focusing on early sepsis diagnosis, risk stratification, and treatment.
- Ensure quality sepsis care and proper sepsis documentation that maximizes bundle adherence and accurate data abstraction for publicly reported quality measures.
- Provide consultations that are consistent with current literature and established institutional sepsis protocols, including familiarity with local resources and the local formulary.

Clinical Educator The clinical educator serves as the program's trainer, researcher, and content expert. In concert with the medical director, the clinical educator develops diagnostic and care protocols and ensures they are both accurate and current. Clinical educator roles include:

- Develop, continuously maintain, and disseminate evidence-based sepsis clinical care protocols for diagnosis, telemedicine activation, treatment, and transfer for sepsis patients.
- Lead a team of clinical experts and hub clinician stakeholders to review, support, and endorse sepsis protocols.
- Review sepsis performance and provide provider-specific feedback.
- Provide end-user training in both sepsis care and telemedicine technology.

Administrator The administrator coordinates the managerial and business aspects of the telemedicine program. Administrator roles include:

- Provide oversight of clinical and non-clinical support staff, including managerial support (e.g., hire, evaluate, address problems) and strategic planning (e.g., new business and program opportunities).
- Serve as a liaison to health system administrators, spoke hospital medical directors, and pharmacy and laboratory managers.
- Negotiate agreements and contracts to collaborate and share data for the purposes of clinical care, quality improvement, and process development.
- Understand telemedicine policy issues and advocate for sustainable telemedicine policy.

Marketing Specialist The marketing specialist focuses on understanding local sepsis care and developing a marketing and sales strategy to align the sepsis program with local needs. Marketing specialist roles include:

- Develop a list of potential telemedicine sites.
- Develop a communication plan and telemedicine promotional materials.
- Develop and implement stakeholder-specific marketing plans (e.g., for hospital board, medical directors, community partners, etc.) and communications plans.
- Promote the telemedicine program through directed marketing and mass media venues.

Data Analyst The data analyst collects, analyzes, and disseminates telemedicine clinical and financial performance. Data analyst roles include:

- Develop and implement data collection tools to collect clinical performance, financial performance, and risk-adjustment factors, and provide care quality and financial performance reports.
- Collaborate with external groups conducting program evaluations, as appropriate.

User Stakeholder The user stakeholder (selected from the user base) is a critical component of the sepsis telemedicine leadership team, and this individual participates in program clinical design, implementation, and administration. User stakeholder roles include:

- Contributes to the design and evaluation of clinical sepsis telemedicine protocols.
- Provide ongoing performance improvement feedback to program leaders, including evaluating user feedback and aggregate clinical outcomes data.

Sepsis Protocol Development

Central to the care of patients with sepsis are screening and treatment protocols. These resuscitation protocols have been developed for decades, and one successful "bundle" of care was associated with a 35% decrease in mortality in a randomized clinical trial published by Rivers in 2001 [13, 64]. These bundles have been revised since that time, and protocolized care has been well established as a strategy to facilitate guideline implementation and improved clinical care [12]. Even in the context of recent trials questioning the utility of the protocol originally published by Rivers in 2001 [65–67], many institutions continue to standardize local care through protocols.

Sepsis telemedicine programs are often built upon protocol development and performance tracking. These protocols are local or regional applications of the *Surviving Sepsis Guidelines*, adapting these guidelines for local formulary issues and systems of care and to standardize documentation [14]. These protocols are also designed to meet the elements of the SEP-1 process metric [19].

In addition, telemedicine networks should apply additional guidance that addresses [1] when telemedicine consultation should be activated, [2] how the telemedicine hub provider will collaborate with local medical staff, [3] what data the telemedicine provider might access, [4] triggers for inter-facility transfer (along with destination selection), and [5] facility-specific treatment protocols.

Consultation Triggers

One significant challenge to telemedicine use is identifying which patients benefit from telemedicine activation and consultation. The threshold for activation should be dictated by the specific problem for which the sepsis telemedicine intervention was designed. Networks that are trying to improve sepsis detection may design consultation triggers differently from those that are trying to improve antibiotic selection in patients with septic shock only. Sepsis diagnosis can be challenging, and selecting very sensitive consultation triggers (e.g., all patients with fever) will necessarily involve telemedicine consultation more frequently than selecting very specific consultation triggers (e.g., only patients with fever who are hypotensive). These consultation triggers can either be provider-directed or automated (initiated by software screening clinical data), and although automated triggers are preferred, technical challenges have made these triggers challenging to implement.

Another important aspect of consultation trigger development is [1] accurate projection of telemedicine network capacity and [2] stakeholder involvement. Accurately projecting telemedicine volume capacity will prevent implementation of a consultation trigger that will overwhelm existing consultation resources. Stakeholder involvement remains critical to facilitating local buy-in of the sepsis program. Figure 15.1 shows one example of an ED-based sepsis consultation trigger used in rural hospitals in one telemedicine network.

Treatment Pathways

In conjunction with the stakeholder group, developing robust sepsis treatment pathways should be designed to address the specific identified clinical problem (e.g., delayed antibiotic administration). Sepsis treatment pathways should adhere to accepted and up-to-date treatment guidelines, and they should consist of a checklist or computer-assisted tool to [1] accurately identify sepsis severity, [2] list the interventions required based on sepsis severity, and [3] guide a provider or monitor through an algorithm of treatment. These tools can also provide clinical documentation and become part of the medical record to meet SEP-1 bundle documentation requirements. Figure 15.2 shows one sample flowsheet that is used in a tele-ICU network for diagnosis and management of sepsis.

Clinician Adoption

For telemedicine to improve sepsis outcomes, telemedicine protocols must be designed with thoughtful end-user input and then be utilized consistently and appropriately. Telemedicine support of sepsis care requires a deep understanding of the local challenges surrounding sepsis care. Thus, careful consideration of users' perceptions of clinical need and usefulness is mandatory for program success [68].

Specific program policies can improve clinician adoption of a sepsis telemedicine program. A local sepsis telemedicine champion should be identified both at the telemedicine hub and at each participating spoke hospital. Involving end users in protocol development can increase use and improve adherence. It also allows hub

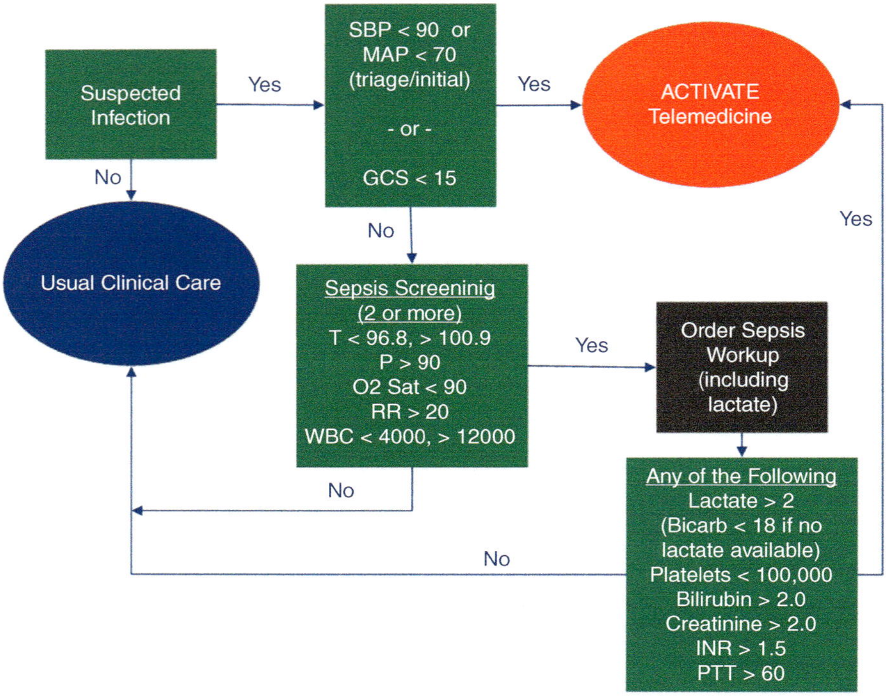

Fig. 15.1 Telemedicine sepsis screening algorithm (Used with permission by Avera eCARE and the Rural Telehealth Research Center) [39]. This flowsheet clarifies sample criteria for activating a telemedicine consultation in an emergency department-based sepsis telemedicine program

clinicians insight into local sepsis culture, drug selection and formulary issues, diagnostic test availability, and existing protocols – all of which help integrate telemedicine into local medical care. Incorporating a sepsis program into an existing telemedicine program can be one strategy to overcome technical barriers to use, and incorporating processes that encourage telemedicine use for non-sepsis cases increases comfort with the telemedicine platform. Some programs improve familiarity with telemedicine with daily camera checks, quality improvement programs that require telemedicine consultation, and provider education using the telemedicine platform. Using telemedicine as a solution to a local problem can also facilitate adoption because users are more invested in program success. Additionally, a bidirectional formal post-consultation feedback process can provide metrics to monitor and gauge program success, allowing for continuous quality improvement for program staff (Table 15.3).

PATIENT NAME: ______________________ MRN: ______________________
DATE/TIME: ______________________ Telemed RN: ______________________
AQOP RN: ______________________ Intensivist: ______________________
Presentation Time: __________ **3 Hour Deadline:** __________ **6 Hour Deadline:** __________
*These are the CMS timelines established and certain interventions are required to be done by the 3 & 6 hour mark

1. Circle the identified severity of sepsis: a. *sepsis* b. *severe sepsis* c. *septic shock*
   a. If *b* or *c* selected, continue the form. If *a* selected, the form is complete at this point.
2. Identify *Presentation Time (time zero)*: (date/time) ______________________
3. Has the patient had blood cultures drawn within the last 24 hours? **YES** **NO** If yes, when: ______________________
   a. If NO, escalate to Intensivist to order.
   b. If YES, proceed to question 4.
4. Have antibiotics been ordered or is patient currently on them? **YES** **NO**
   a. If no, escalate to Intensivist to order.
   b. If YES, have they been given? **YES** **NO** List the abx: ______________________
   c. Date/Time 1st Dose Given of Each: ______________________
5. What is the initial lactic acid level?: __________ mmol/L
   a. If none ordered, escalate to Intensivist to order. (Must be drawn within 3 hours of presentation time)
   b. If initial ≥ 2.0, has a repeat lactic acid level been ordered within 6 hours from presentation time? **YES** **NO** **N/A**
      i. If no, escalate to Intensivist to order. The 2nd lactic acid lab MUST be within 6 hours of presentation time.
6. Has the patient been: hypotensive? Had a lactate ≥ 4? Physician documented septic shock? **YES** **NO**
   a. If No, checklist is complete, escalate all missed measures to Intensivist at this time.
   b. If YES, assess fluids. Continue to question 7.
7. Fluid Volume Resuscitation Assessment
   a. Calculate required fluid volume: pt weight __________ kg X 30mL = __________ mL
   b. Determine how much volume the patient has received already: __________ mL
   c. Determine how much volume the patient WILL receive per orders: __________ mL
   d. Will the patient receive the required 30mL/Kg fluid volumeAND within 6 hour window? **YES** **NO**
      i. If NO, escalate to Intensivist for more fluid orders or increase in rate in order for patient to receive necessary volume within 6 hours from Presentation Time. Provide specific volume needed to total required mL.
      ii. If YES, move to item 8.
8. Schedule the "Acute Sepsis 6 Hr Volume Reassessment"within 6 hours from *Presentation Time.*
   a. Date/Time completed by Intensivist: __________. *Ensure this is done in the window
9. Does the patient have new/persistent hypotensionafter/during volume resuscitation? **YES** **NO**
   a. If yes, escalate to Intensivist to evaluate and order appropriate IV vasopressor. Drug ordered: __________
   b. If no, this form is complete.
   c. TIP:Continue to monitor for hypotension after arriving to ICU! May still need vasopressors!

Fig. 15.2 Sample sepsis telemedicine treatment algorithm (Used with permission by Avera eICU)

Technology Considerations

The technology required for a sepsis tele-ED or tele-ICU program does not differ from other telemedicine uses and in many cases will be built in an existing functional network. The program requires a high-speed, real-time, high-definition audio-video telecommunication connection. Single-button activation of the telemedicine consultation facilitates rapid and straightforward telemedicine consultations and interactions. The technology should be monitored and tested regularly to ensure reliable operation. To reduce the risk of operator error, local spoke hospital staff should be trained in proper equipment use and should routinely apply procedures

Table 15.3 Bidirectional post-consultation feedback is an important component of a sustainable sepsis telemedicine program

Telemedicine hub to user communication
Appropriateness of diagnosis
Time-to-treatment targets
Local and national peer comparisons
Timeliness of telemedicine activation
Protocol adherence
User to telemedicine hub communication
Helpfulness of telemedicine provider
Comfort with recommendations
Appropriateness of communications with provider and patient

that reinforce technology familiarity (e.g., weekly educational interactions or daily camera testing). Finally, hub telemedicine center technical specialists should ensure compliance with pertinent patient data protection regulations and be available 24 hours daily for technical support.

System Integration

A key component of successful telemedicine implementation is to utilize a telemedicine platform that can integrate with clinical electronic medical records (EMRs). Many health systems are transitioning to a uniform EMR, but legacy EMRs may limit the full functionality of telemedicine provider access. EMR uniformity will help a telemedicine provider improve patient care and document patient encounters. Until full EMR interoperability exists, telemedicine providers must have adequate training and experience with participating hospital EMRs to be able to efficiently access data, order therapy, and make recommendations.

In tele-ICU environments, remote physiologic monitoring software provides real-time vital sign monitoring and can identify short- and medium-term trends. Staff are alerted to changes that might reflect clinical deterioration and can provide specific dedicated evaluation. This software-based clinical support system is vital to a telemedicine program.

Lab interfacing is also critical in a tele-ICU system. Providers should be alerted to abnormal lab results promptly. If the lab result demonstrates an issue that needs intervention, the telemedicine provider will notify the bedside provider and intervene.

Telemedicine documentation is a desirable aspect of a sepsis telemedicine program. The ability to record interventions, observations, and justifications not only contributes to safe clinical care but also can satisfy elements of sepsis quality bundles. This collaborative documentation should be designed during program implementation and will clarify the telemedicine provider's role in ongoing clinical care.

Funding

Although a sepsis telemedicine program may be initially funded as part of a larger telemedicine initiative, a business plan should still be developed when adding a new service line. Some telemedicine grant programs may provide funding to expand an existing telemedicine network or develop a new service. In many cases, though, the economic driver for development of a sepsis program is improved quality of care, with savings realized through [1] lower hospital costs (e.g., shorter length-of-stay and improved clinical outcomes) or [2] improved reimbursement through pay-for-performance contracts. Although the SEP-1 sepsis quality measure does not currently influence reimbursement, including sepsis quality measures into future incentive payment structures seems likely. Private and community partnerships can also be a successful financial sustainability option [69].

Rural Hospital Considerations

The rural hospital considering telemedicine access (to provide sepsis care and other consultations) should develop a business plan that projects program cost and benefit. Financial pro forma variables might include telemedicine program service fees, telemedicine equipment and connectivity costs, staff time and compensation, and indirect revenue from additional ancillary services and avoided transfers. Telemedicine may also reduce the need for physician backup for advanced practice providers staffing the rural ED [58]. Nonfinancial business plan variables might include sepsis case volume (and other clinical volumes that might use telemedicine), current sepsis performance, hospital clinician willingness to use telemedicine, hospital clinician willingness to allow protocol-driven telemedicine activation, additional data collection or reporting requirements, additional opportunities for telemedicine-based services (e.g., education, administration, record-keeping), and availability of dedicated fiber or T1 line access.

What Questions Should a Hospital Leader Ask Before Implementing a Tele-sepsis Solution?

- How much will a sepsis telemedicine program cost (incremental cost)?
- How much time will my staff spend administering the program?
- Will I be able to use existing telemedicine resources, or is sepsis telemedicine a new program implementation?
- What is my total sepsis case volume within the proposed network?
- What are my current sepsis outcomes, and what problem is our telemedicine solution intended to solve?

- Do local clinicians consider telemedicine an opportunity to improve care quality and professional collegiality, or do local clinicians consider telemedicine to be an intrusion into their clinical autonomy?
- If sepsis care protocols already exist, do they need to be adapted for telemedicine use?
- What data are to be collected to demonstrate the utility of the telemedicine intervention, and what is the data collection burden for my staff?
- What training will be required for successful implementation of the entire program?
- Do I have sufficient technical support and high-speed Internet bandwidth for the sepsis program?

Potential Pitfalls

What Potential Pitfalls Should Be Considered when Implementing a Sepsis Telemedicine Program?

- Develop a sepsis telemedicine program that is not targeted at specific clinical quality outcomes.
- Implement a sepsis telemedicine program that is not financially sustainable for the health system or for the end users.
- Implement an expensive, time-consuming, or onerous telemedicine program to address a very rare clinical situation that is not valued by the end users [39].
- Overextend hub physicians by requiring telemedicine consultations concurrent with direct patient care.
- Neglect physician or patient discomfort with telemedicine technology [70].
- Develop a sepsis telemedicine program as a stand-alone service, without considering other clinical and non-clinical uses of the technology.
- Fail to develop strong trust, partnership, and collaboration between hub and spoke clinicians [71].
- Employ disrespectful, condescending, or unprofessional hub clinicians.
- Underestimate the clinical importance of standardized sepsis screening and management outside the telemedicine program [52].
- Fail to include all stakeholder groups in sepsis protocol development, review, and updates.
- Neglect to account for local hospital capabilities (e.g., diagnostic, treatment protocols, hospital formulary) during protocol development.
- Rely on an outdated evidence-based sepsis protocol or quality measure.
- Use an incomplete protocol dissemination and implementation process.
- Do not plan for regular sepsis protocol updates.
- Inadequately support the role of the program clinical educator.
- Develop a program that does not facilitate regular and constructive communication between hub and spoke providers.

- Do not design and implement a bidirectional performance feedback process.
- Implement a program without a mechanism of tracking quality, clinical, and financial endpoints.

Future Directions

The role of telemedicine in the future delivery of care for critical illness seems certain, because telemedicine is one solution to the persistent challenge of rapidly bringing expertise to the point of care. Centralization, a term used to describe moving critically ill patients to high-volume centers best equipped to care for them [72], is one solution to improving care for those with emergency care-sensitive conditions in remote areas [73, 74], but telemedicine enables a counter-narrative. While many historic attempts to improve care for rural patients focused on rural hospital bypass or rapid transfer of complex patients to regional centers, telemedicine enables a system of keeping patients in facilities near their homes while maintaining care quality. Centralizing care in referral centers leads both to overwhelmed tertiary centers and also to skill atrophy in smaller facilities. Ultimately, the erosion of capabilities at these smaller hospitals risks the future of these facilities and can force hospital closures, a phenomenon that has become prevalent [75]. These closures can make patients' preferences to be treated locally [76, 77] impossible to accommodate and can wreak havoc on local economies [78]. Bypass of local facilities can strip communities of medical capabilities, increase the burden of transport for emergency medical services, and lead to delays in care for time-sensitive conditions. Telemedicine offers the possibility of delivering the right care at the right time in the right place and also matching patient needs with hospital capacity – a growing problem in an increasingly centralized medical system [79].

Despite the promise of telemedicine, significant barriers remain before sepsis telemedicine programs are fully mainstreamed. One of the most pressing policy challenges is establishing viable financial models. While billing codes exist for telemedicine consultation, significant geographic limitations may be applied, and heterogeneity between payers and state policies still exists [80]. This policy may limit telemedicine innovation in long-term care facilities and non-rural areas. Many telehealth programs operate on a flat monthly fee or at a financial loss as a strategy to capture downstream revenues.

On balance, the future of telemedicine for time-sensitive emergency conditions like sepsis is bright. CMS has highlighted both the importance of improving sepsis outcomes and the broadening of telemedicine payment policy as strategic goals [81]. The Office of the National Coordinator has made interoperability a priority [82], and many companies are developing technical and organizational solutions such as advanced software tools and artificial intelligence to support the detection and resuscitation of patients with sepsis [83, 84]. As the US health-care system pivots toward improving the health and health outcomes of the population in a connected world, the virtual presence of experts at the bedside is likely to become an expanding aspect of high-quality health-care delivery.

Case Studies

Rural Hospital: Case #1

A 78-year-old man with a history of congestive heart failure and chronic kidney disease who lives in a local nursing facility presents to a rural critical access hospital ED with mental status changes and fever. His vital signs in the ED reveal temperature 38.4 degrees Celsius, pulse 102 beats per minute, blood pressure 128/74 mmHg, and oxygen saturation 97% on room air. Laboratory evaluation is remarkable for elevated creatinine at 2.3 mg/dL (baseline 1.6 mg/dL), pyuria present on urinalysis, and elevated lactate at 2.8 mmol/dl. Ceftriaxone was initiated in the ED and the patient was admitted to the general medicine service.

> Telemedicine Perspective: This patient was evaluated quickly in a rural ED, but several elements of the CMS sepsis bundle were missed: no blood cultures were drawn before the initiation of antibiotics and "time zero" was not clearly documented. Because of those deficiencies, this case did not meet the criteria for credit for the SEP-1 CMS quality metric. Further, the antibiotic selected would be appropriate for treatment of community-acquired pneumonia, but his residence in a nursing facility puts him at risk for drug-resistant pathogens. These elements could have been identified by a telemedicine provider and addressed.

Time: 3 hours 35 minutes after arrival
Upon arrival to the medical floor (no ICU was available in this rural hospital), a local family physician reviews the case and identified blood cultures were not yet drawn. He appropriately orders them, but antibiotics have already been given. He documents in his note that time zero was the time of presentation with mental status changes, and he notes that systolic blood pressure is 104 mmHg.

> Telemedicine Perspective: In this case, the admitting provider recognized the importance of documenting time zero, but he applied the old criteria in identifying that time (a time much earlier than would have been required). The elevated lactate was not recognized, so no repeat lactate was performed, and fluid resuscitation was delayed. These management and documentation aspects could have been identified and completed by a telemedicine provider.

Time: 4 hours 56 minutes after arrival
The patient's mental status remains poor and he is increasingly confused. His systolic blood pressure drops to 82 mmHg, and fluid resuscitation is initiated with a 500 mL bolus. The treating physician feels that his severity of illness exceeds the rural hospital capability and initiates transfer to a larger community hospital. Before transfer, a repeat lactate is ordered.

> Telemedicine Perspective: In this case, the local clinician rapidly recognized clinical deterioration and initiated resuscitation. This patient may benefit from more aggressive fluid

resuscitation, and this more aggressive fluid management is now a quality measure in the SEP-1 bundle (for hypotension). In this case, the clinician spends significant time arranging transfer, which could otherwise be done remotely by a telemedicine provider while the local provider is providing ongoing care.

Time: 5 hours 11 minutes after arrival

The transporting ambulance arrives to pick up the patient, but the orders that the admitting physician had written have not all been completed (repeat lactate had not been sent). The blood pressure improved slightly with the small fluid bolus but quickly returned to a systolic blood pressure of 84 mmHg. The family physician is concerned about starting aggressive fluids en route and does not feel he should delay transfer to place a central venous line for vasopressor therapy. The patient continues to get more lethargic but will still respond to painful stimulus. Oxygen saturation is now 92% on 2 L by nasal cannula, so local staff clear the patient for inter-hospital transfer.

Telemedicine Perspective: As this patient is clinically deteriorating, he has quickly exceeded the comfort and capacity of the local hospital. This patient may now remain hypotensive for the duration of the 90-minute transport without having received adequate fluid resuscitation or hemodynamic support. Telemedicine could have provided expert consultation with a critical care physician who could have suggested additional elements of resuscitation prior to transfer and recommended ongoing therapy during the transport period. The telemedicine physician can also provide additional communication with the receiving hospital to ensure that records are transferred appropriately and that critical elements of the resuscitation are completed. Finally, a telemedicine provider could have performed nursing documentation so that the single bedside nurse can complete elements of care prior to transfer.

Time: 7 hours and 14 minutes after arrival

En route to the community hospital, dopamine infusion was initiated by the transferring paramedic and is being infused at 10 mcg/kg/min by peripheral IV. One additional liter of fluid was administered. Blood pressure is now 92/54 and oxygen has been titrated up to 5 L per minute. Repeat laboratory evaluation is performed and another liter of fluid is given. A central venous line and arterial line are placed, and dopamine is replaced with norepinephrine.

Telemedicine Perspective: This patient was transferred at a period in his disease when he was very unstable. Ideally, resuscitation and stabilization, including central venous line placement and likely intubation, could have occurred prior to transfer. Telemedicine can provide expert evaluation and recommendations that might have led to completion of his resuscitation sooner, and may prevent subsequent organ failure and deterioration.

Time: 8 hours 32 minutes after arrival at the first hospital

New laboratory studies demonstrate a lactate of 4.6 mmol/dL, creatinine of 3.1, and white blood cell count of 16.2×10^3 cells/mL. Antibiotics administered prior to transfer were unclear in the paperwork that accompanied the patient, so vancomycin and piperacillin/tazobactam are initiated and norepinephrine is weaned to 8 mcg/min after additional fluid resuscitation. The patient's mental status and oxygen exchange improve, but hemodynamic indices suggest that fluid resuscitation should continue.

Telemedicine Perspective: In retrospect, this patient decompensated from inadequate early management. Unfortunately, he had persistent kidney injury and a prolonged ICU stay, although he did not require intubation. Outcomes in sepsis are strongly related to the timeliness of early resuscitation, which in this case was delayed over 8 hours. Telemedicine is one solution to identify and intervene on these patients earlier and provide expert consultation, documentation assistance, and transfer assistance in a low-resource setting already stretched to provide very complicated medical care.

Key Issues

1. In this case, inadequate early resuscitation contributed to clinical deterioration which necessitated emergency transfer.
2. Information was lost through transitions of care and led to duplicate therapy.
3. Documentation elements required for quality metrics change, and the treating clinician was using an outdated definition for a condition that he treats infrequently.
4. Rural hospital staff had too much to do to complete all tasks prior to transfer. Offloading documentation and arranging for emergency transfer to a telemedicine provider can aid local clinicians in focusing on patient care.
5. Increased variability and lack of protocolization in care contributed to missing standard elements of early sepsis resuscitation.
6. Delays in resuscitation did not meet the elements of guideline-adherent sepsis care.

Tertiary Hospital: Case Study #2

A 78-year-old female with a past medical history of end-stage renal disease, type II diabetes mellitus, rheumatoid arthritis, and dementia presents to a tertiary hospital emergency department from an outpatient dialysis center with hypotension, fever, and lethargy. She just started hemodialysis 3 weeks ago and had not missed any sessions until today, when her hemodialysis session was aborted because her initial blood pressure was 87/42. She has been dialyzed through a tunneled dialysis catheter, but the entry site is now erythematous, and the dialysis technician expressed pus from the insertion site. A 500 mL fluid bolus was initiated prior to ambulance transfer, and paramedics initiated bilevel positive airway pressure (BiPAP) for an oxygen saturation of 88%.

On arrival in the ED, her vital signs include temperature 38.3 degrees Celsius, heart rate 114 beats per minute, blood pressure 88/40 mmHg, respiratory rate 26 breaths per minute, and oxygen saturation 86% on room air. Her laboratory evaluation is remarkable for white blood cell count of 3.2×10^3 cells/mL, pCO_2 68 mmHg, and lactate of 4.2 mmol/L. Her chest x-ray is notable for moderate bilateral pleural effusions. She was restarted on BiPAP for volume overload with hypoxic and hypercapnic acute respiratory failure. Blood, urine, and sputum cultures were sent and ceftriaxone and azithromycin were administered intravenously. The treating emergency physician documented time zero as the time the lactate resulted. Vital signs improved after one liter of normal saline bolus and the patient was admitted to the intensive care unit. A second liter of fluid was ordered, but had not been administered prior to ICU transfer.

Telemedicine Perspective: This patient was evaluated very quickly, but several elements of the CMS sepsis bundle were missed or documented inappropriately. First, time zero was inappropriately recorded as the time the lactate resulted, but criteria were actually met on arrival since the patient was on BiPAP. Additionally, while antibiotic coverage for community acquired pneumonia was initiated, this dialysis patient with evidence of line infection should have been administered broad-spectrum antibiotics with coverage for drug-resistant organisms.

Time: 3 hours and 26 minutes after arrival

Upon arrival to the ICU, the patient's blood pressure was 96/54 mmHg with a mean arterial pressure of 68 mm/Hg. The patient was reported by the ED provider to have received 2.5 liters of normal saline (30 mL/kg). Antibiotics had been administered and blood cultures were drawn before antibiotics had been given. Repeat lactate had not yet been drawn. This patient no longer appeared able to protect her airway and the attending intensivist decided to intubate her.

Telemedicine Perspective: Although the care provided in the ED was very complete, the communication between the ED and the ICU was incomplete. The volume of fluid administered was reported to be adequate, but the reported volume was higher than was actually given. Vital signs are improving.

Time: 4 hours and 9 minutes after arrival

After successful intubation, the chest x-ray demonstrated diffuse pulmonary edema consistent with volume overload and correct placement of the endotracheal tube. The patient's blood pressure remained low after intubation (62/30 mmHg). Norepinephrine infusion was initiated; a triple lumen central venous line and arterial catheter were placed.

Telemedicine Perspective: The bedside provider is still not aware that fluid resuscitation is likely inadequate, which a telemedicine provider with continuity would be able to document and report.

Time: 5 hours and 32 minutes after arrival

Central venous line placement was difficult and took longer than expected. After catheters had been placed, the provider reviewed the medical record and realized that the second liter of normal saline had been ordered but not administered. The provider ordered another liter of normal saline to infuse over the next hour to meet the 6-hour bundle criteria.

Telemedicine Perspective: When this case was abstracted for the SEP-1 measure, the documentation suggested that care was not in compliance with the bundle because time zero was not correctly identified and fluid resuscitation was delayed. A telemedicine provider or nurse could have prompted the physician to complete fluid resuscitation earlier, identify sepsis earlier, and the telemedicine provider could have documented additional elements to support the clinical documentation.

Key Issues

1. In this case, resuscitation performance was very good, but a simple miscommunication between providers led to failure on the SEP-1 metric.
2. In many tertiary care centers, staff physicians are providing care alongside residents, students, and other care team members. Ensuring that all of those team members are educated in the documentation required for SEP-1 bundle compliance (especially with trainees rotating through the hospital) can be difficult, and telemedicine solutions can help to standardize the care provided and the documentation of that care.
3. Staff physicians may also have other responsibilities outside the ICU (clinic, procedures, etc.), so providing minute-by-minute monitoring to evaluate response to care may not be available without a telemedicine network.
4. Bundle criteria could have been met if time zero were identified correctly.

Conflicts of Interest EKH and BS work for Avera eCARE, a provider of ED-based and ICU-based telemedicine services. BGC serves as a senior policy advisor for the US Department of Health & Human Services. The views here do not necessarily represent those of the US Government.

References

1. Steinman M, Morbeck RA, Pires PV, Abreu Filho CA, Andrade AH, Terra JC, Teixeira Junior JC, Kanamura AH. Impact of telemedicine in hospital culture and its consequences on quality of care and safety. Einstein (Sao Paulo). 2015;13:580–6.
2. Liu V, Escobar GJ, Greene JD, et al. Hospital deaths in patients with sepsis from 2 independent cohorts. JAMA. 2014;312:90–2.
3. Elixhauser A, Friedman B, Stranges E. Septicemia in US Hospitals, 2009: Statistical Brief #122. In: Healthcare Cost and Utilization Project (Hcup) Statistical Briefs. Rockville: Agency for Healthcare Research and Quality (US); 2006.
4. Angus DC, Linde-Zwirble WT, Lidicker J, Clermont G, Carcillo J, Pinsky MR. Epidemiology of severe sepsis in the United States: analysis of incidence, outcome, and associated costs of care. Crit Care Med. 2001;29:1303–10.
5. Torio CM, Moore BJ. National Inpatient Hospital Costs: the most expensive conditions by payer, 2013: statistical brief #204. In: Healthcare Cost and Utilization Project (Hcup) statistical briefs. Rockville: Agency for Healthcare Research and Quality (US); 2006.
6. Stevenson EK, Rubenstein AR, Radin GT, Wiener RS, Walkey AJ. Two decades of mortality trends among patients with severe sepsis: a comparative meta-analysis. Crit Care Med. 2014;42:625–31.
7. Hall MJ, Williams SN, DeFrances CJ, Golosinskiy A. Inpatient care for septicemia or sepsis: a challenge for patients and hospitals. NCHS Data Brief. 2011:1–8.
8. Mayr FB, Talisa VB, Balakumar V, Chang CH, Fine M, Yende S. Proportion and cost of unplanned 30-day readmissions after sepsis compared with other medical conditions. JAMA. 2017;317:530–1.
9. Kent N, Fields W. Early recognition of Sepsis in the emergency department: an evidence-based project. J Emerg Nurs. 2012;38:139–43.
10. Kumar A, Roberts D, Wood KE, Light B, Parrillo JE, Sharma S, Suppes R, Feinstein D, Zanotti S, Taiberg L, Gurka D, Kumar A, Cheang M. Duration of hypotension before initiation of effective antimicrobial therapy is the critical determinant of survival in human septic shock. Crit Care Med. 2006;34:1589–96.

11. Gaieski DF, Mikkelsen ME, Band RA, Pines JM, Massone R, Furia FF, Shofer FS, Goyal M. Impact of time to antibiotics on survival in patients with severe sepsis or septic shock in whom early goal-directed therapy was initiated in the emergency department. Crit Care Med. 2010;38:1045–53.
12. Rivers EP. Point: adherence to early goal-directed therapy does it really matter? Yes. After a decade, the scientific proof speaks for itself. Chest. 2010;138:476–80.
13. Rivers E, Nguyen B, Havstad S, Ressler J, Muzzin A, Knoblich B, Peterson E, Tomlanovich M, EG-DT C. Early goal-directed therapy in the treatment of severe sepsis and septic shock. N Engl J Med. 2001;345:1368–77.
14. Rhodes A, Evans LE, Alhazzani W, Levy MM, Antonelli M, Ferrer R, Kumar A, Sevransky JE, Sprung CL, Nunnally ME, Rochwerg B, Rubenfeld GD, Angus DC, Annane D, Beale RJ, Bellinghan GJ, Bernard GR, Chiche J-D, Coopersmith C, De Backer DP, French CJ, Fujishima S, Gerlach H, Hidalgo JL, Hollenberg SM, Jones AE, Karnad DR, Kleinpell RM, Koh Y, Lisboa TC, Machado FR, Marini JJ, Marshall JC, Mazuski JE, McIntyre LA, McLean AS, Mehta S, Moreno RP, Myburgh J, Navalesi P, Nishida O, Osborn TM, Perner A, Plunkett CM, Ranieri M, Schorr CA, Seckel MA, Seymour CW, Shieh L, Shukri KA, Simpson SQ, Singer M, Thompson BT, Townsend SR, Van der Poll T, Vincent J-L, Wiersinga WJ, Zimmerman JL, Dellinger RP. Updated bundles in response to new evidence. Surviving Sepsis Campaign. 2015. Available from: http://www.survivingsepsis.org/SiteCollectionDocuments/SSC_Bundle.pdf. Accessed 26 Oct 2018.
15. Dellinger RP, Levy MM, Rhodes A, Annane D, Gerlach H, Opal SM, Sevransky JE, Sprung CL, Douglas IS, Jaeschke R, Osborn TM, Nunnally ME, Townsend SR, Reinhart K, Kleinpell RM, Angus DC, Deutschman CS, Machado FR, Rubenfeld GD, Webb SA, Beale RJ, Vincent JL, Moreno R. Surviving sepsis campaign: international guidelines for management of severe sepsis and septic shock: 2012. Crit Care Med. 2013;41:580–637.
16. Dellinger RP, Levy MM, Carlet JM, Bion J, Parker MM, Jaeschke R, Reinhart K, Angus DC, Brun-Buisson C, Beale R, Calandra T, Dhainaut J-F, Gerlach H, Harvey M, Marini JJ, Marshall J, Ranieri M, Ramsay G, Sevransky J, Thompson BT, Townsend S, Vender JS, Zimmerman JL, Vincent J-L. Surviving sepsis campaign: international guidelines for management of severe sepsis and septic shock: 2008. Intensive Care Med. 2008;34:17–60.
17. Dellinger RP, Carlet JM, Masur H, Gerlach H, Calandra T, Cohen J, Gea-Banacloche J, Keh D, Marshall JC, Parker MM, Ramsay G, Zimmerman JL, Vincent JL, Levy MM. Surviving sepsis campaign guidelines for management of severe sepsis and septic shock. Crit Care Med. 2004;32:858–73.
18. Levy MM, Evans LE, Rhodes A. The surviving sepsis campaign bundle: 2018 update. Crit Care Med. 2018;46:997–1000.
19. Severe Sepsis and Septic Shock, Sepsis Bundle Project (Sep-1), National Hospital Inpatient Quality Measures. Specifications Manual for National Hospital Inpatient Quality Measures. Vol 5.3. Baltimore: Center for Medicare & Medicaid Services; 2017. p. 1–60.
20. Faust JS, Weingart SD. The past, present, and future of the Centers for Medicare and Medicaid Services Quality Measure Sep-1: The Early Management Bundle for Severe Sepsis/Septic Shock. Emerg Med Clin North Am. 2017;35:219–31.
21. Claypool S. Hospital compare lifts the veil on sepsis care. Check your hospital's score. Stat. 26 Jul 2018.
22. Levy MM, Dellinger RP, Townsend SR, Linde-Zwirble WT, Marshall JC, Bion J, Schorr C, Artigas A, Ramsay G, Beale R, Parker MM, Gerlach H, Reinhart K, Silva E, Harvey M, Regan S, Angus DC. The surviving sepsis campaign: results of an international guideline-based performance improvement program targeting severe sepsis. Intensive Care Med. 2010;36:222–31.
23. Miller RR 3rd, Dong L, Nelson NC, Brown SM, Kuttler KG, Probst DR, Allen TL, Clemmer TP. Multicenter implementation of a severe sepsis and septic shock treatment bundle. Am J Respir Crit Care Med. 2013;188:77–82.
24. Levy MM, Rhodes A, Phillips GS, Townsend SR, Schorr CA, Beale R, Osborn T, Lemeshow S, Chiche JD, Artigas A, Dellinger RP. Surviving sepsis campaign: association between performance metrics and outcomes in a 7.5-year study. Intensive Care Med. 2014;40:1623–33.

25. Gao F, Melody T, Daniels DF, Giles S, Fox S. The impact of compliance with 6-hour and 24-hour sepsis bundles on hospital mortality in patients with severe sepsis: a prospective observational study. Crit Care. 2005;9:R764–70.
26. Levy MM, Artigas A, Phillips GS, Rhodes A, Beale R, Osborn T, Vincent JL, Townsend S, Lemeshow S, Dellinger RP. Outcomes of the surviving sepsis campaign in intensive care units in the USA and Europe: a prospective cohort study. Lancet Infect Dis. 2012;12:919–24.
27. Damiani E, Donati A, Serafini G, Rinaldi L, Adrario E, Pelaia P, Busani S, Girardis M. Effect of performance improvement programs on compliance with sepsis bundles and mortality: a systematic review and meta-analysis of observational studies. PLoS One. 2015;10:e0125827.
28. Venkatesh AK, Slesinger T, Whittle J, Osborn T, Aaronson E, Rothenberg C, Tarrant N, Goyal P, Yealy DM, Schuur JD. Preliminary Performance on the New Cms Sepsis-1 National Quality Measure: Early Insights from the Emergency Quality Network (E-Qual). Ann Emerg Med. 2018;71:10–15.e11.
29. Knowles M. Hospital compare spotlights hospitals' sepsis performance. Becker Hospital Review. 27 Jul 2018.
30. Yealy DM, Huang DT, Delaney A, Knight M, Randolph AG, Daniels R, Nutbeam T. Recognizing and managing Sepsis: what needs to be done? BMC Med. 2015;13:98.
31. Mohr NM, Collier J, Hassebroek E, Groth H. Characterizing critical care physician staffing in rural America: a description of Iowa intensive care unit staffing. J Crit Care. 2014;29:194–8.
32. Ferrer R, Martínez ML, Gomà G, Suárez D, Álvarez-Rocha L, de la Torre MV, González G, Zaragoza R, Borges M, Blanco J, Herrejón EP, Artigas A. Improved empirical antibiotic treatment of sepsis after an educational intervention: the Abiss-Edusepsis study. Crit Care. 2018;22:167.
33. Seymour CW, Gesten F, Prescott HC, Friedrich ME, Iwashyna TJ, Phillips GS, Lemeshow S, Osborn T, Terry KM, Levy MM. Time to treatment and mortality during Mandated Emergency Care for Sepsis. N Engl J Med. 2017;376:2235–44.
34. Gaieski DF, Edwards JM, Kallan MJ, Mikkelsen ME, Goyal M, Carr BG. The relationship between hospital volume and mortality in severe sepsis. Am J Respir Crit Care Med. 2014;190:665–74.
35. Kocher KE, Haggins AN, Sabbatini AK, Sauser K, Sharp AL. Emergency department hospitalization volume and mortality in the United States. Ann Emerg Med. 2014;64:446–457.e446.
36. Faine BA, Noack JM, Wong T, Messerly JT, Ahmed A, Fuller BM, Mohr NM. Interhospital transfer delays appropriate treatment for patients with severe sepsis and septic shock: a retrospective cohort study. Crit Care Med. 2015;43:2589–96.
37. Mohr NM, Harland KK, Shane DM, Ahmed A, Fuller BM, Torner JC. Inter-hospital transfer is associated with increased mortality and costs in severe sepsis and septic shock: an instrumental variables approach. J Crit Care. 2016;36:187–94.
38. Mohr NM, Harland KK, Shane DM, Ahmed A, Fuller BM, Ward MM, Torner JC. Rural patients with severe sepsis or septic shock who bypass rural hospitals have increased mortality: an instrumental variables approach. Crit Care Med. 2017;45:85–93.
39. Mohr NM, Brian Skow M, Wittrock A, Bell A, McDanel J, Fuller BM, Simpson S, Ward MM. Improving access to high quality Sepsis Care in a South Dakota Emergency Telemedicine Network. Research Policy Brief. 2017:1–4.
40. Heath B, Salerno R, Hopkins A, Hertzig J, Caputo M. Pediatric critical care telemedicine in rural underserved emergency departments*. Pediatr Crit Care Med. 2009;10:588–91.
41. Hicks LL, Boles KE, Hudson ST, Madsen RW, Kling B, Tracy J, Mitchell JA, Webb W. Using telemedicine to avoid transfer of rural emergency department patients. J Rural Health. 2001;17:220–8.
42. Duchesne JC, Kyle A, Simmons J, Islam S, Schmieg REJ, Olivier J, McSwain NEJ. Impact of telemedicine upon rural trauma care. J Trauma Acute Care Surg. 2008;64:92–8.
43. Ricci MA, Caputo M, Amour J, Rogers FB, Sartorelli K, Callas PW, Malone PT. Telemedicine reduces discrepancies in rural trauma care. Telemed J E Health. 2003;9:3–11.

44. Mohr NM, Harland KK, Chrischilles EA, Bell A, Shane DM, Ward MM. Emergency department telemedicine is used for more severely injured rural trauma patients, but does not decrease transfer: a cohort study. Acad Emerg Med. 2017;24:177–85.
45. Van Oeveren L, Donner J, Fantegrossi A, Mohr NM, Brown CA 3rd. Telemedicine-assisted intubation in rural emergency departments: a National Emergency Airway Registry Study. Telemed J E Health. 2017;23:290–7.
46. Cho OM, Kim H, Lee YW, Cho I. Clinical alarms in intensive care units: perceived obstacles of alarm management and alarm fatigue in nurses. Healthcare Informatics Research. 2016;22:46–53.
47. Westbrook JI, Duffield C, Li L, Creswick NJ. How much time do nurses have for patients? A longitudinal study quantifying hospital nurses' patterns of task time distribution and interactions with health professionals. BMC Health Serv Res. 2011;11:319.
48. Potter P, Wolf L, Boxerman S, Grayson D, Sledge J, Dunagan C, Evanoff B. Understanding the cognitive work of nursing in the acute care environment. J Nurs Adm. 2005;35:327-335.
49. Nemati S, Holder A, Razmi F, Stanley MD, Clifford GD, Buchman TG. An interpretable machine learning model for accurate prediction of sepsis in the Icu. Crit Care Med. 2018;46:547–53.
50. Rincon TA, Manos EL, Pierce JD. Telehealth intensive care unit nurse surveillance of sepsis. Comput Inform Nurs. 2017;35:459–64.
51. Agarwal AK, Gaieski DF, Perman SM, Leary M, Delfin G, Abella BS, Carr BG. Telemedicine resuscitation and arrest trial (treat): a feasibility study of real-time provider-to-provider telemedicine for the care of critically ill patients. Heliyon. 2016;2:e00099.
52. Rincon TA, Bourke G, Seiver A. Standardizing sepsis screening and management via a tele-Icu program improves patient care. Telemed J E Health. 2011;17:560–4.
53. Loyola S, Wilhelm J, Fornos J. An innovative approach to meeting early goal-directed therapy using telemedicine. Crit Care Nurs Q. 2011;34:187–99.
54. Machado SM, Wilson EH, Elliott JO, Jordan K. Impact of a telemedicine Eicu cart on sepsis management in a community hospital emergency department. J Telemed Telecare. 2018;24:202–8.
55. Morrison JL, Cai Q, Davis N, Yan Y, Berbaum ML, Ries M, Solomon G. Clinical and economic outcomes of the electronic intensive care unit: results from two community hospitals. Crit Care Med. 2010;38:2–8.
56. Breslow MJ, Rosenfeld BA, Doerfler M, Burke G, Yates G, Stone DJ, Tomaszewicz P, Hochman R, Plocher DW. Effect of a multiple-site intensive care unit telemedicine program on clinical and economic outcomes: an alternative paradigm for intensivist staffing. Crit Care Med. 2004;32:31–8.
57. Kumar G, Falk DM, Bonello RS, Kahn JM, Perencevich E, Cram P. The costs of critical care telemedicine programs: a systematic review and analysis. Chest. 2013;143:19–29.
58. MacKinney AC, Ward MM, Ullrich F, Ayyagari P, Bell AL, Mueller KJ. The business case for tele-emergency. Telemed J E Health. 2015;21:1005–11.
59. Lopez-Magallon AJ, Otero AV, Welchering N, Bermon A, Castillo V, Duran A, Castro J, Munoz R. Patient outcomes of an international telepediatric cardiac critical care program. Telemed J E Health. 2015;21:601–10.
60. Amalfitano E. Don't Get Left Behind: Three Critical Questions for Mastering Sep-1 Core Measure Compliance. Action for Better Healthcare. 14 Jul 2016.
61. Mackay F, Roy A, Schorr C, Crabtree P, Puri N. 1471: Cms Sep-1 measure start time. Do We Agree? A Comparison of Clinicians Versus Quality Staff. Crit Care Med. 2018;46:719.
62. Taylor MJ, McNicholas C, Nicolay C, Darzi A, Bell D, Reed JE. Systematic review of the application of the plan-do-study-act method to improve quality in healthcare. BMJ Qual Saf. 2014;23:290–8.
63. MacKinney AC, Mohr NM. Case 446: chest pain in a rural hospital. AHRQ PSNet WebM&M. 2018.

64. Gattinoni L, Brazzi L, Pelosi P, Latini R, Tognoni G, Pesenti A, Fumagalli R. A trial of goal-oriented hemodynamic therapy in critically ill patients. N Engl J Med. 1995;333:1025–32.
65. ProCESS Investigators, Yealy DM, Kellum JA, Huang DT, Barnato AE, Weissfeld LA, Pike F, Terndrup T, Wang HE, Hou PC, LoVecchio F, Filbin MR, Shapiro NI, Angus DC. A randomized trial of protocol-based care for early septic shock. N Engl J Med. 2014;370:1683–93.
66. ARISE Investigators, ANZICS Clinical Trials Group, Peake SL, Delaney A, Bailey M, Bellomo R, Cameron PA, Cooper DJ, Higgins AM, Holdgate A, Howe BD, Webb SA, Williams P. Goal-directed resuscitation for patients with early septic shock. N Engl J Med. 2014;371:1496–506.
67. Mouncey PR, Osborn TM, Power GS, Harrison DA, Sadique MZ, Grieve RD, Jahan R, Harvey SE, Bell D, Bion JF, Coats TJ, Singer M, Young JD, Rowan KM. Trial of early, goal-directed resuscitation for septic shock. N Engl J Med. 2015;372:1301–11.
68. Zapka J, Simpson K, Hiott L, Langston L, Fakhry S, Ford D. A mixed methods descriptive investigation of readiness to change in rural hospitals participating in a tele-critical care intervention. BMC Health Serv Res. 2013;13:33.
69. Latifi R, Hadeed GJ, Rhee P, O'Keeffe T, Friese RS, Wynne JL, Ziemba ML, Judkins D. Initial experiences and outcomes of telepresence in the management of trauma and emergency surgical patients. Am J Surg. 2009;198:905–10.
70. Leong JR, Sirio CA, Clinical RAJEPFA, Outcomes E. Crit Care. 2005;9:E22.
71. Nguyen YL, Kahn JM, Angus DC. Reorganizing adult critical care delivery: the role of regionalization, telemedicine, and community outreach. Am J Respir Crit Care Med. 2010;181:1164–9.
72. Feazel L, Schlichting AB, Bell GR, Shane DM, Ahmed A, Faine B, Nugent A, Mohr NM. Achieving regionalization through rural Interhospital transfer. Am J Emerg Med. 2015;33:1288–96.
73. IOM. Future of Emergency Care. Hospital based emergency care. Washington, DC: National Academies; 2006.
74. Carr BG, Conway PH, Meisel ZF, Steiner CA, Clancy C. Defining the emergency care sensitive condition: a health policy research agenda in emergency medicine. Ann Emerg Med. 2010;56:49–51.
75. Holmes GM, Kaufman BG, Pink GH. Financial distress and closure of rural hospitals [webinar]. Chapel Hill: North Carolina Rural Health Research Program; 2017.
76. Finlayson SR, Birkmeyer JD, Tosteson AN, Nease RF Jr. Patient preferences for location of care: implications for regionalization. Med Care. 1999;37:204–9.
77. Mohr NM, Wong TS, Faine B, Schlichting A, Noack J, Ahmed A. Discordance between patient and clinician experiences and priorities in rural Interhospital transfer: a mixed methods study. J Rural Health. 2016;32:25–34.
78. Holmes GM, Slifkin RT, Randolph RK, Poley S. The effect of rural hospital closures on community economic health. Health Serv Res. 2006;41:467–85.
79. Martinez R, Carr B. Creating integrated networks of emergency care: from vision to value. Health Aff. 2013;32:2082–90.
80. Telehealth and remote patient monitoring use in Medicare and Selected Federal Programs (report Gao-17-365). Washington, DC: United States Government Accountability Office; 2017.
81. Cms proposes historic changes to modernize medicare and restore the doctor-patient relationship [press release]. Washington, DC: Centers for Medicare and Medicaid Services; 2018.
82. Interoperability. Washington, DC: Office of the National Coordinator for Health Information Technology; 2018.
83. Miliard M. With Ehr-based sepsis detection, Epic and Cerner have different approaches. Healthcare IT News. 2017.
84. Colorafi K, Jang B, Quinones E. Fighting Sepsis Your Way: Using the Decisioinsight® Clinical Dashboard to Improve Early Sepsis Diagnosis and Surviving Sepsis Campaign (Ssc) Egdt Bundle Compliance. Houston: Decisio Health; 2018.

Chapter 16
Prehospital Telemedicine and EMS Integration

Haydon M. Pitchford, Marcus C. Divers, Sherita N. Chapman, and Andrew M. Southerland

Introduction

Providing the most appropriate care to patients wherever they are and as soon as they access the medical system is the goal of prehospital medicine. The last 50 years has seen a drastic evolution of prehospital medicine in the United States. Gone are the days of unregulated transport of the sick and injured, having been replaced by a new paradigm of bringing the hospital to the patient and providing interventions at the site of illness. The evolution of prehospital medicine has been in tandem with the evolution of various technologies used by prehospital personnel to communicate with base hospital staff. Prehospital telecommunication originated with basic telemetry and radio designed to allow physicians more clear information on a patient's condition prior to their arrival at the hospital. Today, telemedicine has evolved with the potential to provide real-time audiovisual communications in the prehospital setting with applications in stroke, transport destination and diversion, and community paramedicine among others.

Developing and implementing a telemedicine program in the prehospital environment pose a number of unique challenges. Communication infrastructure, availability of resources, provider training for both in and out of hospital personnel, mobility, and experience are of specific concern. Successful programs are tailored to the workflows of the existing prehospital system, simultaneously addressing a

The authors would like to thank J. Aaron Matthews, MSN, RN, CEN, for his significant contributions to the development of this publication.

H. M. Pitchford · M. C. Divers · S. N. Chapman · A. M. Southerland (✉)
Department of Neurology and Karen S. Rheuban Center for Telehealth, University of Virginia Health System, Charlottesville, VA, USA
e-mail: hmp4yf@virginia.edu; md9da@virginia.edu; sc2bd@virginia.edu; as5ef@virginia.edu

M. A. Koenig (ed.), *Telemedicine in the ICU*,
https://doi.org/10.1007/978-3-030-11569-2_16

local healthcare need while remaining aware of possible local constraints and limitations. In this chapter we will discuss the varying needs, challenges, and successful methods for integrating telemedicine in the prehospital environment. For the purpose of clarity, prehospital herein refers to any encounter prior to arrival at the final receiving hospital or facility.

Background

The need for prehospital emergency medical services (EMS) personnel to contact hospital-based physicians has always been present but limited by environment and technology. EMS personnel cannot operate under their own certification or licenses in the field without express consent from a physician operational medical director (OMD) who determines the scope of clinical practice and provides medical control. OMDs often utilize both "online medical control" for direct patient care orders and "off-line medical control" where the EMS provider is able to perform interventions without direct authorization using predetermined protocols [77]. Therefore, it has always been necessary for EMS personnel to have a way to contact a physician for orders regarding patient care, typically via phone or radio communications, to the receiving or base hospital. As the complexity of hospital care has advanced, so has the need for more advanced technology in prehospital communication.

One of the first examples of prehospital telemedicine was the need to transmit electrocardiography from the field to assist in the early identification of patients who would benefit from advanced coronary care [82]. This technology was later popularized by the television show *Emergency!* in the 1970s during which paramedic firefighters contacted the fictional hospital often while transmitting telemetry. This was accomplished by using a device called a "biophone" (see Fig. 16.1), which

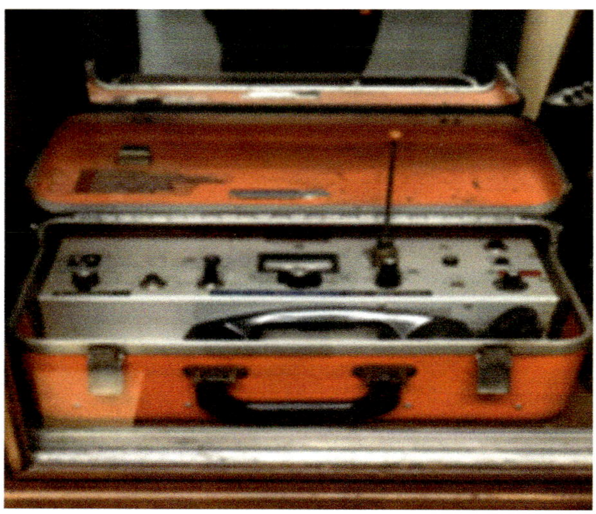

Fig. 16.1 Early BioPhone [94]

was capable of transmitting both radio communications and telemetry at the same time in a portable kit [92]. The original BioPhone used in the television series was later donated and displayed at the Smithsonian Institution's National Museum of American History [32].

Case Study

One high-profile case of an early prehospital telemetry system was when former President Lyndon Johnson suffered a myocardial infarction while visiting his daughter Lynda, in Charlottesville, Virginia. On April 6, 1972, President Johnson awoke in the middle of the night complaining of chest pain. Johnson had experienced a near fatal heart attack before, so he quickly recognized the need for immediate medical attention. The emergency department at the University of Virginia hospital was contacted, and cardiologist Dr. Richard S. Crampton was alerted, who then contacted the Charlottesville-Albemarle Rescue Squad. Dr. Crampton requested that the rescue squad first travel to the hospital to collect both himself and the mobile telemetry and defibrillation device before responding to the former president's location. With this portable equipment, Dr. Crampton performed an electrocardiogram on the former president in the home before personally transporting him directly to the coronary care unit at the University of Virginia [51].

President Johnson did not stay in the hospital for long, however. After just 5 days, Johnson was transferred home to his ranch in Texas, with his electrocardiogram monitored remotely by Dr. Crampton throughout the entire flight. It is believed that this made former President Johnson the first patient to be transferred by an airborne coronary care unit [2]. Once arriving home, physicians continued to monitor the former president's electrocardiogram reading remotely. Following these events President and Mrs. Johnson helped provide financial support for further prehospital cardiac research enabling greater access to the advanced clinical tools the former president benefited from [20].

As late as the 1970s, the training of ambulance attendants in the United States was largely unregulated, and most training was largely limited to a Red Cross first aid course at most [27]. Prior to this period, the focus of EMS was transport and not the provision of direct medical care. Therefore, the ability to transmit and interpret telemetry was a significant development, opening the door for EMS providers to deliver meaningful medical care rather than just transport. The entire field soon underwent massive changes, requiring more structured training programs and standards. Compared to today, the National EMS Scope of Practice model considers electrocardiographic monitoring and interpretation an essential skill [59].

Use Cases for Prehospital Telemedicine

Prehospital Telestroke

Acute stroke is a critically time-sensitive disease in which shorter times from stroke onset to treatment are associated with better patient outcomes [22]. Delays in acute stroke treatment manifest as increased long-term disability and death with corresponding burden and costs for the individual, family, and society at large. A number of factors, both pre- and in-hospital, play a role in the delay to treatment. While efforts to improve in-hospital workflows with the goal of decreasing performance metrics such as door-to-needle time have been successful, improving the prehospital portion of the acute stroke continuum poses unique challenges. Augmenting the interaction between EMS and hospital providers via telemedicine offers an opportunity to address a number of these challenges.

The widespread successful application of telestroke in the emergency room setting throughout the world has led a number of programs to explore a range of services and delivery models including mobile ambulance-based telestroke (see Table 16.1). The ambulance-based application of telestroke was initially pioneered by the TeleBAT group at the University of Maryland in the early 2000s. The TeleBAT telemedicine platform consisted of commercial components with a parallel array of four digital cellular phones using 2G cellular network transmitting data in a store and forward method. The study demonstrated a high-inter-rater reliability and reduction in time to treatment. However, notable limitations included instability of transmission, actor scenarios rather than real patient encounters, and comparison of treatment time with historic control patients.

In 2009, the AHA/ASA scientific statement reviewing the evidence for telestroke models hypothesized that providing stroke expertise to an ambulance via teleconferencing technology could increase diagnostic accuracy, provide earlier resource mobilization, and increase appropriate triage for timelier stroke treatment. However, there was not sufficient evidence for a specific recommendation that time [69]. Since that time, there have been a number of studies evaluating the feasibility and reliability of ambulance-based telestroke. Early research yielded conflicting results on feasibility, but wireless cellular technologies and teleconferencing applications have advanced substantially in the last several years and continue to improve. As seen from table 16.1, the feasibility of ambulance-based telestroke has improved with the support of current cellular technologies (e.g., 4G network, portable mobile devices, and advanced mobile video conferencing platforms). These results, while preliminary, demonstrate that commercially available and widespread mobile devices could be readily incorporated into a mobile, ambulance-based telemedicine program with a secure teleconferencing platform.

Triage of patients to appropriate facilities and early activation or "prenotification" or "prealert" of in-hospital specialty teams is a key function of emergency medical services personnel for time-critical illnesses and injuries. EMS prenotification is associated with more rapid hospital diagnosis, improved quality metrics, and

Table 16.1 Chronology of ambulance-based telestroke

Author	Type of study	Telemedicine platform	Data network	Data transmission method
LaMonte et al. 2000 North America [41]	Pilot feasibility study – simulation and real-time patient	Existing open system commercial components with parallel array of four digital cellular phones	2G	Store and forward
LaMonte et al. 2004 North America [42]	Simulation feasibility study	Existing open system commercial components with parallel array of four digital cellular phones	2G	Store and forward
Liman et al. 2012 Europe [47]	Simulation feasibility study	Prototype mobile telemedicine device (VIMED CAR)	3G	Mobile, real-time audio-video
Bergrath et al. 2012 Europe [7]	Prospective pilot feasibility study	Portable data transmission unit (peeg-box) with four parallel data channels connected to video camera and audio communication devices	2G and 3G	Real-time audio-video and still pictures
Van Hooff et al. 2013 Europe [93]	Pilot feasibility simulation study	Commercially available hardware with web-based telemedicine platform	4G	Mobile, real-time audio-video
Wu et al. 2014 North America [90]	Pilot feasibility simulation study	Existing portable telemedicine unit – RP-Xpress system, zoom camera and microphone with speakers, Verizon 4G LTE jetpack	4G	Mobile, real-time audio-video
Eadie et al. 2014 Europe [55]	Pilot feasibility simulation study	Omni-hub communications system, tablet-based, Verizon SIM card, MotionX GPS, antennae	2G and 3G	Mobile, real-time audio-video
Lippman et al. 2016 North America [48]	Technical observational study	Off-the-shelf, tablet-based telemedicine system, Cisco jabber	4G	Mobile, real-time audio-video
Chapman et al. 2016 North America [75]	Pilot feasibility simulation study	Off-the-shelf, tablet-based telemedicine system, Cisco jabber	4G	Mobile, real-time audio-video
Itrat et al. 2016 North America [35]	Prospective observational study	Existing portable telemedicine unit – RP-Xpress system Mobile CT scanner	4G LTE	Mobile, real-time audio-video
Espinoza et al. 2016 Europe [23]	Pilot feasibility simulation study	Prototype platform using laptop, Mobotix camera, and IXSyS software	4G	Mobile, real-time audio-video

(continued)

Table 16.1 (continued)

Author	Type of study	Telemedicine platform	Data network	Data transmission method
Belt et al. 2016 North America [5]	Prospective pilot feasibility study	Existing portable telemedicine unit – InTouch Xpress system	4G	Mobile, real-time audio-video
Barrett et al. 2017 North America [4]	Proof-of-concept feasibility study	Off-the-shelf, tablet-based telemedicine system	4G LTE	Mobile, real-time audio-video
Chapman Smith et al. 2018 North America [74]	Pilot feasibility and usability simulation study	Off-the-shelf, tablet-based telemedicine system with PTZ camera and microphone with speaker	4G LTE	Mobile, real-time audio-video

better patient outcomes [9, 43, 53, 67]. Additionally, over and under triage can have deleterious effects clinically and financially for patients and health systems [49, 66]. Patients transported to a facility that cannot effectively manage their condition place a resource burden on that facility while care is initiated and interfacility transport is coordinated. Patients *overtriaged* to a specialty center instead place excess strain on limited resources that may need to be redirected elsewhere. This leaves emergency medical services personnel in the position of needing to make the decision of which facility to transport a patient to with limited information and assessment capability.

Many times the first people to respond to a 911 call will be individuals that are trained to the EMT Basic level and perform as such on a volunteer basis [83]. Imagine an EMT Basic in a rural area who volunteers for 12 hours a week at an agency that averages 700 calls for service a year. They were dispatched along with a CPR certified driver to assess a patient presenting with an altered level of consciousness, the only paramedic staffed unit in the region is on another call for service and not available to assist. The EMT basic performs a Cincinnati Prehospital Stroke Scale and finds the patient is experiencing left arm weakness, slurred speech and was last known to be well less than four hours prior. This EMT Basic then has the responsibility to make the determination of whether or not to transport this patient 30 minutes by ground to the Acute Stroke Ready Hospital or to activate critical care air medical services for expedited transport to a Comprehensive Stroke Center. In this scenario, inappropriate triage is a very real concern.

If this patient is transported by ground to the ASRH hospital and is then found to have been a candidate for thrombectomy, there is a significant increase in the amount of time until they reach definitive treatment with delays nearing 100 minutes. Further, this delay both reduces the chances the patient would be a candidate for endovascular therapy and reduces the likelihood of benefit. Conversely, if this patient is evacuated by an air medical team to the comprehensive stroke center only to later find that she was not a candidate for thrombectomy or was experiencing a stroke mimic, she will suffer consequences as well. This includes responsibility for the heavy financial burden of an air ambulance fee, combined with the increased risk that is innate to helicopter transport.

A good physical assessment is key in early identification of a patient experiencing a critical pathology and this is especially true in stroke. Several scales have been designed and validated to help providers recognize stroke in the field (See Table 16.2) [65]. Unfortunately, the sensitivity for EMS provider impression of stroke ranges anywhere from 44% to 91%, with diagnostic accuracy affected by presence of motor symptoms and whether or not a scale was utilized [11]. Additionally, rural emergency medical services personnel are less likely to use or be familiar with one of these scales compared to urban services [52]. With recent literature emphasizing the benefit of thrombectomy for patients suffering from large vessel occlusions, a high-quality assessment is needed to ensure these patients receive maximum benefit [8].

This scenario is not uncommon in the United States prehospital system for both stroke and other pathologies. It is established that utilization of critical care helicopter transport can be beneficial for carefully selected patients, especially for those with long transport times to specialty centers [81]. There is a problem with identification and therefore overutilization, however, with Sequeira et al. finding that as much as 32 percent of scene flights requested for stroke from the field were for mimics [71].

With the tension between early activation of specialized resources to ensure as many eligible patients receive treatment as possible and reducing costly overutilization of these same limited specialty resources, there is an opening for decision support tools. In the realm of prehospital telestroke, there are two primary forms, a dedicated mobile stroke unit or MSU that is often staffed in a single central location by specially trained staff or is facilitated through telemedicine equipped general service ambulances.

It is feasible to perform an NIH Stroke Scale with off-the-shelf technology through a video telemedicine link facilitated by equipment kept in a single kit and not necessarily hardwired into the ambulance itself. In this paradigm, EMS providers were guided through the NIHSS assessment with a vascular neurologist on the other end of the feed at a remote location [75]. Since the time of that study, at least one program has operationalized this into clinical practice [45].

It shows that it is not necessary for a stroke-trained physician to be present in the ambulance at the time of the assessment and that the assessment performed is highly correlated with that of the one performed upon arrival at the receiving facility. While treatment with IV tPA could not be safely administered without further imaging, destination triage, alerting of the receiving stroke team, and guidance in the management of both stroke and other neurological conditions mimicking stroke are not out of the realm of possibility. A further advantage to this setup is that the applications would go beyond telestroke. In the past few years, a number of portable telemedicine kits have been made available for a variety of purposes.

Table 16.2 Characteristics of prehospital stroke scales for large vessel occlusion identification

	Characteristics of prehospital stroke scales for large vessel occlusion identification					
Scale and score	Sample size	Components	Study setting	Sensitivity	Specificity	Accuracy
Cincinnati prehospital stroke severity scale ≥2 [37]	624 in derivation data set, 303 in validation data set	2 points for presence of conjugate gaze (NIHSS≥1); 1 point for presence of arm weakness (NIHSS≥2); and 1 point for presence abnormal level of consciousness commands and questions (NIHSS level of consciousness≥1 each)	Derived from two National Institute of Neurological Disorders and Stroke tissue-type plasminogen activator stroke study trials and validated using interventional Management of Stroke III cohorts	0.83	0.40	0.89
Los Angeles motor scale (LAMS) ≥ 4 [8]	119	Facial droop absent 0, present 1; arm drift absent 0, drifts down 1, falls rapidly 2; grip strength normal 0, weak grip 1, no grip 2	Sample drawn from two database sources from the UCLA Stroke Center between 1996 and 2006	0.81	0.85	0.84
Stroke vision, aphasia, neglect (VAN) positive [80]	62	Positive or negative assessment, initially limb weakness, if positive continue to assessment of visual disturbance, aphasia, or neglect	Single center emergency department	1.0	0.90	0.92
Rapid arterial occlusion evaluation (RACE) ≥ 5 [64]	654 retrospective 357 prospective	Facial palsy (scored 0–2), arm motor function (0–2), leg motor function (0–2), gaze (0–1), aphasia or agnosia (0–2)	Retrospective cohort scored on admission. Prospective cohort scored in field by EMS	0.85	0.68	0.72
Field assessment stroke triage for emergency destination (FAST-ED) ≥ 4 [46]	741	Facial palsy [scored 0–1], arm weakness [0–2], speech changes [0–2], time [documentation for decision-making but no points], eye deviation [0–2], and denial/neglect [0–2	Two university-based hospitals	0.61	0.89	0.79

Mobile CT Stroke Units

The first clinical trials of mobile stroke units (MSU) were in Germany with a trial published by Walter et al. finding that it was feasible to provide guideline-adherent and etiology-specific treatment of acute stroke at the site of the emergency [87]. In addition to standard ambulance equipment, this original mobile stroke unit contained a lead-shielded computed tomography unit, a system allowing for transmission of imaging to the base hospital, and point-of-care testing. The unit itself was staffed by a paramedic and a physician trained in stroke medicine. Following the results of the German trial, mobile stroke units were developed and implemented in other areas with a number of mobile stroke units now operating in the United States. Follow-up studies show that mobile stroke units are both feasible and that tPA and other stroke-specific treatment can be initiated earlier with their utilization [26]. While mobile stroke units are becoming more common, questions remain about patient-centered outcomes, rural versus urban implementation, and overall cost-efficiency [40, 76]. There are a number of ongoing studies powered to assess patient outcomes and cost-effectiveness whose results will inform the expansion of mobile stroke unit programs [10].

While MSUs advance the concept of "bringing the hospital to the patient," this is not without cost. A mobile stroke unit may cost anywhere from 500,000 to 1000,000 to develop and an addition 950,000 to 1200,000 to operate per year [12]. Most early studies involved a neurologist or some other stroke-trained physician on board the mobile stroke unit, but several studies show that using mobile telemedicine improves cost-efficiency [76]. Houston, Texas, found that a telemedicine-based assessment by a vascular neurologist is reliable and accurate when compared to one on board the MSU itself [91].

Community Paramedicine and Mobile Integrated Healthcare

Community paramedicine or mobile integrated healthcare is a model of healthcare delivery where EMS providers take on an expanded role to fill local healthcare gaps. There are various levels of EMS providers with different scopes of practice and training (see Table 16.3). Given the ubiquity of emergency medical services even where access to healthcare is scarce, EMS providers are in the unique position to provide expanded access to community health resources. These programs are gaining in popularity, but questions remain both regarding the safety and liability and legality of expanding the role of EMS providers. Some programs have successfully utilized telemedicine to address these concerns, providing needed oversight and support. Groups such as the National Rural Health Association and the National Association of EMS Physicians have issued position statements supporting community paramedicine implementation, with appropriate oversight [89].

Table 16.3 Overview of emergency medical technician (EMT) training and scope of practice [59, 84, 86]

	Emergency medical responder and EMT[a]	Advanced EMT or EMT intermediate[a]	Paramedic[a]
Level of training	Basic	Intermediate	Advanced
Approximate hours of training	120–150 hours	1000 hours	1200–1800 hours
Medication training	Oxygen, may assist patient with certain medications already prescribed to them, like oral glucose, nitroglycerin, and epinephrine auto injectors	Protocolized administration of certain medications including some narcotics, narcotic antagonists, nitroglycerine, intramuscular epinephrine, intravenous glucose, and nebulized medications	Expanded list of medication defined by local operational medical director. Includes intravenous and intraosseous medication, vasoactive medications, blood products, and thrombolytics
Interventions and psychomotor skills	Fundamental assessment, airway adjuncts, bag mask ventilation, splinting, basic bandaging, spinal immobilization	Advanced assessment, airway management with multi-lumen airways. In some areas, EMT-Is are eligible for advanced training such as ACLS and are trained to perform endotracheal intubation	Advanced assessment; EKG interpretation; definitive airway management including tracheal intubation, cricothyroidotomy; needle decompression; management of certain medical devices like central lines, BiPAP, and capnography; and blood chemistry analysis

[a]Local regulation may reference prehospital providers' level of responsibility by different names; this chart is to serve as a general overview with the understanding there may be significant variation at the local level

Programs have addressed some of the inherent oversight problems with community paramedicine by utilizing telemedicine. According to a survey published by the National Association of Emergency Medical Technicians in April of 2018, 26% of programs surveyed reported using telemedicine technology in some way to facilitate the goals of their local program [30]. Though most data available is still in the preliminary phase, it appears that the use of telemedicine for this purpose is both feasible and results in adequate patient satisfaction [33]. Real-time AV connections between a paramedic and advanced practice provider help bring a connected care team to communities that need more access to providers.

Alternate Destinations and Emergency Department Avoidance

A complex issue facing both community paramedicine and conventional 911 emergency medical services is how to handle patients that have activated 911 with a condition where transport by ambulance to the emergency department is not necessary.

For much of its existence, the paradigm of emergency medical services and prehospital care within the United States involved transport of the patient to the emergency department of a local hospital by necessity. The "you call, we haul" version of prehospital medicine was further entrenched with a number of state regulatory bodies mandating that transport to an emergency department is required for any patient who has activated 911. This combined with increasing call volumes and an increase in non-emergent calls has put significant strain on EMS systems and emergency departments nationwide with one study by Weaver et al. finding a 31% increase in unnecessary calls for service from 1997 to 2007 [54]. As the population of the United States increases and ages, calls for service, both necessary and unnecessary, should be expected to increase. A position paper by the National Association of EMS Physicians and American College of Emergency Physicians states that it may be appropriate to transport non-emergent patients via alternate methods to alternate locations [57].

Reducing the number of unnecessary ambulance transports and emergency department visits could have significant public health benefits. Alternative dispositions for these patients include anything from the patient remaining at their residence with the responding crew assisting with setting up a follow-up appointment later or diverting to another outpatient site of care such as a primary care office via ambulance or taxi rather than the emergency department. Unfortunately, there is not currently enough evidence to say that EMS providers can make the determination of whether or not these alternate destinations are safe for the patient to be transported to on their own [68]. Historical trends show a disparity in EMS provider impression of patient's need to be seen in the emergency department when compared to either emergency physician or admissions statistics, with further review being needed to make a determination one way or another [18]. In the same NAEMSP/ACEP paper referenced prior, it lists oversight by the agency medical director, appropriate training of providers and assurances that whatever alternate destination is chosen is done so with medical necessity in mind [68]. One solution to these conditions is to use telemedicine to help guide destination determination, thus allowing additional oversight and safety.

ETHAN Program Case Study (Alternative Destination)

The city of Houston, Texas, has successfully implemented and published on their experience in addressing this problem. Dubbed the Emergency Telehealth and Navigation (ETHAN) program, and with partnerships between the Houston Fire Department, the University of Texas Health Sciences Center, and other stakeholders, the program brings decision support directly into the scene of an emergency call [29]. Using a tablet that is stocked on every ambulance and emergency vehicle, a paramedic is able to contact an emergency physician by way of a HIPAA compliant video feed. The emergency physician on the other end of the call is then able to access the patient's field medical record created by the paramedics and provide guidance on disposition. Depending on the outcome of the assessment, several options are available ranging from the emergency physician scheduling an appointment at a community primary care clinic and scheduling a taxi to referring the patient to the ED with the originally dispatched ambulance crew [29]. In the first 12 months of the program being implemented, they found a 56% reduction in the number of patients transported to the emergency department when compared to the control group, without a significant difference in patient satisfaction [44]. In recent studies, 58% of patients have approved of EMS transporting to alternative destinations for lower acuity issues and 86% want EMS to have better access to their health records [56, 57].

Interfacility Transport

Interfacility transport is another area where the unique challenges of out of hospital medicine could be addressed with telemedicine. Patients are often transported between hospital facilities when they require a higher level of care or specialty care not offered at the primary facility. These patients may be on medications or need monitoring of parameters that are outside of the normal scope or comfort zone of EMS providers. Interfacility transport teams may consist of a variety of crew compositions, such as utilizing nurses, respiratory therapists, or even physicians to facilitate specialty transport for specific patient populations. Transport duration is an independent predictor of patient safety events [72, 79]. Therefore providing support and oversight to these transport teams is necessary for patient safety. The National Association of EMS Physicians states that interfacility transport requires oversight by a supervision physician, which can be challenging in resource-limited areas and during long geographic transports [73]. Telemedicine offers a way to provide medical oversight for interfacility transport from a central supervising provider in a tertiary location.

Despite this patient population being more complex and often requiring advanced intervention, it is not always necessary for a physician to be physically present for the transport itself. In 1989 McCloskey et al. published a series of 166 cases with a physician-staffed pediatric critical care transport team, finding that physician-only procedures were performed only in 9% of cases, and the transporting physician believed that the transport would have been successful without a physician present for 46% of cases [36]. In 2018 Kawaguchi et al. published an article with similar findings, showing that there was not a significant difference in patient outcomes with an increased use of physicians for transport in pediatric patients [38].

Arkansas Children's Hospital Case Study (Interfacility Transport)
As non-physician specialty teams gain in experience and are able to function with more autonomy without physicians at the bedside, they will still need access to medical control for especially complex cases and to give patient update reports. This may be more difficult than conventional medical control given a patient's complex presentation, limitations of voice contact and the medical control physician may be from a specialty without specific expertise in transport medicine. Research on utilizing advanced telemedicine during specialty care transports is limited. Stroud and Moss from Arkansas Children's Hospital's pediatric transport team Angel found that by utilizing native iPad software FaceTime© between the transport team and receiving PICU physician, significantly more interventions were performed in the FaceTime© group than in the standard phone call group. Although not statistically significant, there was also a decrease in PICU admissions in the FaceTime© group [78]. More research is needed, but there is potential for application into other

specialty care groups to provide support to transport teams in complicated cases, while reducing the need to utilize physicians for transports unless absolutely necessary.

Summary of Current Prehospital Use Cases Utilizing Telemedicine (*Table 16.4*)

Program type	Use case/ studies	Purpose	Potential benefits	Key barriers
Prehospital mobile telestroke	iTREAT, [75] MSU [10, 91]	Improve prehospital diagnosis, routing triage, and treatment times for acute stroke patients	- Early identification of stroke - Early activation of specialty resources - Faster onset to definitive treatment times - Telemedicine-only systems have relatively low start-up cost	- Reimbursement for in ambulance telemedicine treatment - Advanced systems have large start-up cost - Prehospital agency buy-in
Community paramedicine	Supporting on-call primary care physician [16]	Enables EMS providers to use telemedicine for increased oversight in order to improve access to primary care services in low access areas	- Increase access to healthcare services among underserved populations - Give PCPs the ability to serve a larger geographical area	advanced paramedicine training needed improved autonomy for trained EMS provider
Alternative destinations	Project ETHAN [29]	Reduce non-emergency transport to emergency departments and proper triage for appropriate treatment	Reduced unnecessary transports Reduced emergency medical service system burden Improve access to appropriate healthcare resources	Large prehospital presence involvement required by health system
Interfacility	Neonatal transport [78]	Provide up-to-the-minute guidance for complex pathology during transport	Provide support to transport teams managing complex patients	Technology considerations, communication in aircraft is difficult

Implementing a New Telemedicine Program for Prehospital Consultation Within a Healthcare System

In order to properly implement a prehospital telemedicine program, several key factors should be considered when deciding how to scale a program to fit your needs and size. Shown in Table 16.4 are examples of current programs using prehospital telemedicine and should be considered when implementing a program. Top barriers for an organization implementing new telemedicine-based programs tend to be cost, effectiveness, efficiency, and workflow, and all these barriers should be addressed prior to implementation, during the planning and consideration phase [57]. We will go over ways to address these issues as well as others that might come up when planning a prehospital telemedicine program for your organization or institution. After an organization assesses the need for a prehospital telemedicine program, one needs to exam several main considerations: program model, staffing, provider adoption, best-fit technology, start-up, and ongoing funding and regulations.

Staffing Considerations

Hospital systems developing a prehospital telemedicine program need to consider the added burden these programs would have on their current workflow and staffing. An in-depth service analysis should be done to determine the approximate volume of patients being transported by ambulance who would utilize the service and factor that with the increase in time consulting tele-providers would need to properly perform an en route assessment. For instance, emergency medicine physicians are 3 times more likely than the average provider to develop burnout, so having a firm grasp on the extra burden that could be placed on the system is a good way to avoid resistance and improve the effectiveness of the implementation process [6]. A proper physician to patient ratio is also needed in the critical care environment to ensure safety and quality of care [88].

Pilot testing with smaller populations will also give a better representation of the utilization of the new service. Pilot testing is a great tool to confirm the need for a prehospital telemedicine program by looking at utilization rates by EMS agencies and patient outcomes before scaling up to a fully functioning program. Since EMS systems are widely disparate, personalizing implementation to one's specific area and workforce is crucial.

In addition to being familiar with levels of EMS certification (see Table 16.2), it is also important to be familiar with system staffing models. While the majority are fire department based, others may be operated by the municipality, law enforcement, a local health system, or a private third-party vendor. Whichever agency provides EMS for an area will possess a unique history and relationship with the local health systems that must be considered when developing a program. In the case of third-party EMS agencies, for example, there may be additional legal considerations depending on the terms of their contract.

Prehospital staffing models pose unique considerations. In most areas ambulances are only staffed with two personnel, one driver, and one provider of varying levels of training. More resource-rich areas may dispatch a fire department apparatus along with an ambulance, providing extra staff to assist with care. Other departments may only send a single ambulance staffed with two providers regardless of the type of call for service. In the latter case, a program will need to use a telemedicine system that is easy to deploy, low maintenance, and portable to facilitate efficient prehospital care.

Contrast this with a more resource-rich system with a fire department apparatus responding with an ambulance to every call with as many as six paramedics on the scene. While it is still necessary for the telemedicine application to be low maintenance, larger and better staffed departments will have more well-trained individuals to assist with the logistics of deploying the technology while simultaneously administering patient care.

Provider Adoption

Another vital staffing component is having a clinical and/or an administrative "champion(s)" for prehospital telemedicine [16]. Having a champion in each participating department, both in hospital and out, is an important factor for a telemedicine start-up program [14]. Some of the top barriers for staff adoption of telemedicine are technically challenged staff, resistance to change, and poor program design [70]. While having a champion in each department may help alleviate some of these obstacles, one should also administer an extensive training program for new sand current staff to ease program implementation [39].

A key point to remember when implementing a program in the prehospital realm is that the initial release of the program will conflict with standard workflows and protocols and may be seen as extra work for field providers. While most EMS providers feel a video link would be a helpful tool during transports, ease of use remains a high priority [17, 60]. To address this component, successful start-up requires input shared between program developers and the target prehospital providers. For instance, many hospitals have dedicated prehospital liaisons managing EMS education and outreach who should be included in start-up. If an organization does not have a specific prehospital liaison, one should identify an individual with the target prehospital agency to participate in start-up and rollout. Ultimately, emergency responders utilizing the program should be able to provide nuanced feedback on implementation and adoption strategies before and after implementation in the field.

Technology Considerations

Prehospital medicine necessitates time and efficiency more than any other aspect along the continuum of care. Regardless of the purpose of a prehospital telemedicine program, the technology needs to be easy to use and quick to deploy and should require minimal troubleshooting during regular use. This is especially true for a new program, where complicated technology and maintenance requirements may alienate EMS providers from participating in the new workflow. For instance, telemedicine equipment chosen for a prehospital program should be rugged, portable, and compact. In one study, the Mayo Clinic consolidated their various telemedicine platforms and saw improvements in provider satisfaction and decreased reported technical issues by 24% [39].

When choosing the components for a prehospital telemedicine platform, existing stationary systems may not easily translate to the ambulance environment. For instance, there may be local or state EMS regulations limiting the type of equipment that can be deployed in an ambulance. This may require consulting with various telemedicine vendors and testing multiple setups in order to arrive at an acceptable mobile telemedicine platform.

Successful prehospital telemedicine necessitates a high fidelity, live stream audiovisual connection that can be maintained during ambulance transport. As the ambulance is traveling, the connection will need to jump from one cellular tower to another. This can result in data loss and a reduction in feed quality (i.e., jitter). Some private companies have developed software solutions that help maintain *session persistence*, which is the seamless transition between data connections. Essential to a successful start-up, extensive testing should be done on the connectivity in an EMS network service area prior to clinical implementation [49, 74]. This testing may require partnership with local cellular and wireless providers to develop a coverage map along EMS routes, particularly in rural areas [48].

A further consideration is the availability of useable cellular infrastructure and bandwidth. While a coverage area may be adequate for everyday civilian use, networks may become saturated during high-density events slowing data transfer (i.e., packet loss). One solution to this problem is a recently developed program called FirstNet designed for first responders and safety personnel such as police, fire, and EMS. FirstNet is an independent authority within National Telecommunications and Information Administration (NTIA) that "will enable robust data communications between all members of the EMS team in the field and in facilities, and the use of sophisticated diagnostic, treatment and remote medical consultation devices for emergency, non-emergency transport, and community paramedicine care" [60]. The FirstNet network currently runs off the existing AT&T network, where it can provide "preemption" or prioritization for designated devices when the network is otherwise saturated. First responder initiatives like FirstNet will further enable the implementation and expansion of prehospital telemedicine programs [60].

Lastly, national programs to expand broadband coverage such as the Federal Communications Commission's 5G FAST Plan and Connected Care Pilot

Program will further accelerate infrastructure development for prehospital telehealth [24, 25].

Start-Up Funding/Ongoing Funding Models

In addition to technological innovation, implementation of prehospital telemedicine programs requires innovation in funding models to support sustainability. Many early pilot programs have relied on grant funding to establish feasibility, particularly in rural areas, such as from the Health Resources and Services Administration (HRSA) and the Federal Communications Commission (FCC). Expensive initiatives like mobile stroke units equipped with CT scanners may be cost prohibitive, particularly for smaller, rural hospitals and EMS agencies in limited-resource health systems [11, 15, 76].

Even with low-cost models and more competition among telemedicine vendors, clinical implementation and further expansion will require legislation and policy amendments to support prehospital telemedicine as a billable service for participating providers and hospitals. Of great import for the expansion of telestroke programs, the Furthering Access to Stroke Telemedicine (FAST) Act adopted by Congress in 2018 expands the definition of the geographical originating site for billable telestroke encounters [1]. Additionally, a recent policy proposal issued by CMS sought public comment on expanding the originating site for telestroke encounters to "mobile stroke units" [15]. In the current schema, reimbursement for prehospital teleconsultation in the ambulance requires that the hub tele-provider must be the emergency physician at the receiving facility in order to bill for the encounter.

Even with the potential lack of reimbursement, several studies have been done to show a cost-benefit of a functioning prehospital telemedicine program either for stroke care or ED diversion [11, 17]. As telemedicine is more widely adopted and implemented broadly, newer billing models should be available with innovation in physician fee schedules. Importantly, this also requires physicians and professional organizations to publish about the evidence base and consensus regarding the impact of prehospital telemedicine on better patient outcomes and resultant cost savings.

Regulations

Regulations that govern interaction between hospital and emergency medical services personnel depend on the context of the interaction, with medical direction being one of the most important aspects to consider in the context of a prehospital telemedicine program. EMS providers attain cognitive and psychomotor knowledge through the completion of education programs that are based off published standards. The two primary frameworks are the National EMS Scope of Practice and the National Registry of Emergency Medical Technicians [59, 61]. Completion of these programs does not denote the capability to operate autonomously but illustrates a baseline knowledge. Instead, certification and licensure occur at a state level with credentialing of providers taking place at a local agency level. Emergency medical service providers practice with the authorization of a physician medical director and cannot operate without this authorization. The operational medical director (OMD) provides direct and indirect oversight of clinical operations. Indirect oversight, or "off-line" medical direction, is conducted through a detailed set of standardized protocols, which the physician develops, reviews, and publishes in conjunction with agency leadership. On occasion, an EMS provider will need to perform a procedure or administer a medication that falls outside of those agency protocols. On those occasions, the provider will call either the OMD or a surrogate, usually another emergency physician, and get "online" medical direction.

Per federal law, in order for an EMS provider to administer any class of controlled substance in the course of their clinical care outside the physical presence of a medical director, a standing order must be issued that is adopted by one or more medical directors of that particular agency [34]. In the current paradigm of emergency medical services within the United States, physician medical directors are generally, but not exclusively, emergency physicians that have experience in the prehospital environment. Requirements vary from state to state, with most requiring the physician to be Board eligible or certified in emergency medicine or else be actively involved in the provision of emergency care of patients and the completion of an EMS medical direction course [62, 63, 85]. Both the American College of Emergency Physicians (ACEP) and the National Association of EMS Physicians (NAEMSP) have published position papers denoting the importance of physician medical direction [3, 58].

As the role of both telemedicine and prehospital medicine expands, providers from specialties other than emergency medicine will be in positions to offer medical direction to prehospital personnel. Thus it is worth mentioning that EMS personnel are not restricted to only receiving medical direction from their agency's operational medical director. Since it is necessary for prehospital providers to have the ability to contact medical direction for consultation or orders outside standard protocols at all times, most agencies have specific base stations that have been selected by that agency's medical director as an approved source of online medical direction. A base station is defined as a hospital emergency department or healthcare facility that is designated to provide EMS personnel with direct medical oversight [19]. These base stations can be contacted by EMS personnel for direct medical oversight as a surrogate for the agency's operational medical director. The use of any one receiving facility as a base station is variable at the local level. Some agencies will use one central facility as a base station for all online medical direction, while others will designate all receiving facilities as base stations.

Providing medical direction may create a liability exposure for medical directors or their surrogates, but there is little case law on the subject. Possible avenues of liability could come from instructing EMS providers to operate outside their scope of practice, beyond their level of training or deviating from the standard of care [31].

There are a variety of relevant laws and state statutes that provide a degree of immunity to both EMS providers and medical direction physicians, often with the caveat being willful or wanton misconduct [21]. California state code 1799.104 reads that "(a) No physician or nurse, who in good faith gives emergency instructions to an EMT-II or mobile intensive care paramedic at the scene of an emergency, shall be liable for any civil damages as a result of issuing the instructions. (b) No EMT-II or mobile intensive care paramedic rendering care within the scope of his duties who, in good faith and in a non-negligent manner, follows the instructions of a physician or nurse shall be liable for any civil damages as a result of following such instructions" [13, 21]. Additionally, most states have "Good Samaritan" laws that offer a degree of protection to those offering emergency medical assistance [50].

As specialties outside of emergency medicine begin to have more interaction with field providers via telemedicine, it is imperative that individuals providing medical direction are aware of the specific capabilities and limitations of those they are working with. Developing a relationship with the receiving emergency department and individual agency operational medical directors can facilitate safe and effective medical direction. Establishing good relations with your area EMS agencies is a key to making sure all parties know their role in caring for patients in emergency situations.

Beyond medical direction, different state regulations may exist that can limit the scope of a prospective prehospital telemedicine program because prehospital medicine is evolving faster than regulations can keep up with. Community paramedicine provides a clear illustration of this problem, where language in statutes may prevent expanding prehospital provider's scope of practice or function. The result has been a discordance in legal regulations, program aims, and even officials' understanding of the regulations themselves. A 2018 review of state regulations on community paramedicine and survey of emergency medical services officials in each state found a disparity between regulation and survey answers. Of their predefined survey of community paramedicine skills, the concordance of survey responses between EMS providers and regulation ranges from 13% to 96% depending on the skill [28]. This disparity highlights a mixture of factors ranging from inadequate knowledge of state regulation among EMS providers and the simple fact that regulation has not yet caught up to this rapidly expanding subfield.

These issues will likely fade with time as prehospital medicine becomes a more established paradigm, but until then careful consideration of applicable laws and regulations is prudent.

Mount Sinai Visiting Doctors Case Study (Expanded Role of EMS Providers to Augment System Resources with Telemedicine)

Many states have strict definitions of what an EMS provider's scope of practice is and whether it may be expanded, with some states limiting the care that EMS is able to provide to only acute and emergency care. New York is one such state [39]. Nevertheless, there are still ways to make expanded use of EMS even where conventional community paramedicine programs would not be feasible. The Mount Sinai Visiting Doctors program in New York City did so by integrating non-911

EMS units into their workflow by providing a 16-hour training course to paramedics and additional training on medical direction to primary care physicians in the program [16].

When a patient calls in requesting assessment, the on-call physician may opt to send a non-911 ambulance to the patient's home to facilitate a remote assessment and treatment. Upon arrival at the patient's home, the EMS providers perform a patient assessment with a real-time telemedicine link to the MSVD physician, and because the paramedic's scope of practice is not changed, regulatory challenges were avoided. After the assessment the patient and healthcare providers make a shared decision about appropriate disposition. The program has shown early success with high patient and provider satisfaction and a reduction in patients being sent to the emergency department.

Conclusion

As the clinical paradigm for emergency care evolves in parallel with a vast expanse in access to mobile health technology, we will continue to see a growth in applications of prehospital telemedicine in a wide range of clinical fields such as stroke, neonatal care, and trauma among others. The future success of these novel telemedicine programs requires thoughtful integration with emergency medical systems and a nuanced understanding of available mobile technology, broadband infrastructure, and pertinent protocols and regulations. Ultimately, the sustainability and growth of prehospital telemedicine will depend on innovation in funding models that support reimbursement for ambulance-based encounters that will incentivize hospitals and providers to expand new programs. Hopefully, prehospital telemedicine will continue to grow as another method of delivering resources and expertise beyond the walls of the hospital, to patients all along the continuum of care.

References

1. 114th United States Congress. Fixing America's Surface Transportation Act, An Act to authorize funds for Federal-aid highways, highway safety programs, and transit programs, and for other purposes Pub.L. 2015:114–94.
2. Altman L. Johnson gets digitalis after second heart attack to pump enough blood. New York Times. 1972:20.
3. American College of Emergency Physicians. The role of the Physician Medical Director in emergency medical services leadership. Ann Emerg Med. 2018;71:e39–40.
4. Barrett KM, Pizzi MA, Kesari V, TerKonda SP, Mauricio EA, Silvers SM, Habash R, Brown BL, Tawk RG, Meschia JF, Wharen R, Freeman WD. Ambulance-based assessment of NIH stroke scale with telemedicine: a feasibility pilot study. J Telemed Telecare. 2017;23:476–83. https://doi.org/10.1177/1357633X16648490.
5. Belt GH, Felberg RA, Rubin J, Halperin JJ. In-transit telemedicine speeds ischemic stroke treatment: preliminary results. Stroke. 2016;47:2413–5.

6. Berger E. Physician burnout. Ann Emerg Med. 2013;61:A17–9. https://doi.org/10.1016/j.annemergmed.2013.01.001.
7. Bergrath S, Reich A, Rossaint R, Rörtgen D, Gerber J, Fischermann H, Beckers SK, Brokmann JC, Schulz JB, Leber C, Fitzner C, Skorning M. Feasibility of prehospital teleconsultation in acute stroke – a pilot study in clinical routine. 2012;7:1–9.
8. Beume L, Hieber M, Kaller CP, Nitschke K, Bardutzky J, Urbach H, Weiller C, Rijntjes M. Large vessel occlusion in acute stroke cortical symptoms are more sensitive prehospital indicators than motor deficits. Stroke. 2018;49:2323–9.
9. Bijen N, Sidney S, Liebeskind DS, Bruce O, Doojin K, Nerses S, Latisha A, Brian B, Pablo V, Fernando V, Gary D, Reza J, Saver JL. A brief prehospital stroke severity scale identifies ischemic stroke patients harboring persisting large arterial occlusions. Stroke. 2008;39:2264–7. https://doi.org/10.1161/STROKEAHA.107.508127.
10. Bowry R, Parker S, Wu T, Noser E, Jackson K, Rajan SS, Yamal J, Persse D, Richardson L, Grotta JC. Benefits of stroke treatment using a Mobile stroke unit compared with standard management the BEST-MSU study run-in phase. Stroke. 2015;46:3370–4.
11. Brandler E, Gropen TI, Janjua N, Levine SR, Poleshuck R, Spencer J, Gokaldas R, Szarek M, Brandler ES. Factors related to the sensitivity of emergency medical service impression of stroke. Prehosp Emerg Care. 2014;18:387–92.
12. Bukata R. Are Mobile CT Stroke Units Worth the Price Tag?. Emergency Physician's Monthly: 10/31/2018. 2017.
13. California Health and Safety Code. DIVISION 2.5. EMERGENCY MEDICAL SERVICES [1797–1799.207] (Division 2.5 added by Stats. 1980, Ch. 1260.) CHAPTER 9. Liability Limitation [1799.100–1799.112]. 1980.
14. California Telehealth Resource Center. The CTRC Telehealth Program Developer Kit, A Roadmap for Successful Telehealth Program Development. 2014.
15. Centers for Medicare and Medicaid Services. Medicare Physician Fee Schedule CY 2019 CMS-1693-P. 2019.
16. Chellappa DK, DeCherrie LV, Escobar C, Gregoriou D, Munjal KG. Supporting the on-call primary care physician with community paramedicine. Intern Med J. 2018;48:1261–4.
17. Clark W, Chiota-McCollum NA, Cote J, Schneider BJ, Pitchford H, Gunnell BS, Lindbeck GM, Perina DG, O'Connor Robert E, Chapman Smith S, Solenski NJ, Worrall BB, Southerland AM. Abstract TP246: Emergency Medical Services Survey of a Low-cost, Ambulance-based System for Mobile Neurological Assessment: The iTREAT Study. Stroke. 2016;48:ATP246. https://doi.org/10.1161/str.48.suppl_1.tp246.
18. Cone D, Brown LH, Greenberg B, Richards ME, Hubble MW, Cone DC, Millin MG, Schwartz B, Patterson PD. Paramedic determinations of medical necessity: a meta-analysis. Prehosp Emerg Care. 2009;13:516–27.
19. Cone DC, Brice JH, Delbridge TR, Myers JB, Ebook Central – Academic Complete, Wiley Online Library UBCM All Obooks. Medical oversight of EMS systems in: Anonymous emergency medical services: clinical practice and systems oversight. 2nd ed. Chichester/Hoboken: Wiley; 2015 Bass RR, Lawner B, Lee D, Nable JV. Medical oversight of EMS systems. In: Cone DC, Brice JH, Delbridge TR, Myers JB, editors. Emergency medical services: clinical practice and systems oversight; (2015). https://doi.org/10.1002/9781118990810.ch82.
20. Crampton RS, Aldrich RF, Gascho JA, Miles JR Jr, Stillerman R. Reduction of prehospital, ambulance and community coronary death rates by the community-wide emergency cardiac care system. Am J Med. 1975;58:151–65. https://doi.org/10.1016/0002-9343(75)90564-1.
21. Delaware Code TITLE 16 Health and Safety CHAPTER 68. EXEMPTIONS FROM CIVIL LIABILITY Subchapter I. Immunity for Rendering Emergency Care § 6801 Persons rendering emergency care exempt from liability.
22. Donnan G, Bastianello S, Buchan A, Bladin C, D'este C, Attia J, Davis S, Parsons M, Hankey G, Vanhooren G, LEYS D, Kaste M, Lees KR, Bluhmki E, Von Kummer R, Brott TG, Toni D, Grotta JC, Albers GW, Hamilton SA, Marler JR, Tilley BC, Davis SM, Donnan GA, Hacke W. Time to treatment with intravenous alteplase and outcome in stroke: an updated pooled analysis of ECASS, ATLANTIS, NINDS, and EPITHET trials. Lancet. 2010;375:1695–703.

23. Espinoza AV, Van Hooff R, De Smedt A, Moens M, Yperzeele L, Nieboer K, Hubloue I, De Keyser J, Convents A, Tellez HF, Dupont A, Putman K, Brouns R. Development and pilot testing of 24/7 in-ambulance telemedicine for acute stroke: prehospital stroke study at the Universitair Ziekenhuis Brussel-project. Cerebrovasc Dis. 2016;42:15–22.
24. Federal Communications Commission. Carr Announces $100 million 'Connected Care Pilot Program'. 2018.
25. Federal Communications Commission. The FCC's 5G FAST Plan. 2018. https://www.fcc.gov/document/fccs-5g-fast-plan. Accessed 1 Nov 2018.
26. Fiebach JB, Grittner U, Ebinger M, Winter B, Wendt M, Weber JE, Waldschmidt C, Rozanski M, Kunz A, Koch P, Endres M, Audebert HJ, Gierhake D, Villringer K, Kellner PA, Hartmann A, Mackert B. Effect of the use of ambulance-based thrombolysis on time to thrombolysis in acute ischemic stroke a randomized clinical trial. JAMA. 2014;311:1622–31.
27. Gaston SR. Accidental death and disability: the neglected disease of modern society. A progress report. J Trauma Acute Care Surg. 1971;11:195–206.
28. Glenn M, Zoph O, Jenkins K, Fisher J, Weidenaar K, Barraza L, Greco W, Paode P. State regulation of community paramedicine programs: a national analysis. Prehosp Emerg Care. 2018;22:244–51.
29. Gonzalez M, Alqusairi D, Jackson A, Champagne T, Langabeer J II, Persse D. Houston EMS advances mobile integrated healthcare through the ETHAN program. JEMS. 2015;40:11. Accessed 6 Feb 2019.
30. National Association of Emergency Medical Technicians. Second mobile integrated healthcare and community paramedicine national survey report. 2018;13
31. Hindmand R, Maggiore AW. Medical control of emergency medical services. J Health Life Sci Am Health Lawyers Assoc. 2011;4:65–94.
32. Holland C. Reality Plus Drama Equals "EMERGENCY!". Smithsonian Institute's The National Museum of American History. 2015. http://americanhistory.si.edu/blog/reality-plus-drama-equals-emergency. Accessed 08/2018.
33. Howard J, Jensen AM, Ence T, Contreras L, Dunford J. 326 Mobile integrated telehealth: a feasibility study with community paramedicine providers and frequent 911 users. Ann Emerg Med. 2017;70:S129.
34. Hudson R (2017) H.R.304 – Protecting Patient Access to Emergency Medications Act of 2017.
35. Itrat A, Taqui A, Cerejo R, Briggs F, Cho S, Organek N, Reimer AP, Winners S, Rasmussen P, Hussain MS, Uchino K, Tre CPAS. Telemedicine in prehospital stroke evaluation and thrombolysis taking stroke treatment to the doorstep. 2016;73:162–8.
36. McCloskey KA, King WD, Byron L. Pediatric critical care transport: is a physician always needed on the team? Ann Emerg Med. 1989;18:247–9.
37. Katz BS, McMullan JT, Sucharew H, Adeoye O, Broderick JP. Design and validation of a prehospital scale to predict stroke severity Cincinnati prehospital stroke severity scale. Stroke. 2015;46:1508–12.
38. Kawaguchi A, Nielsen CC, Saunders LD, Yasui Y, De Caen A. Outcomes/predictions: impact of physician-less pediatric critical care transport: making a decision on team composition. J Crit Care. 2018;45:209–14.
39. Kreofsky BLH, Blegen RN, Lokken TG, Kapraun SM, Bushman MS, Demaerschalk BM. Sustainable telemedicine: designing and building infrastructure to support a comprehensive telemedicine practice. Telemed J E Health. 2018. https://doi.org/10.1089/tmj.2017.0291.
40. Kunz A, Ebinger M, Geisler F, Rozanski M, Waldschmidt C, Weber JE, Wendt M, Winter B, Zieschang K, Fiebach JB, Villringer K, Erdur H, Scheitz JF, Tütüncü S, Bollweg K, Grittner U, Kaczmarek S, Endres M, Nolte CH, Audebert HJ. Functional outcomes of pre-hospital thrombolysis in a mobile stroke treatment unit compared with conventional care: an observational registry study. 2016;15:1035–43.
41. LaMonte MP, Cullen J, Gagliano DM, Gunawardane R, Hu P, Mackenzie C, Xiao Y. TeleBAT: mobile telemedicine for the Brain Attack Team. J Stroke Cerebrovasc Dis. 2000;9:128–35.
42. LaMonte MP, Xiao Y, Hu PF, Gagliano DM, Bahouth MN, Gunawardane RD, MacKenzie CF, Gaasch WR, Cullen J. Shortening time to stroke treatment using ambulance telemedicine: TeleBAT. J Stroke Cerebrovasc Dis. 2004;13:148–54.

43. Langabeer I, James R, DelliFraine J, Fowler R, Jollis JG, Stuart L, Segrest W, Griffin R, Koenig W, Moyer P, Henry TD. Selected topics: prehospital care: emergency medical services as a strategy for improving ST-elevation myocardial infarction system treatment times. J Emerg Med. 2014;46:355–62.
44. Langabeer JR 2nd, Gonzalez M, Alqusairi D, Champagne-Langabeer T, Jackson A, Mikhail J, Persse D. Telehealth-enabled emergency medical services program reduces ambulance transport to urban emergency departments. West J Emerg Med. 2016;17:713–20. https://doi.org/10.5811/westjem.2016.8.30660.
45. Lewis B. Hendricks regional launches telestroke program. Inside Indiana Business Online Video Article. 2017.
46. Lima FO, Silva GS, Furie KL, Frankel MR, Lev MH, Camargo ECS, Haussen DC, Singhal AB, Koroshetz WJ, Smith WS, Nogueira RG. Field assessment stroke triage for emergency destination a simple and accurate prehospital scale to detect large vessel occlusion strokes. Stroke. 2016;47:1997–2002.
47. Liman TG, Winter B, Waldschmidt C, Zerbe N, Hufnagl P, Audebert HJ, Endres M. Telestroke ambulances in prehospital stroke management concept and pilot feasibility study. Stroke. 2012;43:2086–90.
48. Lippman JM, Cote J, Solenski NJ, Worrall BB, Southerland AM, Smith SNC, McMurry TL, Sutton ZG, Gunnell BS, Cattell-Gordon DC, Rheuban KS, Perina DG. Mobile Telestroke During Ambulance Transport Is Feasible in a Rural EMS Setting: The iTREAT Study. 2016;22:507–13.
49. Madiraju SK, Genuit T, Catino J, Kokaram C, Bukur M. In by helicopter out by cab: the financial cost of aeromedical Overtriage of trauma patients. J Surg Res. 2017;218:261–70.
50. Mallery S. Beyond Seinfeld's Good Samaritan Debacle: Protecting Citizens Who Render Care at the Scene of an Accident From Civil Liability. 2010;41:647–54.
51. Maurer D. Yesteryears: part 1: Lyndon Johnson's 1972 visit to Charlottesville brought unexpected drama. The Daily Progress. 2014.
52. McNamara MJ, Oser C, Gohdes D, Fogle CC, Dietrich DW, Burnett A, Okon N, Russell JA, DeTienne J, Harwell TS, Helgerson SD. Stroke knowledge among urban and frontier first responders and emergency medical technicians in Montana. 2008;24:189–93.
53. Meadows-Pitt M, Fields W. Research: the impact of prehospital 12-Lead electrocardiograms on door-to-balloon time in patients with ST-elevation myocardial infarction. J Emerg Nurs. 2014;40:e63–8.
54. Moore C, Weaver MD. Medical necessity in emergency medical services transports. Am J Med Qual. 2012;27:250–5.
55. Mort A, Eadie L, Regan L, Macaden A, Heaney D, Bouamrane M, Rushworth G, Wilson P. Combining transcranial ultrasound with intelligent communication methods to enhance the remote assessment and management of stroke patients: framework for a technology demonstrator. Health Informatics J. 2016;22:691–701. https://doi.org/10.1177/1460458215580353.
56. Munjal KG, Shastry S, Loo GT, Reid D, Grudzen C, Shah MN, Chapin HH, First B, Sirirungruang S, Alpert E, Chason K, Richardson LD. Patient perspectives on EMS alternate destination models. Prehosp Emerg Care. 2016;20:705–11. https://doi.org/10.1080/10903127.2016.1182604.
57. National Association of EMS Physicians/American College of Emergency Physicians. Position paper: National Association of EMS physicians: alternate ambulance transportation and destination. National Association of EMS Physicians/American College of Emergency Physicians Joint Position Paper. 2001;5:289–289.
58. National Association of EMS Physicians/National Registry of Emergency Medical Technicians. Clinical Credentialing of EMS Providers. Prehosp Emerg Care. 2017;21:397–8.
59. National Highway Traffic Safety Administration. DOT HS 810 657 National EMS Scope of Practice Model. p. 31. 2007.
60. National Public Safety Telecommunications Council National Association of State Emergency Medical Services Officials Emergency Medical Services Communications Working Group. EMS telemedicine report prehospital use of video technologies final report. 2016.
61. National Registry of Emergency Medical Technicians The NREMT Certification Eligibility, Discipline and Appeals Policy. 2018

62. Ohio Administrative Code. 4765-3-05 Medical director requirements for each emergency medical services organization. 2014.
63. Pennsylvania Code § 1023.1. EMS agency medical director.
64. Pérez de la Ossa N, Carrera D, Gorchs M, Querol M, Millán M, Gomis M, Dorado L, López-Cancio E, Hernández-Pérez M, Chicharro V, Escalada X, Jiménez X, Dávalos A. Design and validation of a prehospital stroke scale to predict large arterial occlusion: the rapid arterial occlusion evaluation scale. STROKE. 2014;45:87–91.
65. Rudd M, Buck D, Ford G, Price C. A systematic review of stroke recognition instruments in hospital and prehospital settings. Emerg Med J. 2016;33:818.
66. Ryb GE, Cooper C, Waak SM. Delayed trauma team activation: patient characteristics and outcomes. J Trauma Acute Care Surg. 2012;73:695–8.
67. Saver J, Schwamm L, Hernandez AF, Smith E, Lin CB, Peterson ED, Liang L, Xian Y, Olson DM, Shah BR, Smith EE, Saver JL, Schwamm LH, Fonarow GC. Emergency medical service hospital prenotification is associated with improved evaluation and treatment of acute ischemic stroke. Circ Cardiovasc Qual Outcomes. 2012;5:514–22.
68. Sawyer NT, Coburn JD. Community paramedicine: 911 alternative destinations are a patient safety issue. West J Emerg Med. 2017;18:219–21.
69. Schwamm LH, Holloway RG, Amarenco P, Audebert HJ, Bakas T, Chumbler NR, Handschu R, Jauch EC, Knight WA IV, Levine SR, Mayberg M, Meyer BC, Meyers PM, Skalabrin E, Wechsler LR, Council AHAS, Peripher IC. A review of the evidence for the use of telemedicine within stroke systems of care a scientific statement from the American Heart Association/American Stroke Association. Stroke. 2009;40:2616–34.
70. Scott Kruse C, Karem P, Shifflett K, Vegi L, Ravi K, Brooks M. Evaluating barriers to adopting telemedicine worldwide: a systematic review. J Telemed Telecare. 2018;24:4–12. https://doi.org/10.1177/1357633X16674087.
71. Sequeira D, Martin-Gill C, Guyette FX, Kesinger MR, Thompson LR, Jovin TG, Massaro LM. Characterizing strokes and stroke mimics transported by helicopter emergency medical services. Prehosp Emerg Care. 2016;20:723–8.
72. Singh JM, MacDonald RD, Ahghari M. Emergency medical services/original research: critical events during land-based interfacility transport. Ann Emerg Med. 2014;64:9–15.
73. Shelton SL, Swor RA, Domeier RM, Lucas R. Position paper. Medical direction of interfacility transports. Prehosp Emerg Care. 2000;4:361–4.
74. Smith SNC, Brown PC, Waits KH, Wong JS, Bhatti MS, Toqeer Q, Ricks JV, Stockner ML, Habtamu T, Seelam J, Britt RC, Giovia JM, Blankson BK, Bennam P, Gormley MA, Lu J, Ornato JP. Development and evaluation of a user-centered mobile telestroke platform. Telemed J E Health. 2018; https://doi.org/10.1089/tmj.2018.0044.
75. Smith SNC, Padrick MM, Lippman JM, Mehndiratta P, Chee CY, Solenski NJ, Worrall BB, Southerland AM, McMurry TL, Perina DG, Gunnell BS, Cattell-Gordon DC, Govindarajan P, Resler BL, Keenan K, Cahill EA, Dietiker C, Smith WS. A low-cost, tablet-based option for prehospital neurologic assessment: The iTREAT Study. Neurology. 2016;87:19–26.
76. Southerland AM, Brandler ES. The cost-efficiency of mobile stroke units where the rubber meets the road. Neurology. 2017;88:1300–1.
77. State of Virginia 12VAC5-31-590. Operational Medical Director Requirement.
78. Stroud M, Moss M. Tele-transport: combining mobile patient assessment with critical care outside tertiary care centers. Pediatrics. 2017;140:1.. (abstract).
79. Swickard S, Winkelman C, Hustey FM, Kerr M, Reimer AP. Original research: patient safety events during critical care transport. Air Med J. 2018;37:253–8.
80. Teleb MS, Hage AV, Carter J, Jayaraman MV, McTaggart RA. Stroke vision, aphasia, neglect (van) assessment – a novel emergent large vessel occlusion screening tool: pilot study and comparison with current clinical severity indices. 2017;9:122–6.
81. Thomas SH, Blumen I. Review: helicopter emergency medical services literature 2014 to 2016: lessons and perspectives, Part 2—nontrauma transports and general issues. Air Med J. 2018;37:126–30.

82. Uhley HN. Electrocardiographic telemetry from ambulances. A practical approach to Mobile coronary care units. Am Heart J. 1970;80:838–42.
83. United States Department of Transportation, National Highway Traffic Safety Administration. 2011 EMS System Demographics, The 2011 National EMS Assessment DOT HS. 2014;811:723.
84. University of California Los Angeles, Center for Prehospital Care What's the Difference Between an EMT and a Paramedic? https://www.cpc.mednet.ucla.edu/node/27. Accessed 09/08=1 2018.
85. Virginia Administrative Code. 12VAC5-31-1810. Qualifications for EMS Physician Endorsement. 2012;29(01).
86. Virginia Department of Health. Virginia Certification Program Outlines. 2018. http://www.vdh.virginia.gov/emergency-medical-services/virginia-certification-program-outlines/. Accessed 09/01 2018.
87. Walter S, Kostpopoulos P, Haass A, Helwig S, Keller I, Licina T, Schlechtriemen T, Roth C, Papanagiotou P, Zimmer A, Vierra J, Körner H, Schmidt K, Romann M, Alexandrou M, Yilmaz U, Grunwald I, Kubulus D, Lesmeister M, Ziegeler S. Bringing the hospital to the patient: first treatment of stroke patients at the emergency site. PLOS One. 2010;5:1–5.
88. Ward NS, Afessa B, Kleinpell R, Tisherman S, Ries M, Howell M, Halpern N, Kahn J, Members of Society of Critical Care Medicine Taskforce on ICU Staffing. Intensivist/patient ratios in closed ICUs: a statement from the Society of Critical Care Medicine Taskforce on ICU Staffing. Crit Care Med. 2013;41:638–45. https://doi.org/10.1097/CCM.0b013e3182741478.
89. White R, Wingrove G. Principles for Community Paramedicine Programs: a joint position statement of the National Association of EMS Physicians and the National Rural Health Association. p. 4. 2012.
90. Wu T, Nguyen C, Ankrom C, Yang J, Persse D, Vahidy F, Grotta JC, Savitz SI. Prehospital utility of rapid stroke evaluation using in-ambulance telemedicine: a pilot feasibility study. Stroke. 2014;45:2342–7. https://doi.org/10.1161/STROKEAHA.114.005193.
91. Wu T, Parker SA, Jagolino A, Yamal J, Bowry R, Thomas A, Yu A, Grotta JC. Telemedicine can replace the neurologist on a Mobile stroke unit. Stroke. 2017;48:493–6.
92. Yokley R, Sutherland R. Radio equipment. In: Anonymous emergency!: Behind the Scene, Jones & Bartlett Learning. 2007. p. 116–118.
93. Yperzeele L, Van Hooff R, De Smedt A, Valenzuela Espinoza A, Van Dyck R, Van de Casseye R, Convents A, Hubloue I, Lauwaert D, De Keyser J, Brouns R. Feasibility of AmbulanCe-Based Telemedicine (FACT) Study: safety, Feasibility and Reliability of Third Generation in-Ambulance Telemedicine. PLOS One. 2014;9:1–9.
94. Pitchford HM. Early BioPhone, Charlottesville BioPhone found among a collection of other historical items contained at the Charlottesville Albemarle Rescue Squad. 2018.

Chapter 17
Telemedicine Consultation to the General ICU

Mark Romig, Robert Derrett III, Asad Latif, and Adam Sapirstein

Introduction

When the concepts and technology of telemedicine are applied to the aspects of remote care in the ICU, it is called tele-ICU. The idea of using telemedicine to improve the care of critically ill patients was clearly stated as early as 1982 [1]. Arguably, the first major tele-ICU intervention to use modern technology, research design, and demonstrate effectiveness did not take place until 1997 [2]. The results of this study, conducted at a community hospital affiliate of Johns Hopkins, were published by Rosenfeld and colleagues in 2000 and showed reductions in mortality and costs of care [2]. It is clear even in this earliest telemedicine work that tele-ICU care is largely consultative. By using the word consultative, we mean that the tele-ICU is supportive of the work that is performed in the physical ICU. This contrasts with active management of critically ill patients. Indeed, one of the rationales of creating tele-ICU systems is to provide consultative intensivist staffing to under-staffed ICUs. It is the nature of critical care that active management requires

M. Romig (✉) · A. Latif · A. Sapirstein
Johns Hopkins University School of Medicine, Department of Anesthesiology and Critical Care Medicine, Johns Hopkins Medicine, Armstrong Institute for Quality and Patient Safety, Baltimore, MD, USA
e-mail: mromig1@jhmi.edu

R. Derrett III
University of Minnesota, Minneapolis, MN, USA

M. A. Koenig (ed.), *Telemedicine in the ICU*,
https://doi.org/10.1007/978-3-030-11569-2_17

frequent and high-intensity physical interactions. These interactions require the on-site presence of highly trained and experienced nurses and other medical professionals who have the skills and judgment to perform physical exams and procedures. It is possible for tele-ICU clinicians to perform some elements of active management such as documentation, provider safety double checks, family meetings, and order entry. However, the vast majority of activities are consultative in that they require the tele-ICU clinicians to communicate with the ICU team to provide or alter care.

As indicated above, the idea of a tele-ICU consultation is somewhat amorphous and can be a place holder for a large variety of interactions. It is also true that tele-ICU systems are not uniquely defined. However, it is clear that the best functioning of tele-ICU systems manage technology, processes of care, and culture in an established and engineered framework (see, e.g., [3, 4]). It is also clear that in order to provide any sort of telemedicine consultations to critically ill patients, a mature and reliable system must be established. In the current era of telemedicine, it seems unlikely that such a system will be used exclusively for critical care consultations.

There are numerous telemedicine models and almost any of them could be applied to tele-ICU consultation. The gold standard for tele-ICU care is a dedicated in-room audiovisual system with continuous, around-the-clock coverage staffed by physicians and nurses. In contrast, because many highly staffed ICUs have physicians on-site during working hours, they choose to provide tele-ICU services during just the nighttime hours. In these models, the tele-ICU team is dedicated exclusively to the care of ICU patients. Robotic or mobile audiovisual carts are used to provide telemedicine service in units (or locations) where fixed camera installations are impractical or too costly (Fig. 17.1). These mobile solutions are well established as working models for telemedicine consultations [5, 6]. Finally, with the nearly universal deployment of electronic medical records (EMRs), it is possible for a remote intensivist to conduct telephone consultations with on-site providers. This telephone model is not even as robust as the long-standing model of the on-call intensivist, and we will not consider it further in our discussions. We will assume that any meaningful, real-time consultation of critically ill patients will include both audio and visual channels of communication.

The value a tele-ICU system brings to hospital operations is highly dependent on the anticipated use cases for the implementation. Intensivist staffing has been associated with lower general ICU patient mortality [7]. Based on these and other data, it was suggested that tele-ICU should be a standard, when needed, to bolster ICU staffing and improve clinical outcomes [8]. When tele-ICU was implemented for a 16-week period in a surgical ICU, the mortality rate, complication rate, length of stay, and ICU costs all improved [2]. This ICU was considered to be staffed at a low-intensity, as there were no on-site intensivists, and it is unclear if adding tele-ICU to an ICU that is already highly staffed would result in the same reduction in complications. The case for consultative critical care has not been teased out of the complex models that currently exist for tele-ICU.

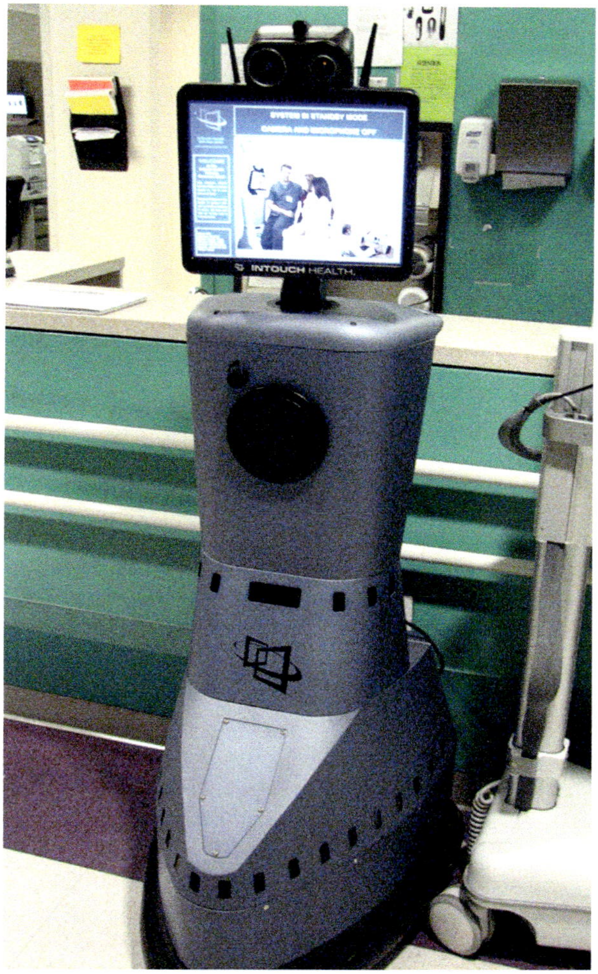

Fig. 17.1 RP-7 Robot (InTouch HealthSanta Barbara, CA). Self-propelled robot with bidirectional audiovisual communication is one method of engaging with patients in tele-ICUs

How Can Telemedicine Facilitate Consultation to Improve Patient Care?

Triage Decisions

Triage decisions can be facilitated and improved using telemedicine when highly specialized care is required. Examples of this exist in neonatology [9], pediatric ICU [10, 11], burn care [12, 13] (where 84% reported using some form of telemedicine usually to improve burn care or triage decisions), and neurology [14]. The body of evidence for using telemedicine in consultation for stroke diagnosis and therapy is the most robust [15].

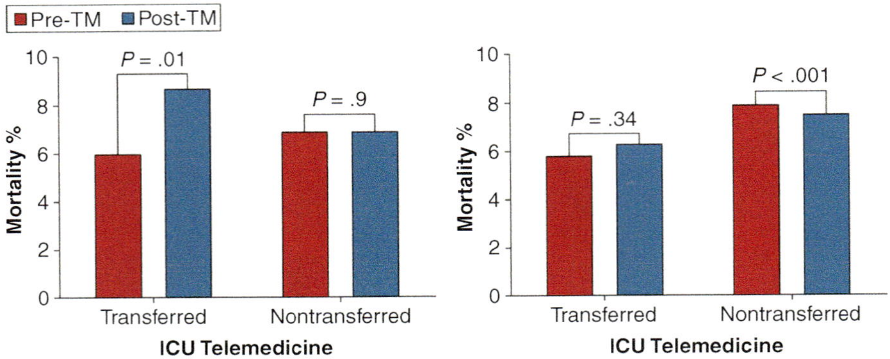

Fig. 17.2 Thirty-day unadjusted mortality in transferred and non-transferred patients in the TM ICU and non-TM ICUs. The comparison between pre-TM and post-TM periods was performed using $\chi 2$ analysis. TM telemedicine. (Reprinted with permission from Fortis et al. [16]. Copyright 2018 by the Elsevier Inc.)

Unnecessary inter-hospital transfers waste healthcare resources, jeopardize patient safety, and may be burdensome to families. Telemedicine deployed across a hospital system or geographic region may give referral centers a means to evaluate patients prior to transfer. Of these patients, a subset may be identified which do not require intensivist care, and thus transfer. Likewise, telemedicine can bring intensivist expertise to the bedside and thus obviate the need for transfer. The Veterans Administration deployed a telemedicine system to provide remote access to patients in 52 small, community, regional ICUs [16]. Over a 4 year period, 97,256 were admitted to these ICUs, and they experienced a reduction in the rate of transfers to their tertiary care center from 3.46% to 1.99% [17]. This reduction was not associated with an increased risk of mortality (Fig. 17.2).

Specialist Consultation

Telemedicine has also been considered as a tool to improve access to subspecialty care in the ICU. Remote neurology consultation and tele-stroke care is a well-established practice to improve the delivery of time-sensitive therapies associated with improved stroke outcomes [15]. This topic is covered in depth in Chap. 12. Infectious disease specialty consultation is common in the ICU, and telemedicine may have a role in improving the access to infectious disease consultation particularly in low-resource environments [18]. The Infectious Disease Society of America supports the use of telemedicine to improve access to infectious disease providers; however there has been no research specifically examining the impact of infectious disease teleconsultation on ICU outcomes [19].

The consultative model of telemedicine is well established at Johns Hopkins through the efforts of Johns Hopkins Medicine International (JHI). JHI focuses on the global expansion of Johns Hopkins Medicine to support care and improvement globally. Using this platform, we have been able to provide specialist consultations to external critical care units across a wide array of disciplines. Typically, a patient has an unexplained clinical condition or is not responding to therapy and is located at an outside ICU that has a relationship with a telemedicine center. In these situations, the background case information is usually transmitted asynchronously to an expert intensivist, surgeon, or medical specialist. This allows the specialist consultant at Johns Hopkins to review the patient's history in detail prior to the actual teleconsultation. With this preparation, the consultant conducts a consultative meeting with the remote team. Traditionally, this sort of consultation was performed over the phone. However, with improved technology, shared medical records platforms, and healthcare systems integration, these consultations can now be performed with synchronous, real-time review of patient data including lab data, radiographic images, and video linkage of physical exams (Fig. 17.3). There is no doubt that this kind of interaction provides a deeper shared understanding of the patient and helps the consultant and ICU team to develop a care plan. While exact data for the Johns Hopkins International experience is not yet published, a survey of activities shows that the majority of consultations are conducted in oncology and a significant fraction take place for neurosurgical or neurological diagnoses (personal communica-

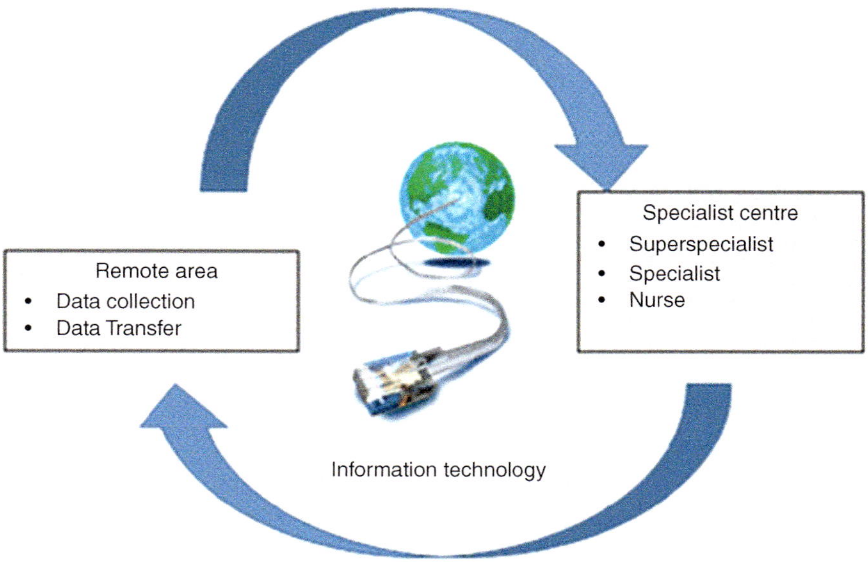

Fig. 17.3 Basic concept of telemedicine: transmitting and receiving data in a healthcare environment. (Reprinted with permission from Hao et al. [45]. Copyright 2014 by the Springer International Publishing.)

tions RD). Other specialty consultations by the Johns Hopkins program include allergy and immunology, endocrinology, dermatology, cardiology, infectious disease, gastroenterology, nephrology, rheumatology, psychiatry, and pulmonology. All of the surgical subspecialties have been able to use this platform to provide consultative care. While JHI consultations are provided on an ad hoc basis, it is important to note the emerging trend of establishing tele-ICU centers that are geographically time shifted from the target ICUs. This allows the tele-ICUs to monitor the remote ICUs at night while it is daytime locally [20].

Bedside psychiatric evaluation of the critically ill patient is challenging. Patients often experience cognitive and behavioral symptoms due to their disease process, such as delirium or traumatic brain injury. Likewise, sedation and analgesic medication regimens can limit the effectiveness of a psychiatric evaluation. These issues are unlikely to be any less of confounders when telemedicine is introduced. The value of telepsychiatry itself remains in question, and the advent of new mobile mental health applications is further challenging this approach [21]. In our opinion, it is unclear whether the telepsychiatry model can or should be translated to the patient in the ICU setting.

Tele-ICU nursing is not generally considered a consultative service because the most common application of a tele-ICU system is to add an additional level of monitoring for all patients within the ICU. Nurses are essential telemedicine staff in this model and clearly function as specialists in the intricacies of critical care nursing. In such a setting, tele-ICU nurses may also provide the most important role in consultative care. These nurses continuously perform virtual rounds for a set of patients, typically 30–35 in number [22]. In addition to monitoring the alerts generated by the tele-ICU system, tele-ICU nurses may monitor compliance with care pathways and quality indicators. Perhaps even more important is the potential of an experienced tele-ICU nurse to provide nursing consultations to the bedside nursing team [23]. As the average experience of a bedside critical care nurse continues to decrease, the value of a nursing consultation is likely to increase over time and could have major impacts on quality of care, nursing satisfaction, and burnout [24, 25]. There is evidence suggesting that bedside critical care nurses feel less anxiety when they have the ability to consult with an experienced tele-ICU nurse, and we will discuss this in greater detail below.

Tele-sitting

The incidence of agitated delirium in the ICU is very high and has a major impact not only on patient outcomes but also ICU operations. The current approach to care of delirious patients is to minimize sedatives and maintain a high nurse-to-patient staffing ratio or employ a bedside sitter to prevent an agitated patient from self-harm. In situations where sitters are not available, patients may be cared for in the ICU setting simply by using a nurse to monitor and intervene during periods of agitation. There is now a growing use of virtual or tele-sitters to remotely monitor multiple, at-risk patients. This simple application of telemedicine systems may have profound impact on ICU throughput and manpower costs [26].

Best Practices Oversight

Failure to provide evidence-based best care practices is a significant contributor to morbidity and mortality in the ICU [27]. Improving the reliable delivery of the processes of care aimed at reducing preventable harm can improve patient morbidity and mortality. Telemedicine may have a role in improving process compliance for best care practices in the ICU. We performed a study of a purely consultative telemedicine care model using an audiovisual tele-ICU implementation. In this study, the tele-ICU team communicated deficiencies in best care practices to the ICU team but did not perform documentation or write any orders. We examined compliance with best practice care processes before and after implementation [28]. The majority of care processes showed a positive trend toward compliance with many reaching statistical significance. Compliance with both mechanical (93.6% to 98.2%) and pharmacologic (80.8% to 88.8%) deep vein thrombosis prophylaxis improved significantly. Daily sedation interruption improved from 69.7% to 85.5% and compliance with an oral care regimen improved from 69.7% to 90.9%, both of which were statistically significant (Fig. 17.4). Most striking, compliance with Joint Commission guidelines for restraints improved significantly from 38.7% to 82.7%. Interestingly, during this same time period, compliance with the head of the bed greater than 30 degrees, regular repositioning, and gastrointestinal ulcer prophylaxis trended down, although this was not significant. This study was performed in a highly staffed ICU

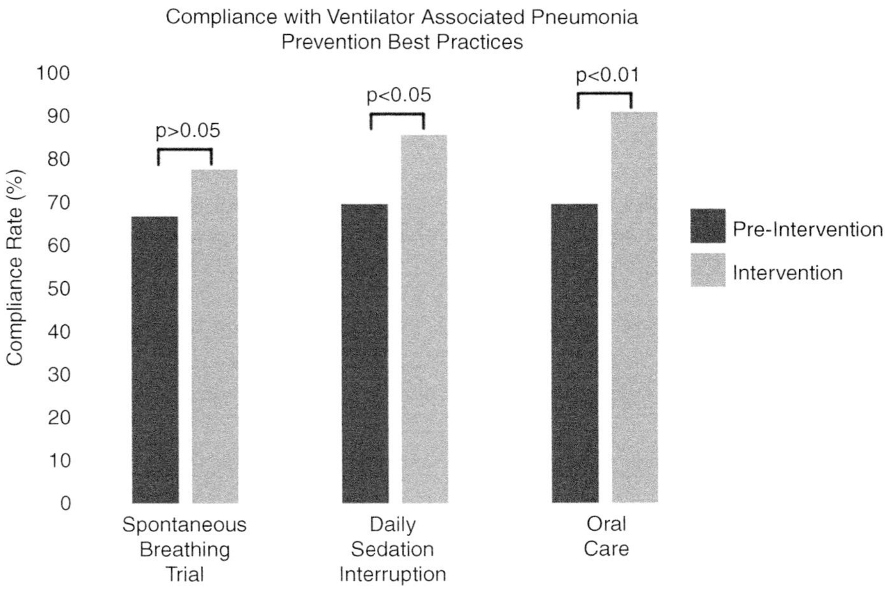

Fig. 17.4 Compliance with Ventilator Associated Pneumonia Prevention Best Practices. Tele-ICU significantly improves compliance with daily sedation interruption (69.7% vs 85.5%, $p < 0.05$) and oral care (69.7% vs 90.9%, $p < 0.01$). The trend toward improvement in daily spontaneous breathing trials was not significant (66.7% vs 77.6%, $p > 0.05$) (unpublished data)

in an academic tertiary center, and we expect the magnitude of these improvements would be even greater in a lower resourced ICU.

The effects of adhering to best practices may be profound in terms of patient outcomes and care efficiency. ICU telemedicine appears to benefit hospital throughput by decreasing length of stay. In a 1 year study, seven academic ICUs were examined using a stepped-wedge design [29]. Patients were allocated to either a pre- or post-tele-ICU intervention group, based on the rollout of the tele-ICU intervention in their ICU. Length of stay was decreased from 13.3 to 9.8 days per patient after the initiation of tele-ICU. Likewise, the mortality rate in this period decreased significantly from 13.6% to 11.8%. These improvements may be the result of improvement in processes of care. Adherence to best practices such as deep vein thrombosis prevention and stress ulcer prophylaxis were improved during this period, which may be the underlying driver for the improvements in length of stay and mortality. The authors of this study also make the case that a proper tele-ICU implementation requires "reengineering" the process of ICU care. This reengineered ICU may lead to improvements that cannot be attributed to any one specific intervention or consultation [29].

Value and Costs of Tele-ICU Implementation and Impact on Consultations

Typically, tele-ICU systems are implemented "on top of" current ICU resources. They require significant capital and operational expenditures which are not offset by a reduction in other fixed costs. Therefore, the economic goal of tele-ICU systems is to achieve a return on investment through reduction of marginal costs by improving patient outcomes and more efficient resource utilization. Improvements in metrics such as length of stay and readmission rates may be associated with significant costs savings to a hospital system. Several research studies have tried to evaluate the savings that may be elicited from a tele-ICU system by extrapolating the deferred costs from a reduced length of stay. One study reported a 10% reduction in length of stay which was extrapolated to a $2.5 million value [30]. Another study employed an independent consulting firm to estimate that their 30–34% ICU length of stay reduction was comparable to a 25–31% reduction in ICU costs and a 12–19% reduction in hospital costs [2]. These cost savings, however, are difficult to generalize as they are financial extrapolations on clinical data and costs may vary across geographic regions. It is important to note that all of the financial analyses of tele-ICU were conducted at a time when there was essentially no reimbursement for telemedicine services. Over recent years, the value of telemedicine consultation is increasingly recognized by insurers, and this appears to be spurring implementation of telemedicine systems and their utilization [31, 32]. Therefore, if current trends in reimbursement continue, we expect that tele-ICUs may be able to provide value not only through cost avoidance but also through recovering costs with billing. The path to billing for specialty consultation appears to be much more clear now.

The costs to start-up a tele-ICU have previously been evaluated in a number of studies and are consistently found between $50 and 100,000 per ICU bed in a closed tele-ICU model with proactive monitoring [33]. The University of Massachusetts Medical Center System has one of the largest and best researched tele-ICU systems. This group provided a detailed cost accounting for both the one-time costs associated with starting a ~ 100-bed tele-ICU and annualized estimate of the recurring costs for maintaining tele-ICU activities [34]. The initial implementation costs were about $7 million, of which approximately 40% were used for physical capital costs. The remainder of the costs can be categorized as software licensing, project management, and consulting fees. These costs are reflective of an era in which integrated EMRs were not typical. Currently, EMR adoption is near universal, and most major EMR vendors are embedding telemedicine capabilities within their systems. These capabilities can be used as part of a tele-ICU system. Thus, in the present day, we expect that some of the software licensing, consulting, and network costs will be reduced by adopting telemedicine components of an existing EMR. Cost accounting based on these new assumptions has not been published and may be difficult to disambiguate from the bundled costs of maintaining multifaceted medical records systems.

However, staffing costs remain the largest component of the ongoing costs of any telemedicine system. The same University of Massachusetts group determined these costs were about 90% of system sustainment. Unlike capital costs, staffing costs are likely to have increased since these estimates were made. Indeed, using the University of Massachusetts data, we estimate that in 2010, each tele-ICU bed will cost approximately $25,000 per year. If the goal of the tele-ICU system is to provide specialist consultation, this will require an additional cost for access and time for specialists.

Barriers to Tele-ICU Consultation

Since the earliest implementation of tele-ICUs, bedside nurses and physicians have demonstrated reluctance to accept the advice of or ask for consultation with tele-ICU clinicians. For example, in a large, comprehensive trial conducted in five different hospitals, physicians granted treatment authority to the tele-ICU for only ~ 30% of the ICU patients [35]. However, this same group compared safety attitudes before and after tele-ICU implementation and found that it improved teamwork and safety climate in some ICUs, especially among nurses [36]. Technology assessment tools have been used to determine the drivers of both physicians' and nurses' attitudes toward the use of tele-ICU. Nurses were influenced by the perceived ease of system use and felt that tele-ICU could be beneficial in ICUs without high levels of physician staffing [37], while physicians were not concerned with ease of use but had attitudes that were driven by their perceptions of the usefulness of the system [38]. These staff perceptions regarding telemedicine implementations may have a number of impacts on successful tele-ICU adoption and staff satisfaction. In a survey of 93 nurses from 3 academic ICUs, 72% of nurses felt that a nocturnal tele-ICU implementation improved patient survival, but only 47% believed that tele-ICU reduced medical errors [39]. A small percentage had concerns that tele-ICU was intrusive (11%) and left staff feeling as if they were being spied on (13%). Most interesting, 61% of nurses reported being more likely to contact the tele-ICU physician if they knew that physician, and 79% felt that it was important to personally know the tele-ICU physician.

Nursing perceptions of the impact of tele-ICU on quality of care and staff satisfaction have also been studied with a prospective, controlled method [40]. Nursing staff in a surgical ICU were surveyed prior to and after a 2-month tele-ICU implementation and found to have improved perceptions of effectiveness, communication, relations, job satisfaction, and burnout. In the same institution, another surgical ICU that was used as a control and completed the survey tool without any intervention did not show the same improvements in perceptions as the study ICU. In this implementation, the tele-ICU was staffed by clinicians that already worked within that ICU and were familiar to the bedside staff.

Job satisfaction and reduced burnout is strongly correlated with improvements in staff retention. Thus, tele-ICU has the potential to indirectly reduce costs associated with staff turnover such as recruitment and training; however, this effect has not been directly studied. It is notable that, in both of these studies, either the bedside staff was familiar with the tele-ICU staff or felt that such a relationship was an important factor in their decision to engage with the tele-ICU. This relationship may be an important and unrecognized factor in successful tele-ICU implementation but has not yet been studied in a controlled manner.

Discussion

There are many factors that are leading inexorably to the expansive development of telemedicine systems. These factors include the adoption of EMRs and the ability to integrate population-based monitoring into this platform, the decreasing costs of hardware for implementation, the building evidence that telemedicine adds value and should be directly compensated by insurers, and the acceptance of extended multidisciplinary care teams for the care of the critically ill patient. Leaders in critical care have recently pronounced that telemedicine will become universally available in the ICU [41].

We can anticipate that, as technical capabilities advance, there will be an associated increase in the demands for critical care telemedicine. These demands are likely to take on forms that are distinct from the customary models of the tele-ICU. It is interesting to consider that the driving force behind the original development of the tele-ICU was that it could mitigate ICU staffing shortages. Over recent years, there is a growing awareness that certain diseases may be detected and treated before they rise to the level of critical illness. Evidence of this phenomenon is seen in the early detection and treatment of sepsis using predictive analytics [42]. Coupled with the awareness that early intervention may forestall the need for ICU admission is the increasing array of remote sensor systems. These systems provide high-fidelity, continuous patient monitoring without the requirement for ICU admission. Thus, we are close to achieving the ability to provide meaningful, routine critical care consultation beyond the ICU. This ability can be used to improve early intervention, limit geographic disparity, and react to disaster situations. The ability to use telemedicine to prevent the need for ICU admissions may be extrapolated from improved outcomes when telemedicine was used in a progressive care unit [43].

Defining the roles and organizational structure for using telemedicine to provide critical care consultation is essential in extending the expertise of the critical care clinicians beyond the walls of the ICU. Technology and telemedicine services can provide consultative care almost anywhere, but alone, they cannot provide critical care. It is important to emphasize the distinction between critical care delivery and critical care consultation. There are essential features of an ICU that are required to provide critical care, and these include a dedicated physical space [44]. We believe that a robust tele-ICU system, staffed by ICU clinicians and overseeing care in the ICU, is needed for the most responsive and impactful telemedicine critical care consult service. Only such a system can assure the full spectrum of consultative activities that we have described. Indeed, this system will be able to leverage investments in telemedicine so that consultations are used to assure timely therapy, appropriate triage, and use of the physical ICU to its maximal capabilities.

References

1. Grundy BL, Jones PK, Lovitt A. Telemedicine in critical care: problems in design, implementation, and assessment. Crit Care Med. 1982;10(7):471–5.
2. Rosenfeld BA, Dorman T, Breslow MJ, Pronovost P, Jenckes M, Zhang N, et al. Intensive care unit telemedicine: alternate paradigm for providing continuous intensivist care. Crit Care Med. 2000;28(12):3925–31.
3. Irwin RS, Flaherty HM, French CT, Cody S, Chandler MW, Connolly A, et al. Interdisciplinary collaboration: the slogan that must be achieved for models of delivering critical care to be successful. Chest. 2012;142(6):1611–9.
4. Lilly CM, McLaughlin JM, Zhao H, Baker SP, Cody S, Irwin RS. A multicenter study of ICU telemedicine reengineering of adult critical care. Chest. 2014;145(3):500–7.
5. Wood D. No longer rocket science: robots have found their place in healthcare. Telemed J E Health. 2011;17(6):409–14.
6. Becevic M, Clarke MA, Alnijoumi MM, Sohal HS, Boren SA, Kim MS, et al. Robotic Telepresence in a Medical Intensive Care Unit – Clinicians' Perceptions. Perspect Health Inf Manag. 2015;1c:12.
7. Pronovost PJ, Angus DC, Dorman T, Robinson KA, Dremsizov TT, Young TL. Physician staffing patterns and clinical outcomes in critically ill patients: a systematic review. JAMA. 2002;288(17):2151–62.
8. Gasperino J. The leapfrog initiative for intensive care unit physician staffing and its impact on intensive care unit performance: a narrative review. Health Policy. 2011;102(2–3):223–8.
9. Fang JL, Collura CA, Johnson RV, Asay GF, Carey WA, Derleth DP, et al. Emergency video telemedicine consultation for newborn resuscitations: The Mayo Clinic Experience. Mayo Clin Proc. 2016;91(12):1735–43.

10. Ellenby MS, Marcin JP. The role of telemedicine in pediatric critical care. Crit Care Clin. 2015;31(2):275–90.
11. Dayal P, Hojman NM, Kissee JL, Evans J, Natale JE, Huang Y, et al. Impact of telemedicine on severity of illness and outcomes among children transferred from Referring Emergency Departments to a Children's Hospital PICU. Pediatr Crit Care Med. 2016;17(6):516–21.
12. Theurer L, Bashshur R, Bernard J, Brewer T, Busch J, Caruso D, et al. American telemedicine association guidelines for Teleburn. Telemed J E Health. 2017;23(5):365–75.
13. Wallace DL, Hussain A, Khan N, Wilson YT. A systematic review of the evidence for telemedicine in burn care: with a UK perspective. Burns. 2012;38(4):465–80.
14. Holt B, Faraklas I, Theurer L, Cochran A, Saffle JR. Telemedicine use among burn centers in the United States: a survey. J Burn Care Res. 2012;33(1):157–62.
15. Ali SF, Hubert GJ, Switzer JA, Majersik JJ, Backhaus R, Shepard LW, et al. Validating the teleStroke mimic score: a prediction rule for identifying stroke mimics evaluated over telestroke networks. Stroke. 2018;49(3):688–92.
16. Fortis S, Sarrazin MV, Beck BF, Panos RJ, Reisinger HS. ICU telemedicine reduces interhospital ICU transfers in the veterans health administration. Chest. 2018;154(1):69–76.
17. Fortis S, Weinert C, Bushinski R, Koehler AG, Beilman G. A health system-based critical care program with a novel tele-ICU: implementation, cost, and structure details. J Am Coll Surg. 2014;219(4):676–83.
18. Parmar P, Mackie D, Varghese S, Cooper C. Use of telemedicine technologies in the management of infectious diseases: a review. Clin Infect Dis. 2015;60(7):1084–94.
19. Siddiqui J, Herchline T, Kahlon S, Moyer KJ, Scott JD, Wood BR, et al. Infectious Diseases Society of America position statement on telehealth and telemedicine as applied to the practice of infectious diseases. Clin Infect Dis. 2017;64(3):237–42.
20. Christenbury J. Emory cares for ICU patients remotely, turning 'night into day' from Australia: Emory University Media Relations; 2018. Available from: https://news.emory.edu/stories/2018/05/buchman-hiddleson_eicu_perth_australia/index.html. Accessed Sept 2018.
21. Hubley S, Lynch SB, Schneck C, Thomas M, Shore J. Review of key telepsychiatry outcomes. World J Psychiatry. 2016;6(2):269–82.
22. American Telemedicine Association TeleICU Practice Guidelines Work Group. Guidelines for TeleICU operations. 2014.
23. Hoonakker PLT, Pecanac KE, Brown RL, Carayon P. Virtual collaboration, satisfaction, and trust between nurses in the tele-ICU and ICUs: results of a multilevel analysis. J Crit Care. 2017;37:224–9.
24. Siffleet J, Williams AM, Rapley P, Slatyer S. Delivering best care and maintaining emotional wellbeing in the intensive care unit: the perspective of experienced nurses. Appl Nurs Res. 2015;28(4):305–10.
25. Khan N, Jackson D, Stayt L, Walthall H. Factors influencing nurses' intentions to leave adult critical care settings. Nurs Crit Care. 2019;24(1):24–32.
26. Kensley A. Patient sitter, meet telesitter [internet]. 2016. Available from: https://www.uchealth.org/today/2016/02/17/patient-sitter-meet-telesitter/. Accessed Sept 2018.
27. Hayward RA, Asch SM, Hogan MM, Hofer TP, Kerr EA. Sins of omission: getting too little medical care may be the greatest threat to patient safety. J Gen Intern Med. 2005;20(8):686–91.
28. Latif A, Romig M, Pronovost P, Sapirstein A. A consultative telemedicine service improves compliance with best practice guidelines in a highly staffed intensive care unit. Crit Care Med. 2010;38(12):U180.
29. Lilly CM, Cody S, Zhao H, Landry K, Baker SP, McIlwaine J, et al. Hospital mortality, length of stay, and preventable complications among critically ill patients before and after tele-ICU reengineering of critical care processes. JAMA. 2011;305(21):2175–83.
30. Breslow MJ, Rosenfeld BA, Doerfler M, Burke G, Yates G, Stone DJ, et al. Effect of a multiple-site intensive care unit telemedicine program on clinical and economic outcomes: an alternative paradigm for intensivist staffing. Crit Care Med. 2004;32(1):31–8.
31. State Telehealth Laws and Reimbursement Policies Report: The Center for Connected Health Polic; 2018. Available from: http://www.cchpca.org/state-telehealth-laws-and-reimbursement-policies-report. Accessed Sept 2018.

32. Neufeld JD, Doarn CR, Aly R. State Policies Influence Medicare Telemedicine Utilization. Telemed J E Health. 2016;22(1):70–4.
33. Chen J, Sun D, Yang W, Liu M, Zhang S, Peng J, et al. Clinical and economic outcomes of telemedicine programs in the intensive care unit: a systematic review and meta-analysis. J Intensive Care Med. 2018;33(7):383–93.
34. New England Health Care Institute. Critical care, critical choices: the case for tele-ICUs in intensive care. Cambridge: New England Healthcare Institute; 2010.
35. Thomas EJ, Lucke JF, Wueste L, Weavind L, Patel B. Association of telemedicine for remote monitoring of intensive care patients with mortality, complications, and length of stay. JAMA. 2009;302(24):2671–8.
36. Chu-Weininger MY, Wueste L, Lucke JF, Weavind L, Mazabob J, Thomas EJ. The impact of a tele-ICU on provider attitudes about teamwork and safety climate. Qual Saf Health Care. 2010;19(6):e39.
37. Kowitlawakul Y. The technology acceptance model: predicting nurses' intention to use telemedicine technology (eICU). Comput Inform Nurs. 2011;29(7):411–8.
38. Hu PJ, Chau PY. Physician acceptance of telemedicine technology: an empirical investigation. Top Health Inf Manag. 1999;19(4):20–35.
39. Mullen-Fortino M, DiMartino J, Entrikin L, Mulliner S, Hanson CW, Kahn JM. Bedside nurses' perceptions of intensive care unit telemedicine. Am J Crit Care. 2012;21(1):24–32.
40. Romig MC, Latif A, Gill RS, Pronovost PJ, Sapirstein A. Perceived benefit of a telemedicine consultative service in a highly staffed intensive care unit. J Crit Care. 2012;27(4):426.e9–16.
41. Vincent JL, Creteur J. The hospital of tomorrow in 10 points. Crit Care. 2017;21(1):93.
42. Taylor RA, Pare JR, Venkatesh AK, Mowafi H, Melnick ER, Fleischman W, et al. Prediction of in-hospital mortality in emergency department patients with sepsis: a local big data-driven, machine learning approach. Acad Emerg Med. 2016;23(3):269–78.
43. Armaignac DL, Saxena A, Rubens M, Valle CA, Williams LS, Veledar E, et al. Impact of telemedicine on mortality, length of stay, and cost among patients in progressive care units: experience from a large healthcare system. Crit Care Med. 2018;46(5):728–35.
44. Marshall JC, Bosco L, Adhikari NK, Connolly B, Diaz JV, Dorman T, et al. What is an intensive care unit? A report of the task force of the World Federation of Societies of Intensive and Critical Care Medicine. J Crit Care. 2017;37:270–6.
45. Hao J, et al. Tele-ICU: the way forward in geriatric care? Aging Clin Exp Res. 2014;26(6):575–82.

Index

M. A. Koenig (ed.), *Telemedicine in the ICU*,
https://doi.org/10.1007/978-3-030-11569-2

U

V

W

Printed by Printforce, the Netherlands